NEURORADIOLOGY SIGNS

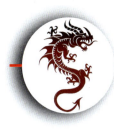

NEURORADIOLOGY SIGNS

Mai-Lan Ho, MD
Fellow in Neuroradiology
University of California, San Francisco
San Francisco, California

Ronald L. Eisenberg, MD, JD
Professor of Radiology
Beth Israel Deaconess Medical Center
Harvard Medical School
Boston, Massachusetts

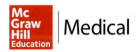 Medical

New York   Chicago   San Francisco   Athens   Lisbon   Madrid
Mexico City   Milan   New Delhi   Singapore   Sydney   Toronto

Neuroradiology Signs

1 2 3 4 5 6 7 8 9 0   CTP/CTP   19 18 17 16 15 14

ISBN 978-0-07-180432-5
MHID 0-07-180432-3

This book was set in Sabon Roman by Thomson Digital.
The editors were Michael Weitz and Brian Kearns.
The production supervisor was Richard Ruzycka.
The illustration manager was Armen Ovsepyan.
Project management was provided by Saloni Narang, Thomson Digital.
The interior designer was Diana Andrews.
The cover designer was Anthony Landi.
China Translation & Printing Services, Ltd. was printer and binder.

This book is printed on acid-free paper.

Library of Congress Cataloging-in-Publication Data

Ho, Mai-Lan, author.
  Neuroradiology signs / Mai-Lan Ho, Ronald L. Eisenberg.
    p. ; cm.
  Includes bibliographical references.
  ISBN 978-0-07-180432-5—ISBN 0-07-180432-3
  I. Eisenberg, Ronald L., author. II. Title.
  [DNLM: 1. Nervous System Diseases—diagnosis. 2. Neuroimaging. WL 141.5.N47]
  RC386.6.N48
  616.8'0475—dc23
                                                          2013043235

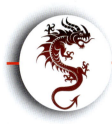

About the Authors

Mai-Lan Ho, MD, is a Fellow in Neuroradiology at the University of California, San Francisco. She completed her residency in diagnostic radiology at Beth Israel Deaconess Medical Center, Harvard Medical School; as well as chemical engineering training at Stanford University and Massachusetts Institute of Technology. Dr. Ho is the recipient of several prestigious radiology awards including the William W. Olmsted Editorial Fellowship for Trainees, Roentgen Resident/Fellow Research Award, and Bracco Diagnostics Research Resident Grant from the Radiological Society of North America; Lucy Frank Squire Award from the American Association for Women Radiologists; and Stephen A. Kieffer Award from the Eastern Neuroradiological Society.

Ronald L. Eisenberg, MD, JD, is a Professor of Radiology at Beth Israel Deaconess Medical Center, Harvard Medical School. He earned his medical degree from the University of Pennsylvania, and residency training at Massachusetts General Hospital and the University of California, San Francisco. Dr. Eisenberg is an internationally renowned radiologist who has authored 21 books in radiology, including the 1984 *Atlas of Signs in Radiology* and the 1994 *Skull and Spine Imaging: An Atlas of Differential Diagnosis*. He is also Section Editor of the "Pattern of the Month" series for the *American Journal of Roentgenology*.

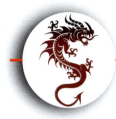

Dedication

To my parents, Huong and Sa Ho, for their love and support;
David Hackney and Hugh Curtin, for their wisdom and guidance;
and Jeff Petrella, for his friendship and inspiration

— Mai-Lan Ho

To Zina, Avlana, and Cherina

— Ronald L. Eisenberg

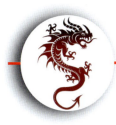

Foreword

It is my pleasure to introduce *Neuroradiology Signs*, the first comprehensive multimodality guide to signs in neuroimaging. The idea for this text came from Dr. Mai-Lan Ho, currently a Fellow in Neuroradiology at the University of California, San Francisco. Inspired by the *Radiology* "Signs in Imaging" series, she began compiling a database of imaging signs as part of her residency training at Beth Israel Deaconess Medical Center, Harvard Medical School. Noticing the scarcity of literature specific to neuroradiology, she teamed up with Dr. Ron Eisenberg, author of the original 1984 *Atlas of Signs in Radiology*. Together they developed the concept for this book, which consists of over 440 spectacular CT, MR, angiography, radiography, ultrasound, and nuclear medicine cases. The text is organized into subspecialty chapters with high-resolution radiologic images, full-color photos, imaging findings, differential diagnosis, discussion, and up-to-date references.

Neuroradiology Signs should benefit any student, resident, or fellow (or staff!) wishing to review imaging features and pathology of the brain, head and neck, and spine. This is a perfect boards study aid, as well as a great reference book for any clinician wishing to refresh or expand their differential diagnosis in neuroimaging.

William P. Dillon, MD
Elizabeth A. Guillaumin Professor of
Radiology, Neurology and Neurosurgery
Executive Vice-Chair and Chief of Neuroradiology
Department of Radiology and Biomedical Imaging
University of California, San Francisco
San Francisco, California

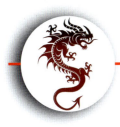

Preface

We have always been fascinated by imaging patterns ranging from pathognomonic "Aunt Minnie" lesions to key findings with focused differential diagnoses. The identification of a specific imaging sign can dramatically alter a radiologist's impression of a case and help clinch the diagnosis. In many cases, it is recognition of these fine details that distinguishes very good readers from truly great ones.

With this book, we aim to fill a relative void in the literature with a review of over 440 signs in neuroradiology across the modalities of computed tomography, magnetic resonance, angiography, radiography, ultrasound, and nuclear medicine. The book is divided into seven chapters: (1) Adult and General Brain; (2) Pediatric Brain; (3) Head, Neck, and Orbits; (4) Vascular; (5) Skull and Facial Bones; (6) Vertebrae; and (7) Spinal Cord and Nerves. All cases have been reviewed by subspecialty experts, and are presented in a comprehensive yet concise fashion.

In each chapter, signs are listed on separate pages and organized in alphabetical order for the convenience of the reader. Each section includes imaging findings, differential diagnosis, discussion, and key references. Furthermore, color photos clarify the etymology of each sign. This novel feature makes the learning process more enjoyable, while also providing "real-world" visual correlation. Imaging modalities for each sign are listed in order of increasing complexity. Readers can refer to the ACR Appropriateness Criteria® for evidence-based guidelines regarding the most suitable imaging examination in a given clinical scenario. For easy reference, the index at the end of the book is organized in three ways: by sign, diagnosis, and modality.

We have designed this book for a wide audience including general and subspecialty neuroradiologists, neuroradiology fellows, and radiology residents; as well as neurologists, surgeons, primary care physicians, technologists, and medical students. As such, it is a handy reference for the bookshelf or reading room, and very high-yield material for board examinations. We hope that you have as much fun reading our book as we did writing it!

— Mai-Lan Ho, MD
— Ronald L. Eisenberg, MD, JD

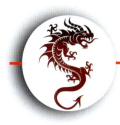

Acknowledgments

This project would not have been possible without the help of Michael Weitz and Brian Kearns at McGraw-Hill, Saloni Narang at Thomson Digital, and our fabulous section editors and contributors. I am grateful to Wikipedia and Microsoft Office Online for their vast collections of open-source stock photography.

To my mother, Huong, and father, Sa: thank you for your eternal love and understanding. Your support helped me get through all those late-night writing sessions! My chemical engineering professor, Channing Robertson: thanks for believing in me and encouraging me to think "outside the box." To Claire Anderson: you introduced me to radiology, and thus changed my life forever. Nahum Goldberg: thanks for discovering me and giving me a chance to be part of something greater. To Alex Bankier: I could not have asked for a better advisor and confidant—together we made the Scholar's Track! Jonny Kruskal and Debbie Levine: thank you for your exemplary mentorship throughout my residency. David Hackney: I owe much of my success to you, and value your opinion above all. Hugh Curtin: what can I say that hasn't already been said? You're a living legend, and like a father to me. Gul Moonis, Rafael Rojas, Rafeeque Bhadelia, and Jim Wu: you are talented, inspirational, and genuine "friends of the resident." Jeff Petrella: thank you for your selfless advice and clarity of insight. A continually positive force in my life, you always bring out the best in me. And finally, I would like to acknowledge all my fantastic teachers, colleagues, and friends at UCSF and our exceptional leader, Bill Dillon, who is the "quintessential" academic neuroradiologist and a true visionary!

— Mai-Lan Ho, MD

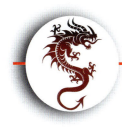

Section Editors

Rafeeque Bhadelia, MD
Clinical Director and Associate Professor
  in Neuroradiology
Beth Israel Deaconess Medical Center
Harvard Medical School
Boston, Massachusetts

Daniel T. Ginat, MD, MS
Assistant Professor in Neuroradiology
University of Chicago
Chicago, Illinois

Amy F. Juliano, MD
Instructor in Radiology
Massachusetts Eye and Ear Infirmary
Harvard Medical School
Boston, Massachusetts

Gul Moonis, MD
Assistant Professor in Neuroradiology
Beth Israel Deaconess Medical Center
Massachusetts Eye and Ear Infirmary
Harvard Medical School
Boston, Massachusetts

Jared A. Narvid, MD
Clinical Instructor in Neuro-Interventional
  Radiology
University of California, San Francisco
San Francisco, California

Sanjay P. Prabhu, MBBS, MRCPCH, FRCR
Assistant Professor in Neuroradiology
Director of Advanced Image Analysis Laboratory
Children's Hospital Boston
Harvard Medical School
Boston, Massachusetts

Rafael Rojas, MD
Assistant Professor in Neuroradiology
Beth Israel Deaconess Medical Center
Harvard Medical School
Boston, Massachusetts

Jim S. Wu, MD
Assistant Professor in Musculoskeletal Imaging
Beth Israel Deaconess Medical Center
Harvard Medical School
Boston, Massachusetts

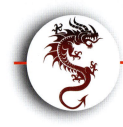

Contributors

Larry Barbaras, BS
Senior Programmer and Analyst in Radiology
Beth Israel Deaconess Medical Center
Harvard Medical School
Boston, Massachusetts

A. James Barkovich, MD
Chief of Pediatric Neuroradiology
University of California, San Francisco
San Francisco, California

Cynthia T. Chin, MD
Professor in Neuroradiology and Neurosurgery
Director of Precision Spine and Peripheral
  Nerve Center
University of California, San Francisco
San Francisco, California

Hugh D. Curtin, MD
Chair of Radiology
Massachusetts Eye and Ear Infirmary
Harvard Medical School
Boston, Massachusetts

Kevin J. Donohoe, MD
Assistant Professor in Nuclear Medicine
Beth Israel Deaconess Medical Center
Harvard Medical School
Boston, Massachusetts

Christopher F. Dowd, MD
Professor in Neuro-Interventional Radiology,
  Neurological Surgery, Neurology,
  and Anesthesia and Perioperative Care
University of California, San Francisco
San Francisco, California

Christine M. Glastonbury, MBBS
Professor in Neuroradiology,
  Otolaryngology-Head and Neck Surgery,
  and Radiation Oncology
University of California, San Francisco
San Francisco, California

David B. Hackney, MD
Chief of Neuroradiology
Assistant Dean for Faculty Development
Beth Israel Deaconess Medical Center
Harvard Medical School
Boston, Massachusetts

Mary G. Hochman, MD, MBA
Chief of Musculoskeletal Imaging
Beth Israel Deaconess Medical Center
Harvard Medical School
Boston, Massachusetts

Jason M. Johnson, MD
Clinical Instructor in Neuroradiology
University of California, San Francisco
San Francisco, California

Michael Larson, MFA
Media Specialist in Radiology
Beth Israel Deaconess Medical Center
Harvard Medical School
Boston, Massachusetts

Deborah Levine, MD
Chief of Obstetric and Gynecologic Ultrasound
Vice Chair for Academic Affairs in Radiology
Beth Israel Deaconess Medical Center
Harvard Medical School
Boston, Massachusetts

William A. Mehan Jr., MD
Assistant Professor in Neuroradiology
Tufts Medical Center
Boston, Massachusetts

J. Anthony Parker, MD, PhD
Associate Professor in Nuclear Medicine
Beth Israel Deaconess Medical Center
Harvard Medical School
Boston, Massachusetts

A. Suresh Reddy, MD
Chief of Interventional Neuroradiology
Beth Israel Deaconess Medical Center
Harvard Medical School
Boston, Massachusetts

Ammar Sarwar, MD
Fellow in Interventional Radiology
Beth Israel Deaconess Medical Center
Harvard Medical School
Boston, Massachusetts

Ajith J. Thomas, MD
Chief of Cerebrovascular Surgery
Beth Israel Deaconess Medical Center
Harvard Medical School
Boston, Massachusetts

Jesse L. Wei, MD
Director of Radiology Informatics
Instructor in Abdominal Radiology
Beth Israel Deaconess Medical Center
Harvard Medical School
Boston, Massachusetts

Carol Wilcox, RT(R), (CT)
Senior Imaging Technologist
Beth Israel Deaconess Medical Center
Harvard Medical School
Boston, Massachusetts

Donna Wolfe, MFA
Medical Editor in Radiology
Beth Israel Deaconess Medical Center
Harvard Medical School
Boston, Massachusetts

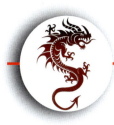

Abbreviations

3D = three-dimensional

ACA = anterior cerebral artery

ACOM = anterior communicating artery

ADC = apparent diffusion coefficient

ADH = antidiuretic hormone

AICA = anterior inferior cerebellar artery

AIDS = acquired immune deficiency disorder

AP = anteroposterior

ASL = arterial spin labeling

AVF = arteriovenous fistula

AVM = arteriovenous malformation

CCA = common carotid artery

CN = cranial nerve

CNS = central nervous system

CSF = cerebrospinal fluid

CT = computed tomography

CTA = computed tomography arteriography

CTP = computed tomography perfusion

CTV = computed tomography venography

dAVF = dural arteriovenous fistula

DTI = diffusion tensor imaging

DTPA = diethylene triamine pentaacetic acid

DVA = developmental venous anomaly

DWI = diffusion-weighted imaging

ECA = external carotid artery

ECD = ethyl cysteinate dimer

EDH = epidural hematoma

FDG = fluorodeoxyglucose

FLAIR = fluid-attenuated inversion recovery

Ga-67, ^{67}Ga = gallium-67

GBM = glioblastoma multiforme

HAART = highly active antiretroviral therapy

HMPAO = hexamethyl propylene amine oxime

I-123, ^{123}I = iodine-123

IAC = internal auditory canal

ICA = internal carotid artery

In-111, ^{111}In = indium-111

MCA = middle cerebral artery

MIP = maximum intensity projection

MMA = middle meningeal artery

MPR = multiplanar reformat

MR = magnetic resonance

MRA = magnetic resonance arteriography

MRP = magnetic resonance perfusion

MRS = magnetic resonance spectroscopy

MRV = magnetic resonance venography

MS = multiple sclerosis

NAA = *N*-acetyl aspartate

NF1 = neurofibromatosis type I

NF2 = neurofibromatosis type II

NM = nuclear medicine

PA = posteroanterior

PCA = posterior cerebral artery

PCNSL = primary central nervous system lymphoma

PCOM = posterior communicating artery

PD = proton density

PET = positron emission tomography

PICA = posterior inferior cerebellar artery

PNET = primitive neuroectodermal tumor

SAH = subarachnoid hemorrhage

SCA = superior cerebellar artery

SDH = subdural hematoma

SPECT = single photon emission computed tomography

STA = superficial temporal artery

STIR = short-tau inversion recovery

SWI = susceptibility-weighted imaging

TB = tuberculosis

Tc-99m, ^{99m}Tc = metastable technetium-99

TOF = time-of-flight

US = ultrasonography

WHO = World Health Organization

XA = angiography

XR = radiography

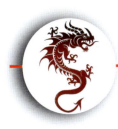

Contents

CHAPTER ONE

ADULT AND GENERAL BRAIN

ACCORDION, BUCKLING

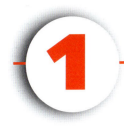

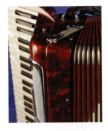

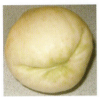

Modalities:
CT, MR

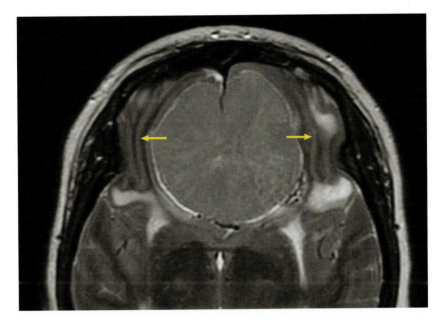

FINDINGS:

Axial T2-weighted MR shows a mass in the anterior interhemispheric fissure, with surrounding T2-hyperintense rim. There is lateral displacement of the frontal lobe gyri (arrows) and mild vasogenic edema.

DIAGNOSIS:

Extraaxial mass (meningioma)

DISCUSSION:

Correct localization of an intracranial mass is crucial for accurate diagnosis and surgical planning. Intraaxial masses expand the brain parenchyma, with surrounding vasogenic edema. Extraaxial masses displace and compress the adjacent brain, with inward bowing of gyri ("accordion" or "buckling" sign) and less edema than intraaxial lesions. Other useful findings of an extraaxial mass include the "CSF cleft" and "dural tail" signs. Meningioma is the most common extraaxial mass, and comprises 15% of all brain tumors.

References:

Drevelegas A. Extra-axial brain tumors. *Eur Radiol.* 2005;15(3):453-467.

George AE, Russell EJ, Kricheff II. White matter buckling: CT sign of extraaxial intracranial mass. *AJR Am J Roentgenol.* 1980;135(5):1031-1036.

AQUEDUCTAL/CSF FLOW VOID, TRUMPET

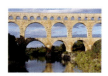

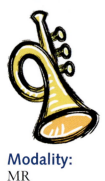

Modality:
MR

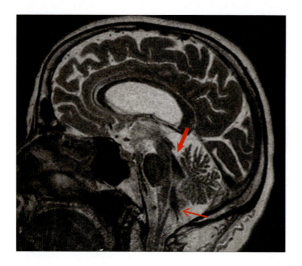

FINDINGS:

Sagittal T2-weighted MR shows signal voids within the aqueduct of Sylvius (thick arrow), fourth ventricle, and cisterna magna (thin arrow). There is mild dilation of the cerebral aqueduct.

DIFFERENTIAL DIAGNOSIS:

- Communicating hydrocephalus
- Intracranial volume loss

DISCUSSION:

Cerebrospinal fluid (CSF) is produced in the choroid plexus of the ventricles, circulates continuously through the brain and spinal cord, and is reabsorbed by arachnoid granulations and/or lymphatic channels. CSF circulation is propagated by the heart in a pulsatile fashion. High-velocity and turbulent flow can produce signal voids within the ventricular system on T2-weighted MR images. Findings are most apparent in and can distend the aqueduct of Sylvius, creating a "trumpet" appearance in conjunction with the fourth ventricle. This is characteristic of normal pressure hydrocephalus (NPH), but may occur with any cause of increased CSF volume, including other forms of communicating (nonobstructive) hydrocephalus and intracranial volume loss. Other imaging signs of NPH include rounding of the frontal and temporal horns, enlarged sylvian fissures, crowding of gyri at the vertex, and upward bowing of the corpus callosum. Quantitative CSF flow imaging using phase-contrast techniques is helpful in assessing the severity of disease and predicting response to CSF shunting.

References:

Bradley WG Jr, Kortman KE, Burgoyne B. Flowing cerebrospinal fluid in normal and hydrocephalic states: appearance on MR images. *Radiology.* 1986;159(3):611-616.

McCoy MR, Klausner F, Weymayr F, et al. Aqueductal flow of cerebrospinal fluid (CSF) and anatomical configuration of the cerebral aqueduct (AC) in patients with communicating hydrocephalus—the trumpet sign. *Eur J Radiol.* 2013;82(4):664-670.

ARC, BROKEN/INCOMPLETE/OPEN RING, CRESCENT, HORSESHOE, LEADING EDGE

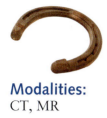

Modalities:
CT, MR

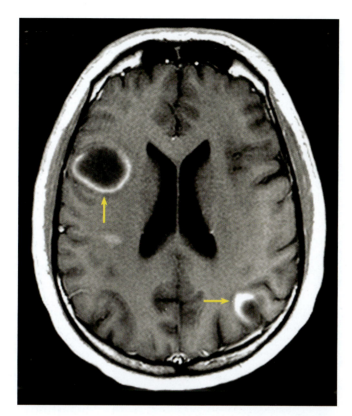

FINDINGS:

Axial contrast-enhanced T1-weighted MR shows multiple enhancing lesions, including the right frontal operculum and left inferior parietal lobule (arrows). These demonstrate curvilinear enhancement, with discontinuity along the superficial margins.

DIFFERENTIAL DIAGNOSIS:

- Demyelinating disease
- Primary tumor
- Lymphoma

DISCUSSION:

Approximately half of tumefactive demyelinating lesions demonstrate pathologic enhancement. "Incomplete ring" enhancement is a relatively specific sign, helping to distinguish active demyelination (particularly multiple sclerosis) from infectious and neoplastic etiologies. The enhancing component represents the active (leading) edge of demyelination and extends toward the white matter. The nonenhancing component represents the inactive (trailing) edge of demyelination and can point toward the gray matter or basal ganglia. A central nonenhancing core may also be present, corresponding to chronic inflammation with gliosis. Vasogenic edema may be present, especially in regions of active disease. The general mnemonic for cerebral ring-enhancing lesions is "MAGIC DR L": metastasis, abscess, glioblastoma multiforme, infarct (subacute), contusion, demyelinating disease, radiation necrosis, and lymphoma. Other than demyelinating disease, incomplete ring enhancement is occasionally seen in low-grade primary tumors and lymphoma affecting immunocompromised patients.

References:

Given CA 2nd, Stevens BS, Lee C. The MRI appearance of tumefactive demyelinating lesions. *AJR Am J Roentgenol.* 2004;182(1):195-199.

Masdeu JC, Quinto C, Olivera C, et al. Open-ring imaging sign: highly specific for atypical brain demyelination. *Neurology.* 2000;54(7):1427-1433.

Smirniotopoulos JG, Murphy FM, Rushing EJ, et al. Patterns of contrast enhancement in the brain and meninges. *Radiographics.* 2007;27(2):525-551.

ASYMMETRIC/ECCENTRIC TARGET

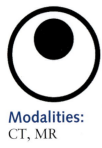

Modalities:
CT, MR

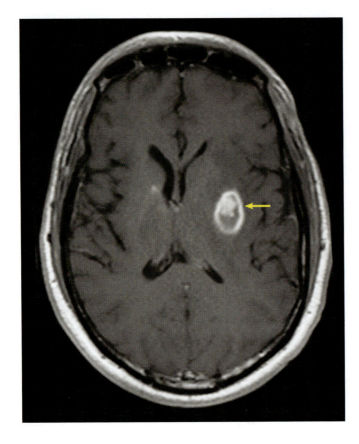

FINDINGS:

Axial contrast-enhanced T1-weighted MR shows a left basal ganglia rim-enhancing lesion with large eccentric nodule (arrow).

DIFFERENTIAL DIAGNOSIS:

- Toxoplasmosis
- Other infection
- Malignancy

DISCUSSION:

Toxoplasmosis refers to infection by the protozoan *Toxoplasma gondii* and occurs from exposure to feces from infected cats, who are the primary hosts; or by ingestion of infected raw meat such as pork. Ingested oocysts from cat feces and tissue cysts from contaminated meat transform into tachyzoites within the bloodstream. These preferentially localize in CNS and muscle tissue, where they develop into cystic bradyzoites. In pregnant women, tachyzoites can also cross the placental barrier and cause neonatal infection. Toxoplasmosis brain lesions are usually multifocal, with rim enhancement and large irregular nodules representing a combination of inflammation, hemorrhage, and necrosis. In the cortex and deep gray matter, the nodules tend to be eccentrically located ("asymmetric target" sign), corresponding pathologically to necrotizing abscesses with penetrating vessels. Deep parenchymal lesions may demonstrate a more concentric appearance ("concentric target" sign), which is more specific for toxoplasmosis and corresponds pathologically to central hemorrhage. In contrast, bacterial abscesses are typically smooth and ring-enhancing without associated nodularity. Neurocysticercosis demonstrates small calcified "dotlike" lesions, corresponding pathologically to parasitic scolices. Primary cystic neoplasms and metastases are usually more heterogeneous in appearance.

References:

Kumar GG, Mahadevan A, Guruprasad AS, et al. Eccentric target sign in cerebral toxoplasmosis: neuropathological correlate to the imaging feature. *J Magn Reson Imaging.* 2010;31(6):1469-1472.

Mahadevan A, Ramalingaiah AH, Parthasarathy S, et al. Neuropathological correlate of the "concentric target sign" in MRI of HIV-associated cerebral toxoplasmosis. *J Magn Reson Imaging.* 2013;38(2):488-495.

BAT, BEARDED SKULL, DRAGON CLAW

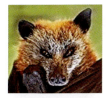

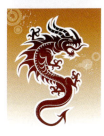

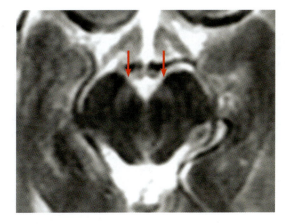

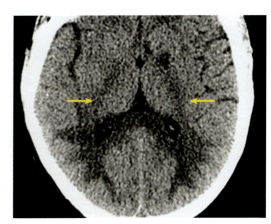

Modalities:
CT, MR

FINDINGS:

- Axial T2-weighted MR reveals edema in the ventral midbrain (arrows) with sparing of the red nuclei.
- Axial CT shows edema in the posterior limbs of the internal capsules (arrows), optic radiations, and splenium.

DIAGNOSIS:

Toxic leukoencephalopathy

DISCUSSION:

Toxic leukoencephalopathy can be caused by drug abuse, environmental toxins, immunosuppressive medications, and cranial irradiation. Classically, there is diffuse supratentorial white matter T2 hyperintensity and reduced diffusion. Selective involvement of the internal capsules and optic radiations produces a "dragon claw" appearance. Infratentorial abnormalities may also occur, particularly in cases of heroin inhalation ("chasing the dragon"). The "bat" sign of the midbrain refers to edema in the medial lemnisci and spinothalamic tracts ("face") with sparing of the substantia nigra and red nuclei ("eyes"). The pontocerebellar "bearded skull" sign represents edema of the corticospinal tracts ("eyes"), medial lemnisci and central tegmental tracts ("mouth"), and cerebellar white matter, sparing the dentate nuclei ("beard"). Findings can be difficult to distinguish from other leukoencephalopathies, and clinical correlation is essential for diagnosis.

Reference:

Keogh CF, Andrews GT, Spacey SD, et al. Neuroimaging features of heroin inhalation toxicity: "chasing the dragon." *AJR Am J Roentgenol.* 2003;180(3):847-850.

BAT WING, BUTTERFLY, TRIDENT

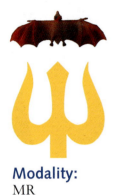

Modality:
MR

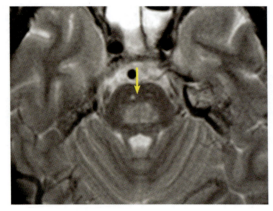
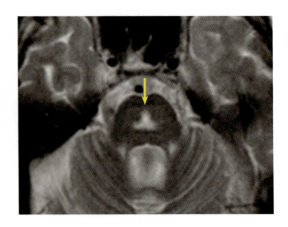

FINDINGS:

Axial T2-weighted MR in two different patients shows central pontine hyperintensities, sparing the tegmentum ventrally and corticospinal tracts laterally.

DIAGNOSIS:

Osmotic demyelination syndrome

DISCUSSION:

Osmotic demyelination syndrome (ODMS), formerly classified into central pontine myelinolysis (CPM) and extrapontine myelinolysis (EPM), refers to acute demyelination caused by rapid changes in serum osmolality. The classic presentation is an alcoholic, hyponatremic patient who undergoes rapid correction of serum sodium levels, resulting in massive fluid efflux from the brain into the serum. Symmetric T2-hyperintense signal and reduced diffusion are seen in the central pons, basal ganglia, and/or cerebral white matter. Mild injury produces signal abnormality in the median raphe and basis pontis, with a bilobed ("bat wing") or triangular ("trident") morphology. More profound injury affects the entire pons with relative sparing of the tegmentum, corticobulbar, and corticospinal tracts ("snake eyes" appearance). In the subacute period, signal changes improve or resolve completely. The differential for central pontine T2 hyperintensity includes infarction, neoplasm, demyelination, infection, metabolic disorders, and radiation. However, combined findings of CPM and EPM are essentially pathognomonic for ODMS.

References:

Ho VB, Fitz CR, Yoder CC, et al. Resolving MR features in osmotic myelinolysis (central pontine and extrapontine myelinolysis). *AJNR Am J Neuroradiol.* 1993;14(1):163-167.

Miller GM, Baker HL Jr, Okazaki H, et al. Central pontine myelinolysis and its imitators: MR findings. *Radiology.* 1988;168(3):795-802.

BLACK/DARK CEREBELLUM

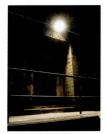

Modality:
MR

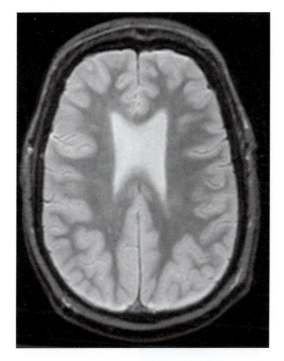

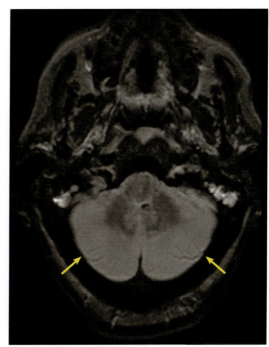

FINDINGS:

- Axial T2-weighted MR of the cerebrum shows diffuse edema with abnormally hyperintense cortex and gyral swelling.
- Axial T2-weighted MR of the cerebellum shows normal signal (arrows), which appears artifactually hypointense relative to the cerebrum.

DIAGNOSIS:

Diffuse cerebral edema

DISCUSSION:

Diffuse cerebral edema occurs in various settings including trauma, hypoxia, ischemia, and infection. There is relative sparing of the basal ganglia, brainstem, and cerebellum. The mechanism is unknown but may represent preferential arterial circulation, delayed venous drainage, or decompression by transtentorial herniation. The preserved cerebellum appears brighter than the edematous cerebrum on CT ("white cerebellum") and darker on T2-weighted MR ("black cerebellum"), which is the reverse of the normal appearance.

References:

Bird CR, Drayer BP, Gilles FH. Pathophysiology of "reverse" edema in global cerebral ischemia. *AJNR Am J Neuroradiol.* 1989;10(1):95-98.

Brant WE, Helms C. *Fundamentals of Diagnostic Radiology*, 3rd ed. Baltimore: Lippincott Williams and Wilkins, 2012.

BLACK HOLE

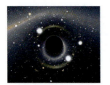

Modalities:
CT, MR

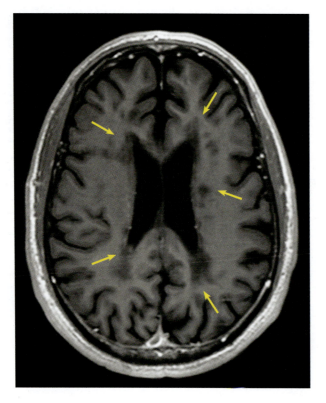

FINDINGS:

Axial contrast-enhanced T1-weighted MR shows multiple T1-hypointense, nonenhancing periventricular foci (arrows).

DIFFERENTIAL DIAGNOSIS:

- Chronic demyelination
- Focal encephalomalacia

DISCUSSION:

Multiple sclerosis (MS) is a chronic demyelinating disorder characterized by spatial and temporal heterogeneity. Acute demyelinating lesions are associated with edema, enhancement, and/or reduced diffusion. In the chronic stage, permanent axonal damage yields gliotic "black holes" that are hypodense on CT, hypointense on T1-weighted MR, and nonenhancing. There is a moderate correlation between the development of "black holes" and the degree of clinical disability in MS. Focal encephalomalacia caused by ischemia, infection, or trauma can demonstrate similar imaging characteristics, though the spatial distribution differs from that of MS.

References:

Bagnato F, Jeffries N, Richert ND, et al. Evolution of T1 black holes in patients with multiple sclerosis imaged monthly for 4 years. *Brain*. 2003;126(pt 8):1782-1789.

Naismith RT, Cross AH. Multiple sclerosis and black holes: connecting the pixels. *Arch Neurol*. 2005;62(11):1666-1668.

BOXCAR VENTRICLES

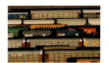

Modalities:
CT, MR

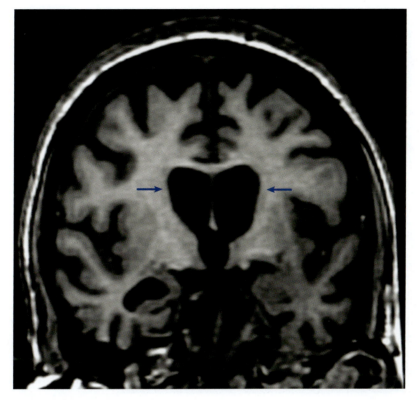

FINDINGS:

Coronal FLAIR MR shows atrophy of the caudate nuclei (arrows) with resulting enlargement and squaring of the frontal horns.

DIFFERENTIAL DIAGNOSIS:

- Huntington disease
- Other neurodegenerative disorders

DISCUSSION:

Huntington disease is an autosomal dominant neurodegenerative disorder with onset in middle age. Symptoms include chorea, psychiatric problems, and progressive cognitive decline. Imaging shows selective atrophy of the basal ganglia, particularly the caudate nuclei. This produces characteristic squaring of the frontal horns ("boxcar ventricles"). Findings may be difficult to distinguish from age-related changes and other dementing disorders, and correlation with clinical symptoms is crucial for diagnosis.

References:

Barra FR, Gonçalves FG, de Lima Matos V, et al. Signs in neuroradiology—part 2. *Radiol Bras.* 2011;44(2):129-133.

Mascalchi M, Lolli F, Della Nave R, et al. Huntington disease: volumetric, diffusion-weighted, and magnetization transfer MR imaging of brain. *Radiology.* 2004;232(3):867-873.

BRIGHT BASAL GANGLIA

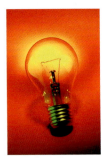

Modality:
MR

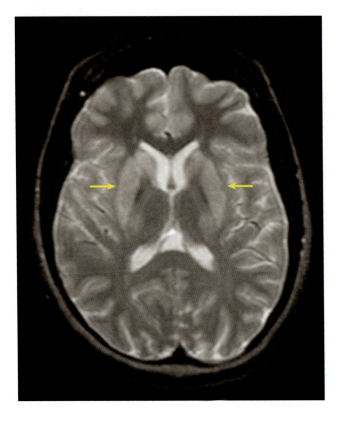

FINDINGS:

Axial T2-weighted MR shows abnormal hyperintense signal in the bilateral caudates and putamina (arrows).

DIFFERENTIAL DIAGNOSIS:

- Toxic poisoning
- Metabolic derangements
- Neurodegenerative disorders
- Vascular conditions
- Inflammation/infection
- Malignancy

DISCUSSION:

The basal ganglia and thalami are paired deep gray matter structures with high metabolic activity, and are susceptible to injury from a number of causes. On MR, hyperintensity on T2- and/or T1-weighted sequences ("bright basal ganglia") can be seen with various etiologies including toxic, metabolic, neurodegenerative, vascular, inflammatory/ infectious, and neoplastic. Toxic etiologies include carbon monoxide, methanol, and cyanide poisoning. Metabolic conditions include liver disease, hyperglycemia, hypoglycemia, hypoxic-ischemic encephalopathy, hemolytic-uremic syndrome, mitochondrial disorders, osmotic myelinolysis, and Wernicke encephalopathy. Neurodegenerative disorders include Huntington disease, dysmyelinating disorders, neurodegeneration with brain iron accumulation (NBIA), Creutzfeldt-Jakob disease, and Fahr disease. Vascular abnormalities include venous thrombosis and arterial infarction. Inflammatory/infectious disorders include viral encephalitides, toxoplasmosis, systemic lupus erythematosus, and Behçet disease. Neoplasms include CNS lymphoma and glioma. Other MR sequences should be reviewed to identify reduced diffusion, hemorrhage, contrast enhancement, and/or mass effect. Clinical history; time course; and additional abnormalities of the thalami, cerebral cortex, corpus callosum, white matter, cerebellum, or brainstem can also help narrow the differential diagnosis.

References:

Hegde AN, Mohan S, Lath N, et al. Differential diagnosis for bilateral abnormalities of the basal ganglia and thalamus. *Radiographics*. 2011;31(1):5-30.

Ho VB, Fitz CR, Chuang SH, et al. Bilateral basal ganglia lesions: pediatric differential considerations. *Radiographics*. 1993;13(2):269-292.

BRIGHT/DENSE/WHITE CEREBELLUM, REVERSAL

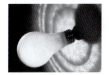

Modality:
CT

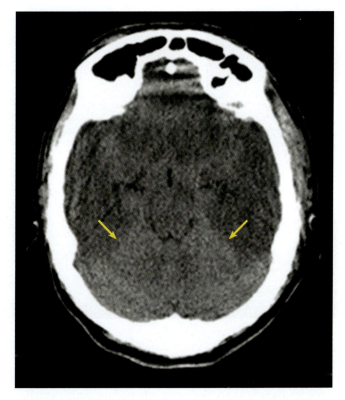

FINDINGS:

Axial CT reveals diffuse cerebral edema with hypoattenuation, sulcal effacement, and loss of gray-white distinction. The cerebellum is preserved and appears relatively hyperdense (arrows).

DIAGNOSIS:

Diffuse cerebral edema

DISCUSSION:

Diffuse cerebral edema occurs in various settings including trauma, hypoxia, ischemia, and infection. There is relative sparing of the basal ganglia, brainstem, and cerebellum. The mechanism is unknown but may be due to preferential arterial circulation, delayed venous drainage, or decompression by transtentorial herniation. The preserved cerebellum appears brighter than the edematous cerebrum on CT ("white cerebellum") and darker on T2-weighted MR ("black cerebellum"), which is the reverse of the normal appearance.

References:

Bird CR, Drayer BP, Gilles FH. Pathophysiology of "reverse" edema in global cerebral ischemia. *AJNR Am J Neuroradiol.* 1989;10(1):95-98.

Brant WE, Helms C. *Fundamentals of Diagnostic Radiology*, 3rd ed. Baltimore: Lippincott Williams and Wilkins, 2012.

BUBBLY, FEATHERY, SOAP BUBBLE, SWISS CHEESE

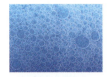

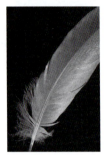

Modalities:
CT, MR

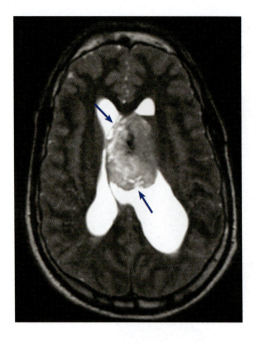

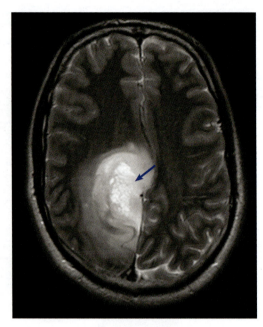

FINDINGS:

- Axial T2-weighted MR in first patient shows a multilocular lesion (arrows) in the left lateral ventricle attached to the septum pellucidum, with blood-fluid level in the left frontal horn.
- Axial T2-weighted MR in second patient shows a multilocular lesion (arrow) in the right cingulate sulcus, with infiltrative surrounding hyperintense signal.

DIFFERENTIAL DIAGNOSIS:

- Central neurocytoma
- Oligodendroglioma

DISCUSSION:

Central neurocytomas and oligodendrogliomas have a similar histological and imaging appearance with T2-hyperintense multilocular "bubbly" contents, variable enhancement, and calcification. However, central neurocytomas occur in younger adults (20-40 years) and are almost always located in the lateral ventricles, abutting the septum pellucidum. Acute symptoms may result from ventricular obstruction and/or hemorrhage. Oligodendrogliomas occur in an older age group (over 50 years) and are located in the cortex and subcortical white matter, most commonly within the frontal lobe. Growth pattern is indolent and may produce pressure erosions of the calvarium.

References:

Koeller KK, Rushing EJ. From the archives of the AFIP: Oligodendroglioma and its variants: radiologic-pathologic correlation. *Radiographics*. 2005;25(6):1669-1688.

Smith AB, Smirniotopoulos JG, Horkanyne-Szakaly I. From the radiologic pathology archives: intraventricular neoplasms: radiologic-pathologic correlation. *Radiographics*. 2013;33(1):21-43.

BULLSEYE, CONCENTRIC TARGET

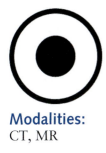

Modalities:
CT, MR

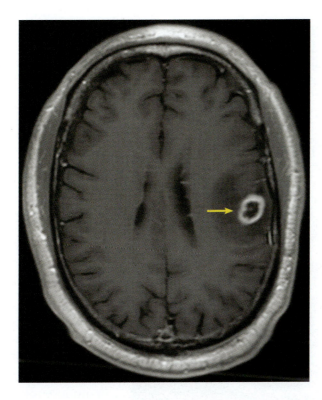

FINDINGS:

Axial contrast-enhanced T1-weighted MR shows a left perirolandic ring-enhancing lesion with central enhancing focus (arrow).

DIFFERENTIAL DIAGNOSIS:

- Tuberculoma
- Toxoplasmosis
- Metastasis

DISCUSSION:

CNS tuberculosis occurs following hematogenous dissemination from the respiratory or gastrointestinal systems. Superficial infection results in meningitis or cerebritis, whereas deep infection produces tuberculoma (caseating granuloma) and liquefied abscess. The "target" appearance reflects a central nidus of granulomatous inflammation, which enhances and may later calcify. However, this appearance is not specific and can be seen with other infections (particularly fungal), tumefactive demyelination (Balo concentric sclerosis), partially thrombosed aneurysms, and metastases. In immunocompromised patients, toxoplasmosis should be a major diagnostic consideration. Toxoplasmosis brain lesions are usually multifocal, with rim enhancement and large irregular nodules representing a combination of inflammation, hemorrhage, and necrosis. In the cortex and deep gray matter, the nodules tend to be eccentrically located ("asymmetric target" sign), corresponding pathologically to necrotizing abscesses with penetrating vessels. Deep parenchymal lesions may demonstrate a more concentric appearance ("concentric target" sign), which is more specific for toxoplasmosis and corresponds pathologically to central hemorrhage.

References:

Bargalló J, Berenguer J, García-Barrionuevo J, et al. The "target sign": is it a specific sign of CNS tuberculoma? *Neuroradiology.* 1996;38(6):547-550.

Bernaerts A, Vanhoenacker FM, Parizel PM, et al. Tuberculosis of the central nervous system: overview of neuroradiological findings. *Eur Radiol.* 2003;13(8):1876-1890.

Mahadevan A, Ramalingaiah AH, Parthasarathy S, et al. Neuropathological correlate of the "concentric target sign" in MRI of HIV-associated cerebral toxoplasmosis. *J Magn Reson Imaging.* 2013 Feb 25.

BUNCH OF GRAPES, GRAPELIKE, RACEMOSE

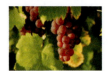

Modalities:
CT, MR

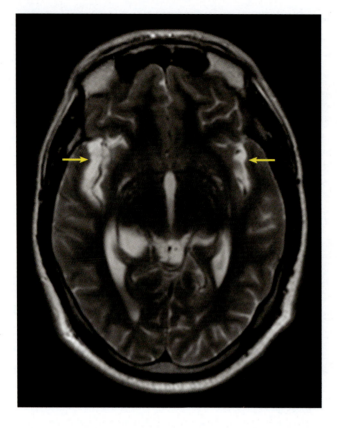

FINDINGS:

Axial T2-weighted MR shows multiple clustered cystic lesions expanding the bilateral sylvian fissures (arrows).

DIAGNOSIS:

Racemose neurocysticercosis

DISCUSSION:

Neurocysticercosis is a neurologic disease caused by the pork tapeworm *Taenia solium*. It is the most common parasitic infection of the CNS, and the leading cause of acquired epilepsy worldwide. Infection occurs by ingestion of larval eggs in raw or undercooked pork. Once the larvae reach the small intestine, they attach to the intestinal wall via scolices and release additional ova. Through fecal-oral contamination, ova are digested in the stomach and release oncospheres. These penetrate the intestinal wall and enter the bloodstream, preferentially depositing in brain, eyes, and muscle. Locations of disease include subarachnoid-cisternal, parenchymal, intraventricular, and spinal. Five stages have been described: noncystic, vesicular, colloidal vesicular, granular nodular, and calcified nodular. Noncystic neurocysticercosis is asymptomatic with no imaging findings. Vesicular neurocysticercosis demonstrates parenchymal and/or subarachnoid cysts with associated scolices ("cyst with dot" appearance) and little or no edema. The racemose variant (Latin for "bunch of grapes") consists of clustered cysts, usually without scolices. These are typically located in the sylvian fissures and basal cisterns. Colloidal vesicular neurocysticercosis is marked by larval disintegration with marked enhancement, edema, and peripheral capsule formation. Granular nodular neurocysticercosis is characterized by cyst retraction and gliosis. Calcified nodular neurocysticercosis is the nonactive stage, in which the lesion has completely involuted and calcified.

Reference:

Kimura-Hayama ET, Higuera JA, Corona-Cedillo R, et al. Neurocysticercosis: radiologic-pathologic correlation. *Radiographics*. 2010;30(6):1705-1719.

BUTTERFLY, HEART

Modality:
NM

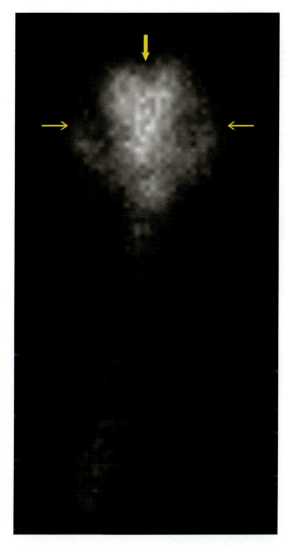

FINDINGS:

Anterior planar In-111 DTPA cisternogram shows slow ascent of tracer from the intrathecal injection site over the cerebral convexities (thin arrows), with reflux into the lateral ventricles (thick arrow).

DIFFERENTIAL DIAGNOSIS:

- Normal pressure hydrocephalus
- Cerebral atrophy

DISCUSSION:

Radionuclide cisternography involves intrathecal injection of a radiolabeled pharmaceutical (usually indium-111 diethylene triamine pentaacetic acid) with sequential imaging to evaluate CSF flow. In a normal patient, tracer ascends up the spinal column to the level of the basal cisterns by 1 hour, the frontal poles and sylvian fissures by 2-6 hours, the cerebral convexities by 12 hours, and the superior sagittal sinus by 24 hours. In patients with normal pressure hydrocephalus (NPH), there is impaired absorption of CSF by the arachnoid granulations. This causes early reflux of tracer into the lateral ventricles ("butterfly/heart" appearance), with little flow over the cerebral convexities at 24-48 hours. Ventricular reflux and delayed ascent of tracer can be seen in cerebral atrophy, but should not persist by 24-48 hours.

Reference:

Chuang TL, Hsu MC, Wang YF. Normal pressure hydrocephalus: scintigraphic findings on SPECT/CT image. *Ann Nucl Med Sci.* 2010;23:169-174.

BUTTERFLY, MIRROR IMAGE

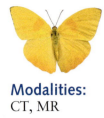

Modalities:
CT, MR

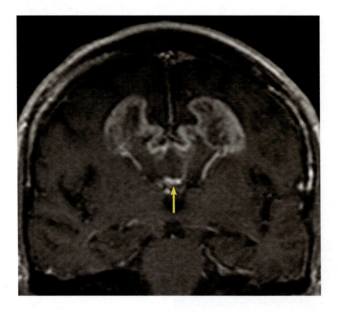

FINDINGS:

Coronal contrast-enhanced T1-weighted MR shows a peripherally enhancing bifrontal mass extending through the corpus callosum (arrow).

DIFFERENTIAL DIAGNOSIS:

- Glioblastoma multiforme
- Lymphoma
- Tumefactive multiple sclerosis

DISCUSSION:

"Butterfly" lesions involve both cerebral hemispheres and the intervening corpus callosum. The compact structure of the corpus callosum generally serves as a barrier to disease spread, except in aggressive lesions such as glioblastoma multiforme (GBM), CNS lymphoma, and tumefactive multiple sclerosis. GBM demonstrates infiltrative margins, with shaggy rim enhancement and internal hemorrhage/necrosis. Tumor behavior is aggressive, with frequent recurrence after surgery and chemoradiation. CNS lymphoma generally demonstrates smoother margins, sometimes with peripheral notching. Due to tumor hypercellularity, lesions are typically hyperdense on CT and hypointense on T2-weighted MR, with reduced diffusion. Tumor hypovascularity is reflected by mild homogeneous enhancement. There is marked improvement or complete resolution with steroid treatment. Tumefactive MS rarely has a butterfly appearance and may demonstrate incomplete "leading edge" enhancement, corresponding to active areas of demyelination. Lesions tend to be disseminated in space and time, and are variably responsive to steroids.

Reference:

Ho ML, Moonis G, Ginat DT, Eisenberg RL. Lesions of the corpus callosum. *AJR Am J Roentgenol.* 2013;200(1):W1-W16.

CALLOSAL-SEPTAL, STACK OF COINS, SUBCALLOSAL STRIATIONS, VENUS NECKLACE

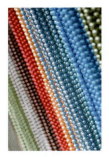

Modality:
MR

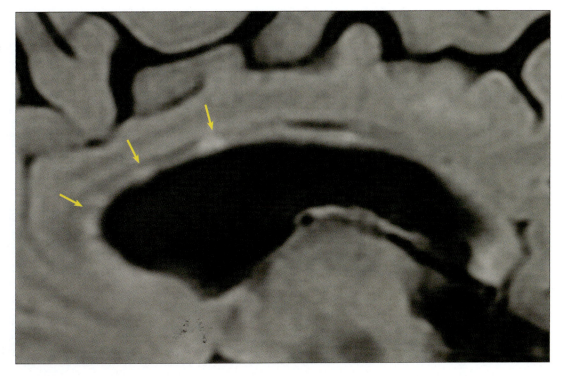

FINDINGS:

Sagittal FLAIR MR shows multiple linear hyperintensities (arrows) at the callosal-septal interface.

DIAGNOSIS:

Multiple sclerosis

DISCUSSION:

Multiple sclerosis (MS) is a chronic demyelinating disorder characterized by spatial and temporal heterogeneity. On thin-section sagittal FLAIR MR, hyperintense foci can be seen along the undersurface of the corpus callosum at its junction with the septum pellucidum (callosal-septal interface). These are oriented perpendicular instead of parallel to the ependyma, creating a "stack of coins" or "Venus necklace" appearance. The mechanism is thought to be perivenular demyelination along subependymal veins, and is highly sensitive and specific for detection of early MS.

Reference:

Palmer S, Bradley WG, Chen DY, et al. Subcallosal striations: early findings of multiple sclerosis on sagittal, thin-section, fast FLAIR MR images. *Radiology*. 1999;210(1):149-153.

CAULIFLOWER, LOBULATED, SCALLOPED

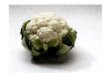

Modalities:
CT, MR

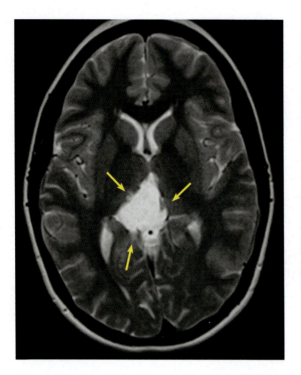 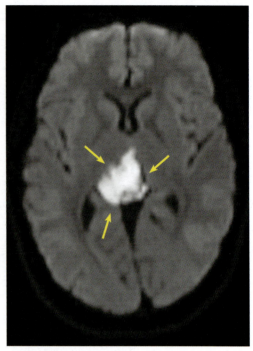

FINDINGS:

Axial T2-weighted and DWI MR show a lobulated pineal region mass (arrows) with T2-hyperintense signal and reduced diffusion.

DIAGNOSIS:

Epidermoid cyst

DISCUSSION:

Epidermoid cysts are rare congenital inclusion cysts that typically occur in extraaxial locations, such as the pineal region and cerebellopontine angles. Lesions demonstrate lobulated "cauliflower" margins with insinuation into adjacent structures and neurovascular encasement, making complete resection difficult. There is continual desquamation of epithelial cells into the cyst, resulting in gradual progressive enlargement. On MR, internal contents are mildly T2-hyperintense to CSF with persistent signal on FLAIR images, reflecting complex fluid contents. Lack of FLAIR suppression and the presence of reduced diffusion enable distinction of epidermoid from arachnoid cysts. Occasionally internal protein, lipid, and/or hemorrhage may produce T1-hyperintense signal, the so-called "white epidermoid."

Reference:

Smith AB, Rushing EJ, Smirniotopoulos JG. From the archives of the AFIP: lesions of the pineal region: radiologic-pathologic correlation. *Radiographics*. 2010;30(7):2001-2020.

CHOROIDAL/HIPPOCAMPAL FISSURE DILATION, CRACKED WALNUT

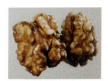

Modalities:
CT, MR

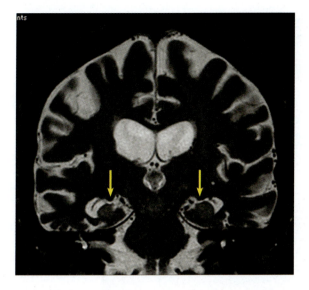

FINDINGS:

Coronal high-resolution T2-weighted MR shows enlargement of the hippocampal and choroidal fissures (arrows). There is diffuse cerebral volume loss with enlargement of sulci.

DIAGNOSIS:

Alzheimer disease

DISCUSSION:

Alzheimer disease (AD) is the most common form of dementia, with abnormal folding of beta-amyloid proteins leading to deposition of senile plaques and neurofibrillary tangles in the brain parenchyma. There is resulting cerebral atrophy, particularly in the temporal and parietal lobes. A reliable early imaging marker for AD is bilateral hippocampal atrophy with resulting dilation of the perihippocampal fissures. The transverse fissures of Bichat extend laterally from the perimesencephalic cisterns. Superolaterally, the choroidal fissures course above the hippocampi. Inferolaterally, the hippocampal fissures extend between the hippocampi and parahippocampal gyri. In advanced disease, there is more widespread atrophy with symmetrically enlarged sulci. This finding is best appreciated along the high cerebral convexities, creating a "cracked walnut" appearance. Findings may be difficult to distinguish from age-related volume loss and other dementing disorders, and correlation with clinical symptoms is crucial for diagnosis.

References:

Holodny AI, George AE, Golomb J, et al. The perihippocampal fissures: normal anatomy and disease states. *Radiographics*. 1998;18(3):653-665.

Li Y, Li J, Segal S, et al. Hippocampal cerebrospinal fluid spaces on MR imaging: Relationship to aging and Alzheimer disease. *AJNR Am J Neuroradiol*. 2006;27(4):912-918.

CIRCLE, OVAL, PERIOD

Modality:
NM

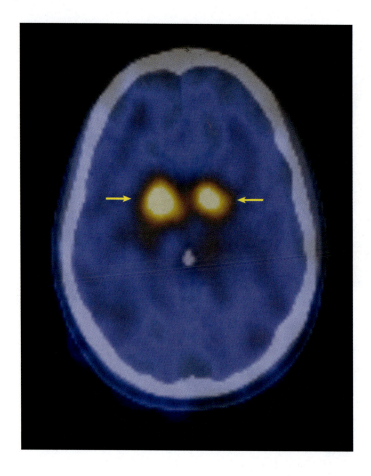

FINDINGS:

I-123 SPECT-CT shows absence of tracer uptake in the putamina and decreased uptake in the caudate nuclei (arrows).

DIAGNOSIS:

Parkinsonian syndromes

DISCUSSION:

Movement disorders and dementia in the elderly population have a variety of etiologies. When there is diagnostic uncertainty between parkinsonian and other disorders, baseline SPECT can be performed with the dopamine transporter ligand ioflupane (iodine-123), commercially known as DaTscan™. An abnormal appearance is absence of putaminal uptake with normal or decreased caudate uptake, which may be unilateral or bilateral ("period" sign). This indicates a nigrostriatal neurodegenerative condition (Parkinson disease, atypical parkinsonism, and Lewy body dementia), for which dopaminergic therapy may be beneficial. Normally there is bilateral symmetric uptake in the caudates and putamina ("comma" sign). This indicates a non-nigrostriatal etiology (Alzheimer dementia, essential tremor, vascular, drug-related), which will not respond to dopaminergic therapy.

References:

Cummings JL, Henchcliffe C, Schaier S, et al. The role of dopaminergic imaging in patients with symptoms of dopaminergic system neurodegeneration. *Brain*. 2011;134(pt 11):3146-3166.

Kupsch AR, Bajaj N, Weiland F, et al. Impact of DaTscan SPECT imaging on clinical management, diagnosis, confidence of diagnosis, quality of life, health resource use and safety in patients with clinically uncertain parkinsonian syndromes: a prospective 1-year follow-up of an open-label controlled study. *J Neurol Neurosurg Psychiatry*. 2012;83(6):620-628.

CLUSTER, DAUGHTER, SECONDARY

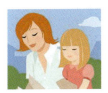

Modalities:
CT, MR

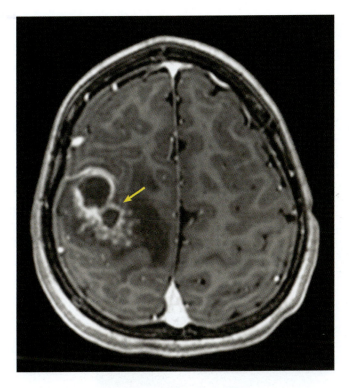

FINDINGS:

Axial contrast-enhanced T1-weighted MR shows two ring-enhancing lesions and several adjacent enhancing nodules in the right precentral gyrus (arrow). There is surrounding vasogenic edema.

DIAGNOSIS:

Cerebral abscess

DISCUSSION:

Cerebral abscesses may result from penetrating trauma, surgery, direct spread of adjacent infection, or hematogenous dissemination. Various bacterial, fungal, and parasitic pathogens have been described. Four stages of evolution have been described at imaging, representing a spectrum from soft tissue phlegmon to liquefied abscess: early cerebritis (days 1-3), late cerebritis (days 4-7), early capsule (days 10-14), and late capsule (> day 14). If untreated, the infection may progress with formation of one or multiple secondary ("daughter") abscesses adjacent to and contiguous with the parent abscess. There is a tendency for evagination toward the deep or ventricular margin ("dimple" sign). The "daughter" appearance should be distinguished from "satellite" lesions seen with brain tumors. These can be remote from the primary lesion, reflecting microscopic tumor infiltration and/or metastatic dissemination. In addition, tumor growth is slow compared to the rapid evolution of cerebral infection.

References:

Britt RH, Enzmann DR. Clinical stages of human brain abscesses on serial CT scans after contrast infusion. Computerized tomographic, neuropathological, and clinical correlations. *J Neurosurg.* 1983;59(6):972-989.

Hsu WC, Tang LM, Chen ST, et al. Multiple brain abscesses in chain and cluster: CT appearance. *J Comput Assist Tomogr.* 1995;19(6):1004-1006.

COMMA, CRESCENT

Modality:
NM

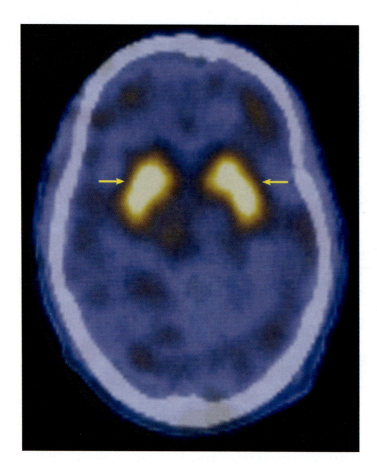

FINDINGS:

I-123 SPECT-CT shows normal bilateral uptake in the caudates and putamina (arrows).

DIAGNOSIS:

Normal I-123 scan

DISCUSSION:

Movement disorders and dementia in the elderly population have a variety of etiologies. When there is diagnostic uncertainty between parkinsonism and other disorders, baseline SPECT can be performed with the dopamine transporter ligand ioflupane (iodine-123), commercially known as DaTscan™. An abnormal appearance is absence of putaminal uptake with normal or decreased caudate uptake, which may be unilateral or bilateral ("period" sign). This indicates a nigrostriatal neurodegenerative condition (Parkinson disease, atypical parkinsonism, and Lewy body dementia), for which dopaminergic therapy may be beneficial. Normally there is bilateral symmetric uptake in the caudates and putamina ("comma" sign). This indicates a non-nigrostriatal etiology (Alzheimer dementia, essential tremor, vascular, drug-related) that will not respond to dopaminergic therapy.

References:

Cummings JL, Henchcliffe C, Schaier S, et al. The role of dopaminergic imaging in patients with symptoms of dopaminergic system neurodegeneration. *Brain.* 2011;134(pt 11):3146-3166.

Kupsch AR, Bajaj N, Weiland F, et al. Impact of DaTscan SPECT imaging on clinical management, diagnosis, confidence of diagnosis, quality of life, health resource use and safety in patients with clinically uncertain parkinsonian syndromes: a prospective 1-year follow-up of an open-label controlled study. *J Neurol Neurosurg Psychiatry.* 2012;83(6):620-628.

CONCENTRIC BANDS/RINGS, LAMELLATED, ONION SKIN

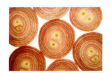

Modality:
MR

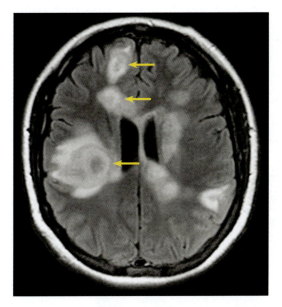
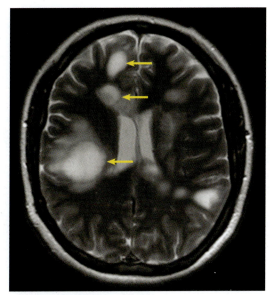

FINDINGS:

Axial FLAIR and T2-weighted MR show multiple rounded areas of white matter hyperintensity with a concentric layered appearance (arrows).

DIAGNOSIS:

Balo concentric sclerosis

DISCUSSION:

Balo concentric sclerosis is a rare and aggressive variant of multiple sclerosis, characterized by concentric layers of demyelination ("onion skin" appearance). It is hypothesized that demyelination spreads centrifugally from a central venule, with multiple episodes of reactivation. On T2-weighted MR, alternating hyperintense and hypointense bands correspond pathologically to demyelinated and myelinated white matter. Although the tumefactive appearance has been confused with neoplasia, the lamellated imaging pattern is pathognomonic for demyelination.

References:

Caracciolo JT, Murtagh RD, Rojiani AM, et al. Pathognomonic MR imaging findings in Balo concentric sclerosis. *AJNR Am J Neuroradiol.* 2001;22(2):292-293.

Karaarslan E, Altintas A, Senol U, et al. Baló's concentric sclerosis: clinical and radiologic features of five cases. *AJNR Am J Neuroradiol.* 2001;22(7):1362-1367.

CORDUROY, LAMINATED, STRIATED, STRIPED, TIGROID

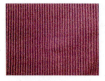

Modalities:
CT, MR

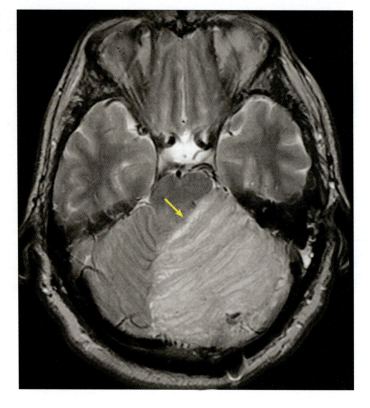

FINDINGS:

Axial T2-weighted MR shows expanded cerebellar folia with alternating hyperintense and hypointense bands in the left cerebellar hemisphere and vermis (arrow).

DIAGNOSIS:

Lhermitte-Duclos disease

DISCUSSION:

Lhermitte-Duclos disease (dysplastic cerebellar gangliocytoma) is a rare hamartomatous lesion of the cerebellum that is characterized by hypertrophy of the stratum granulosum. This results in characteristic disorganization and enlargement of the cerebellar folia, which appear T2-hyperintense to isointense and T1-hypointense to isointense ("corduroy" sign). Lhermitte-Duclos is associated with Cowden (multiple hamartoma) syndrome, caused by loss-of-function mutations in the tumor suppressor gene *PTEN*. Patients with Cowden syndrome exhibit hamartomas of the skin and mucous membranes. There is an increased risk of benign and malignant tumors of various organ systems (breast, thyroid, gastrointestinal, genitourinary, gynecologic).

Reference:

Meltzer CC, Smirniotopoulos JG, Jones RV. The striated cerebellum: an MR imaging sign in Lhermitte-Duclos disease (dysplastic gangliocytoma). *Radiology*. 1995;194(3):699-703.

CORTICAL RIBBON

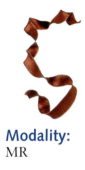

Modality:
MR

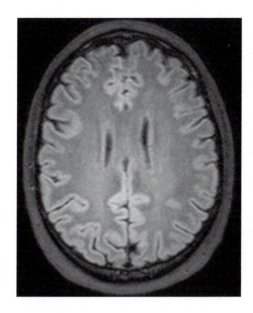
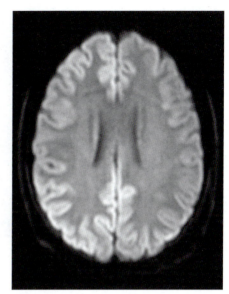

FINDINGS:

Axial FLAIR and DWI MR show hyperintense signal throughout the cerebral cortex.

DIFFERENTIAL DIAGNOSIS:

- Hypoxic-ischemic injury
- Creutzfeldt-Jakob disease
- Meningoencephalitis
- Metabolic disorders
- Postictal state

DISCUSSION:

Cortical gray matter is eight times more metabolically active than the white matter, and is thus highly susceptible to injury from a number of causes. On MR, hyperintense cortical signal on T2-weighted and DWI sequences ("cortical ribbon") can be seen with various etiologies including vascular, toxic/metabolic, postictal, inflammatory/infectious, and neoplastic. Vascular causes include arterial infarct and venous thrombosis. Metabolic conditions include hypoxic-ischemic encephalopathy, drug exposures, hypoglycemia, and mitochondrial disorders. Infectious etiologies include prion, viral, tuberculous, and fungal encephalitides. Neoplastic involvement of the cortex is suggestive of primary glial tumors. Other MR sequences should be reviewed to identify contrast enhancement, hemorrhage, and/or mass effect. Clinical history; time course; and additional abnormalities of the basal ganglia, thalami, corpus callosum, white matter, cerebellum, or brainstem can also help narrow the differential diagnosis.

Reference:

Sheerin F, Pretorius PM, Briley D, et al. Differential diagnosis of restricted diffusion confined to the cerebral cortex. *Clin Radiol.* 2008;63(11):1245-1253.

CORTICAL VEIN

Modalities:
US, CT, MR

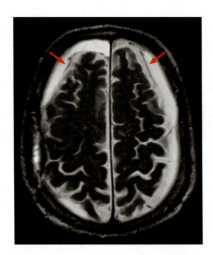 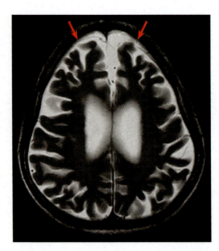

FINDINGS:

- Axial T2-weighted MR in a patient with bilateral subdural hygromas shows inward displacement of cortical veins (arrows) away from the dura.
- Axial T2-weighted MR in a patient with cerebral volume loss shows enlarged subarachnoid spaces with outward displacement of cortical veins (arrows) into the CSF.

DIFFERENTIAL DIAGNOSIS:

- Subdural fluid collections
- Cerebral atrophy

DISCUSSION:

Subdural fluid collections may represent hygromas or hematomas from trauma or surgery, empyemas due to infection, or effusions in intracranial hypotension. Subdural collections can be difficult to distinguish from cerebral atrophy, in which the subarachnoid space is enlarged due to decreased gyral volume. However, identification of cortical veins along the cerebral convexities can help differentiate the subdural and subarachnoid spaces. With subdural collections, the cortical veins are displaced inward and away from the dura. With cerebral volume loss, the cortical veins are displaced outward into the CSF. In infants, identification of cortical veins is also useful in distinguishing external hydrocephalus from subdural collections. External hydrocephalus refers to benign enlargement of the bifrontal subarachnoid spaces, a condition that is self-limiting and resolves by 2-3 years of age. Subdural fluid collections are always abnormal and should raise concern for nonaccidental trauma.

References:

Deltour P, Lemmerling M, Bauters W, et al. Posttraumatic subdural hygroma: CT findings and differential diagnosis. *JBR-BTR*. 1999;82(4):155-156.

McCluney KW, Yeakley JW, Fenstermacher MJ, et al. Subdural hygroma versus atrophy on MR brain scans: "the cortical vein sign." *AJNR Am J Neuroradiol*. 1992;13(5):1335-1339.

CRESCENT, FINGERLIKE, GRANULAR, SCALLOPED

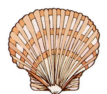

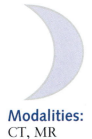

Modalities:
CT, MR

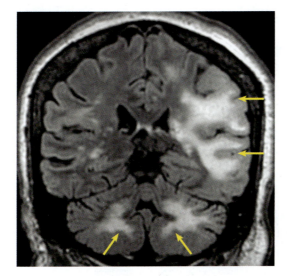

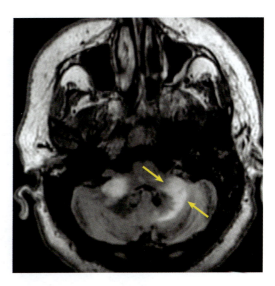

FINDINGS:

- Coronal FLAIR MR shows multifocal hyperintensities in the left temporal/ parietal and cerebellar white matter, with involvement of the subcortical U fibers (arrows).
- Axial FLAIR MR shows hyperintensities in the bilateral brachia pontis and left corpus medullare cerebelli (arrows).

DIAGNOSIS:

Progressive multifocal leukoencephalopathy

DISCUSSION:

Progressive multifocal leukoencephalopathy (PML) is caused by reactivation of the JC virus (JCV) in immunocompromised individuals. Involvement of oligodendrocytes leads to rapidly progressive demyelination that may be solitary, multifocal, or confluent. Classically, there is bilateral asymmetric involvement of the supratentorial white matter, basal ganglia, and thalami. This tends to involve the subcortical U (arcuate) fibers with a "scalloped" appearance, sparing of periventricular white matter, and no significant mass effect. In contrast, HIV encephalopathy causes symmetric periventricular signal abnormality and spares the subcortical U fibers, with associated volume loss. PML can occasionally affect the cerebellum and brainstem, with contiguous involvement of the brachium pontis and corpus medullare cerebelli producing a "crescent" morphology. Atypical imaging manifestations include mildly reduced diffusion, faint peripheral enhancement, hemorrhage, and gray matter involvement. If there is significant contrast enhancement or mass effect, alternative diagnoses such as infectious encephalitis, lymphoma, and acute disseminated encephalomyelitis (ADEM) should be considered.

Reference:

Shah R, Bag AK, Chapman PR, et al. Imaging manifestations of progressive multifocal leukoencephalopathy. *Clin Radiol*. 2010;65(6):431-439.

CRESCENTIC

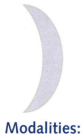

Modalities:
CT, MR

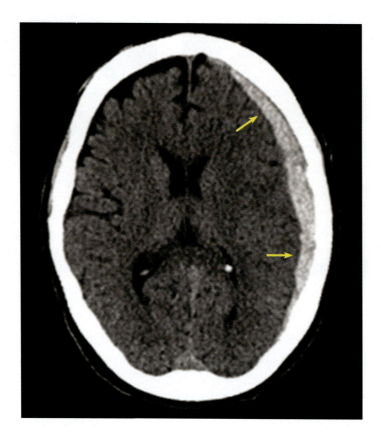

FINDINGS:

Axial CT shows an acute left holohemispheric subdural hematoma (arrows).

DIAGNOSIS:

Subdural hematoma

DISCUSSION:

Subdural hematomas (SDHs) are bleeds between the dura mater and arachnoid mater. These are caused by shear stress on bridging veins due to rotational and/or linear forces, with low-pressure bleeding. In very young, elderly, and alcoholic patients, the presence of enlarged subdural spaces predisposes to SDH with minimal head trauma. Symptoms include gradually increasing headache and confusion. At imaging, SDH is typically crescentic in appearance, tracking along the cerebral convexities. These can cross beneath cranial sutures, stopping only at dural reflections such as the falx cerebri and tentorium cerebelli. The differential for hyperdensity in the subdural space includes infectious (subdural empyema), inflammatory, and neoplastic etiologies, which can readily be distinguished on contrast-enhanced images.

Reference:

Brant WE, Helms C. *Fundamentals of Diagnostic Radiology*, 3rd ed. Baltimore: Lippincott Williams and Wilkins, 2012.

CRUCIFORM, HOT CROSS BUN, MOLAR TOOTH

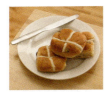

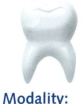

Modality:
MR

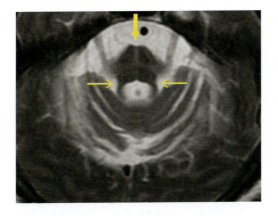

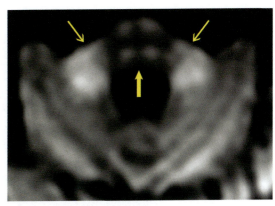

FINDINGS:

- Axial T2-weighted MR shows pontine and cerebellar atrophy with a cruciform appearance (thick arrow). The brachia conjunctivum (thin arrows) are preserved.
- Axial DWI MR shows atrophy and increased signal in the pons (thick arrow) and brachia pontis (thin arrows). The fourth ventricle is dilated.

DIAGNOSIS:

Multiple system atrophy, cerebellar subtype

DISCUSSION:

Multiple system atrophy (MSA) is an adult-onset neurodegenerative disease characterized by parkinsonism, autonomic failure, cerebellar ataxia, and pyramidal signs. Classification is based on the predominant clinical characteristics and includes MSA-P (parkinsonian) or striatonigral degeneration (SND), MSA-C (cerebellar) or olivopontocerebellar atrophy (OPCA), and MSA-A (autonomic) or Shy-Drager syndrome (SDS). MSA-C shows selective atrophy of the pons, cerebellum, and middle cerebellar peduncles. The "cruciform" appearance of the pons results from neuronal degeneration in the pontine raphe and transverse pontocerebellar fibers, with preservation of the pontine tegmentum and corticospinal tracts. Atrophy of the middle cerebellar peduncles and preservation of the superior cerebellar peduncles yields a "molar tooth" appearance, with ballooning of the intervening fourth ventricle. Cerebellar atrophy results in a "fine comb" appearance of the folia and a "fish-mouth" deformity on sagittal images. Spinocerebellar ataxia and vasculitis are other rare causes of spinal cord and cerebellar atrophy.

References:

Huang YP, Tuason MY, Wu T, et al. MRI and CT features of cerebellar degeneration. *J Formos Med Assoc.* 1993;92(6):494-508.

Shrivastava A. The hot cross bun sign. *Radiology.* 2007;245(2):606-607.

(CSF) CLEFT, MENISCUS

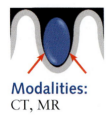

Modalities:
CT, MR

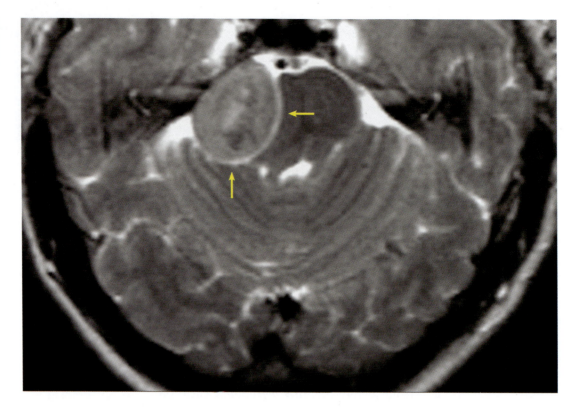

FINDINGS:

Axial T2-weighted MR shows a right cerebellopontine angle mass with surrounding T2-hyperintense rim (arrows). The right pons and brachium conjunctivum are compressed and displaced away from the mass.

DIAGNOSIS:

Extraaxial mass (meningioma)

DISCUSSION:

Correct localization of an intracranial mass is crucial for accurate diagnosis and surgical planning. Extraaxial masses frequently demonstrate a rim of high T2 signal that separates them from subjacent brain. This has been proposed to represent intervening cerebrospinal fluid ("CSF cleft"), dura, vessels, and/or tumor capsule. The classic differential for lesions of the cerebellopontine angle includes meningioma, schwannoma, ependymoma, astrocytoma, metastasis, lipoma, epidermoid cyst, and arachnoid cyst.

References:

Brant WE, Helms C. *Fundamentals of Diagnostic Radiology*, 3rd ed. Baltimore: Lippincott Williams and Wilkins, 2012.

Takeguchi T, Miki H, Shimizu T, et al. Evaluation of the tumor-brain interface of intracranial meningiomas on MR imaging including FLAIR images. *Magn Reson Med Sci.* 2003;2(4):165-169.

CSF/FLAIR/SUBARACHNOID/SULCAL HYPERINTENSITY

Modality:
MR

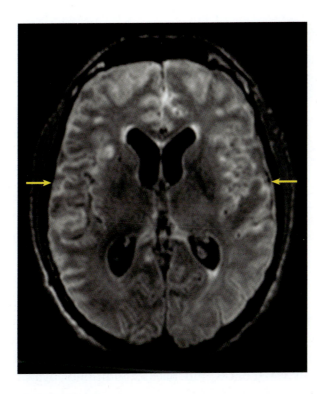

FINDINGS:

Axial FLAIR MR shows diffusely abnormal hyperintense signal within the subarachnoid spaces (arrows).

DIFFERENTIAL DIAGNOSIS:

- Subarachnoid hemorrhage
- Meningitis
- Leptomeningeal carcinomatosis
- Vascular disease
- Supplemental oxygen
- Propofol
- Prior contrast administration
- Artifact

DISCUSSION:

FLAIR MR imaging utilizes an inversion recovery pulse sequence to null the signal from cerebrospinal fluid. Various conditions affecting the leptomeninges, CSF, and/or vasculature can lead to inadequate nulling of subarachnoid signal ("FLAIR hyperintensity" sign). Causes include subarachnoid hemorrhage, meningitis, leptomeningeal carcinomatosis, acute infarct, arterial occlusive disease, supplemental oxygen administration, propofol, prior intravenous contrast administration, and various artifacts (motion, pulsation, susceptibility). The CT correlate of this finding is known as the "pseudo-subarachnoid hemorrhage" sign.

References:

Maeda M, Yagishita A, Yamamoto T, et al. Abnormal hyperintensity within the subarachnoid space evaluated by fluid-attenuated inversion-recovery MR imaging: a spectrum of central nervous system diseases. *Eur Radiol.* 2003;13(Suppl 4):L192-L201.

Stuckey SL, Goh TD, Heffernan T, et al. Hyperintensity in the subarachnoid space on FLAIR MRI. *AJR Am J Roentgenol.* 2007;189(4):913-921.

CYST WITH DOT

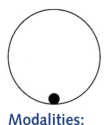

Modalities:
CT, MR

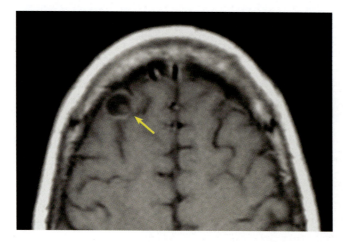

FINDINGS:

Axial contrast-enhanced T1-weighted MR shows a right frontal cystic lesion with enhancing rim and punctate internal focus (arrow).

DIFFERENTIAL DIAGNOSIS:

- Neurocysticercosis
- Toxoplasmosis
- Cystic neoplasms

DISCUSSION:

Neurocysticercosis is a neurologic disease caused by the pork tapeworm *Taenia solium*. It is the most common parasitic infection of the CNS, and the leading cause of acquired epilepsy worldwide. Infection occurs by ingestion of larval eggs in raw or undercooked pork. Once the larvae reach the small intestine, they attach to the intestinal wall via scolices and release additional ova. Through fecal-oral contamination, ova are digested in the stomach and release oncospheres. These penetrate the intestinal wall and enter the bloodstream, preferentially depositing in brain, eyes, and muscle. Locations of disease include subarachnoid-cisternal, parenchymal, intraventricular, and spinal. Five stages have been described: noncystic, vesicular, colloidal vesicular, granular nodular, and calcified nodular. Noncystic neurocysticercosis is asymptomatic with no imaging findings. Vesicular neurocysticercosis demonstrates parenchymal and/or subarachnoid cysts with associated scolices (larval hexacanth and head, forming the "cyst with dot" appearance) and little or no edema. Colloidal vesicular neurocysticercosis is marked by larval disintegration with marked enhancement, edema, and peripheral capsule formation. Granular nodular neurocysticercosis is characterized by cyst retraction and gliosis. Calcified nodular neurocysticercosis is the nonactive stage, in which the lesion has completely involuted and calcified. In contrast, toxoplasmosis lesions typically have larger and more irregular nodules, reflecting associated hemorrhage and inflammation. Cystic neoplasms are usually more heterogeneous in appearance, and may demonstrate an enhancing mural nodule.

Reference:

Kimura-Hayama ET, Higuera JA, Corona-Cedillo R, et al. Neurocysticercosis: radiologic-pathologic correlation. *Radiographics*. 2010;30(6):1705-1719.

CYST WITH NODULE, MURAL NODULE

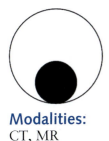

Modalities:
CT, MR

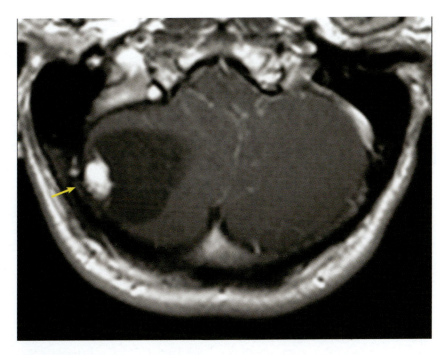

FINDINGS:

Axial contrast-enhanced T1-weighted MR shows a right cerebellar cystic lesion with enhancing mural nodule (arrow).

DIFFERENTIAL DIAGNOSIS:

- Hemangioblastoma
- Infection
- Metastasis

DISCUSSION:

Fluid-secreting tumors have a mixed solid and cystic appearance, with the "mural nodule" representing tumor, and the large adjacent cyst representing reactive fluid. In adults, the most common posterior fossa masses are hemangioblastoma and metastases. The mural nodule of hemangioblastoma is hypervascular, with intense contrast enhancement and flow voids on MR. Infection can also yield solid/cystic lesions, but these are usually multiple and supratentorial in location. Toxoplasmosis and neurocysticercosis lesions tend to have more well-defined, peripherally enhancing cysts surrounding the parasitic organisms ("eccentric/concentric target" and "cyst with dot" signs). Metastases rarely produce the "cyst with nodule" appearance in the setting of internal necrosis, which tends to be more heterogeneous.

References:

Garg A, Suri A, Gupta V. Cyst with a mural nodule: unusual case of brain metastasis. *Neurol India.* 2004;52(1):136.

Lee SR, Sanches J, Mark AS, et al. Posterior fossa hemangioblastomas: MR imaging. *Radiology.* 1989;171(2):463-468.

DAWSON FINGERS, OVOID

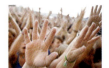

Modality:
MR

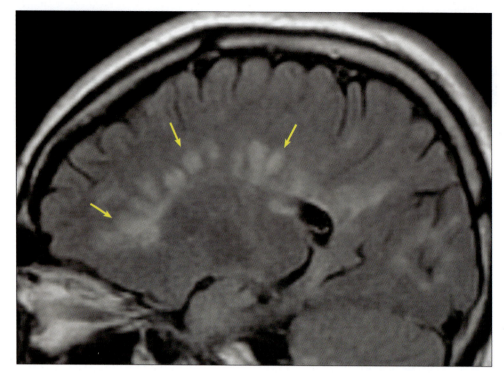

FINDINGS:

Sagittal FLAIR MR shows multiple ovoid hyperintensities (arrows) contacting the corpus callosum and radiating perpendicularly from the lateral ventricles.

DIAGNOSIS:

Multiple sclerosis

DISCUSSION:

Multiple sclerosis (MS) is a chronic demyelinating disorder characterized by spatial and temporal heterogeneity. On T2-weighted and FLAIR MR, characteristic ovoid plaques are seen radiating perpendicularly from the lateral ventricles ("Dawson fingers"). This is thought to represent perivenular inflammation along the courses of the medullary veins, and is both sensitive and specific for MS. Isolated cerebral plaques remote from the ependymal veins are known as "Steiner splashes." The differential includes other demyelinating diseases, such as acute hemorrhagic leukoencephalitis (Weston-Hurst syndrome), in which linear areas of periventricular hemorrhage may be identified on SWI MR. Another possibility is vasculitis, which can be associated with perivenular enhancement and multifocal infarcts.

References:

Horowitz AL, Kaplan RD, Grewe G, et al. The ovoid lesion: a new MR observation in patients with multiple sclerosis. *AJNR Am J Neuroradiol.* 1989;10(2):303-305.

Tan IL, van Schijndel RA, Pouwels PJ, et al. MR venography of multiple sclerosis. *AJNR Am J Neuroradiol.* 2000;21(6):1039-1042.

DIMPLE

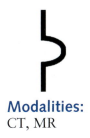

Modalities:
CT, MR

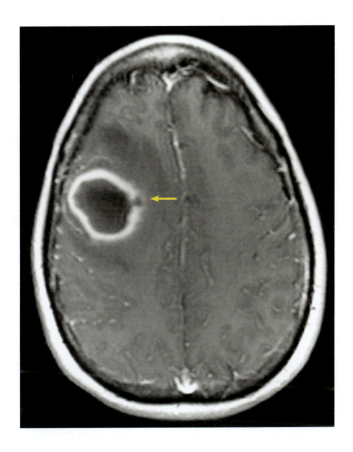

FINDINGS:

Axial contrast-enhanced T1-weighted MR shows a right frontal lobe lesion with peripheral enhancement and focal medial evagination (arrow), as well as surrounding vasogenic edema.

DIAGNOSIS:

Abscess

DISCUSSION:

Cerebral abscesses may result from penetrating trauma, surgery, direct spread of adjacent infection, or hematogenous dissemination. Various bacterial, fungal, and parasitic pathogens have been described. The time for formation of a mature abscess ranges from two weeks to a few months. Organized abscesses demonstrate a smooth peripheral enhancing rim of fibrous collagen. This tends to be slightly thinner on the ventricular side than along the cortical margin, possibly due to differences between white and gray matter perfusion. Over time, the abscess may evaginate or "dimple" toward the ventricular margin. If untreated, there is risk of intraventricular rupture with ependymal spread of infection, which greatly increases morbidity and mortality.

Reference:

Loevner LA, Yousem DM. *Brain Imaging: Case Review Series*, 2nd ed. St Louis, MO: Mosby, 2008.

DISAPPEARING/GHOST/VANISHING TUMOR, SENTINEL LESION

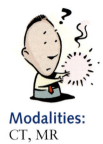

Modalities:
CT, MR

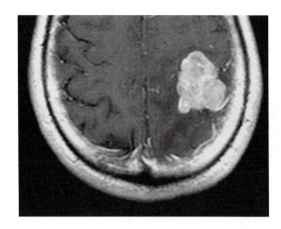 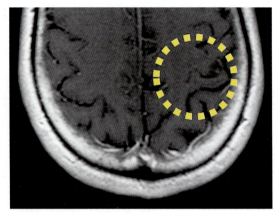

FINDINGS:

Axial contrast-enhanced T1-weighted MR shows a lobulated enhancing left perirolandic mass with surrounding vasogenic edema. Following steroid treatment, there is complete resolution of the mass (dotted circle).

DIFFERENTIAL DIAGNOSIS:

- CNS lymphoma
- Tumefactive demyelination

DISCUSSION:

Primary central nervous system lymphoma (PCNSL) occurs in immunocompromised patients and immunocompetent individuals after the fifth decade. The most common type is non-Hodgkin B-cell lymphoma. Due to tumor hypercellularity, lesions are typically hyperdense on CT and hypointense on T2-weighted MR, with reduced diffusion. The enhancement pattern is homogeneous and solid in immunocompetent patients, but more heterogeneous and ring-enhancing in immunocompromised patients. Lesions can be multifocal and involve the brain parenchyma, vessels, ependyma, and meninges. Lymphoma responds dramatically to steroids and radiation therapy, often disappearing completely on immediate posttreatment imaging ("ghost tumor"). However, this is generally followed by recurrence and systemic involvement within 3 years. Recent studies suggest a minimum of 5-year follow-up to screen for disease relapse. Granulomatous and demyelinating diseases can regress with steroids, but have a different clinical presentation and imaging appearance. Tumors other than lymphoma may decrease in size because of reduced inflammation and edema, but should not disappear completely.

References:

Bromberg JE, Siemers MD, Taphoorn MJ. Is a "vanishing tumor" always a lymphoma? *Neurology.* 2002;59(5):762-764.

Okita Y, Narita Y, Miyakita Y, et al. Long-term follow-up of vanishing tumors in the brain: how should a lesion mimicking primary CNS lymphoma be managed? *Clin Neurol Neurosurg.* 2012;114(9):1217-1221.

DONUT/DOUGHNUT, RIM, RING

Modalities:
CT, MR

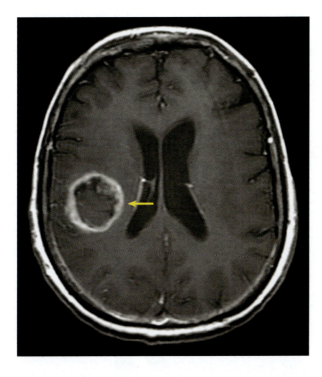

FINDINGS:

Axial contrast-enhanced T1-weighted MR shows a right corona radiata mass (arrow) with complete rim enhancement.

DIFFERENTIAL DIAGNOSIS:

- Metastasis
- Abscess
- Glioblastoma multiforme
- Radiation necrosis
- CNS lymphoma
  (if immunocompromised)
- Toxoplasmosis
  (if immunocompromised)

DISCUSSION:

The classic mnemonic for ring-enhancing lesions is "MAGIC DR L": metastasis, abscess, glioblastoma multiforme, infarct (subacute), contusion, demyelinating disease, radiation necrosis, and lymphoma. Metastases are often multiple and centered at the gray-white junction, with variable internal necrosis that can yield a ring-enhancing pattern. Organized abscesses have smooth rim enhancement with internal reduced diffusion. GBM shows a thick irregular rim with heterogeneous internal enhancement. Infarcts rarely demonstrate ring enhancement, unless located in the deep gray matter. Contusions infrequently have ring enhancement, and may show susceptibility from internal hemorrhage. Tumefactive demyelination demonstrates "incomplete ring" enhancement along the active (leading) edge of disease, and nonenhancement of the inactive (trailing) edge. Radiation necrosis has variable enhancement patterns, with encephalomalacia creating a "soap-bubble" appearance. In immunocompromised patients, the two ring-enhancing lesions suggest CNS lymphoma or toxoplasmosis. Treatment is often empiric, but additional imaging studies that can aid in diagnosis are thallium-201 SPECT (increased uptake in lymphoma, decreased in toxoplasmosis), MR spectroscopy (increased choline in lymphoma, decreased in toxoplasmosis), and MR perfusion (centrally increased cerebral blood volume in lymphoma, decreased in toxoplasmosis).

References:

Chang L, Cornford ME, Chiang FL, et al. Radiologic-pathologic correlation. Cerebral toxoplasmosis and lymphoma in AIDS. *AJNR Am J Neuroradiol.* 1995;16(8):1653-1663.

Smirniotopoulos JG, Murphy FM, Rushing EJ, et al. Patterns of contrast enhancement in the brain and meninges. *Radiographics.* 2007;27(2):525-551.

DOTLIKE, LACY

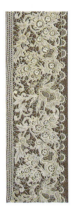

Modality:
MR

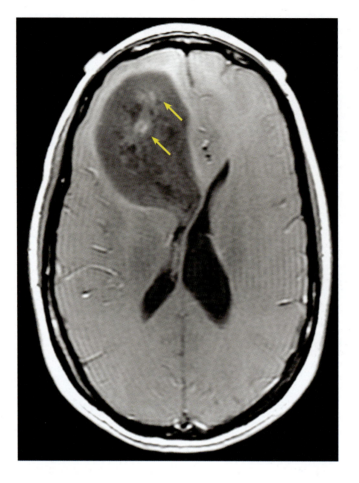

FINDINGS:

Axial contrast-enhanced T1-weighted MR shows a hypointense mass extending from the right frontal horn to the subcortical white matter. There are faint internal foci of enhancement (arrows).

DIFFERENTIAL DIAGNOSIS:

- Oligodendroglioma
- Oligoastrocytoma

DISCUSSION:

Oligodendroglioma is a glial neoplasm that typically affects males in the fourth to seventh decades. The World Health Organization classifies oligodendroglioma into well-differentiated and anaplastic types. In addition, mixed gliomas can occur, with the most common being oligoastrocytoma (oligodendrocytes and astrocytes). The most frequent location is the frontal lobe, followed by the temporal lobe. Lesions tend to be superficial with involvement of the cortex and/or subcortical white matter, often producing scalloping of the overlying calvarium. Margins are generally well-circumscribed, and internal contents are T2-hyperintense and multilocular with a "bubbly" appearance. Internal "dotlike" or "lacy" enhancement is a characteristic feature, though some lesions may not enhance at all. The presence of contrast enhancement indicates a higher tumor grade and worse patient prognosis. Other imaging features include calcification and occasional hemorrhage.

Reference:

Koeller KK, Rushing EJ. From the archives of the AFIP: Oligodendroglioma and its variants: radiologic-pathologic correlation. *Radiographics*. 2005;25(6):1669-1688.

DOVE TAIL

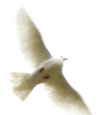

Modalities:
CT, MR

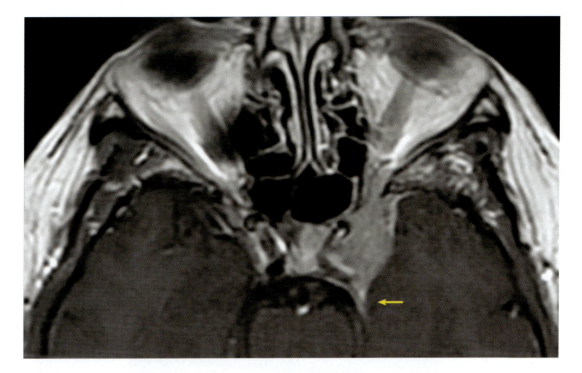

FINDINGS:

Axial contrast-enhanced T1-weighted MR shows an enhancing left cavernous sinus/sellar mass that encases and narrows the cavernous ICA. There is dural extension anteriorly along the left sphenoid wing and posteriorly along the tentorium cerebelli (arrow).

DIFFERENTIAL DIAGNOSIS:

- Meningioma
- Lymphoma
- Granulomatous disease

DISCUSSION:

Cavernous sinus meningiomas may extend posteriorly along the dura with smooth bulging of the tentorium cerebelli, giving a "dove's tail" appearance. Lymphoma and granulomatous disease can occasionally involve the tentorium, but tend to have a more infiltrative growth pattern. Other primary and metastatic tumors in this location usually have a more tumefactive appearance with resultant mass effect.

Reference:

Grossman RI and Yousem DM. *Neuroradiology: The Requisites*, 2nd ed. St. Louis, MO: Mosby, 2003.

DUCKY BREAST, EPSILON, KNOB, KNEE, REVERSE OMEGA, SIGMOID HOOK

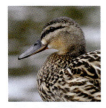

Modalities:
CT, MR

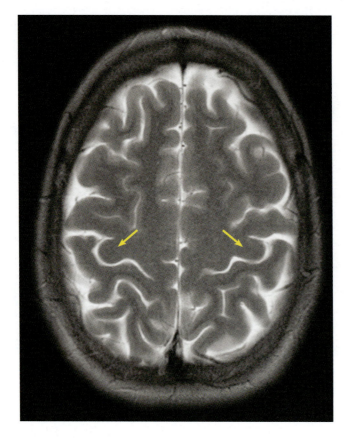

FINDINGS:

Axial T2-weighted MR shows a hooked appearance of the central sulci enclosing the motor hand regions (arrows).

DIAGNOSIS:

Normal central sulcus

DISCUSSION:

The central sulcus is an important landmark of the brain that separates the frontal and parietal lobes, as well as the primary motor and somatosensory cortex. The midportion of the central sulcus is focally indented by the posterior precentral gyrus, which resembles the upside-down Greek letter omega (Ω) in the axial plane, and sigma (ς) in the sagittal plane. When a double gyrus is present, the appearance mimics the letter epsilon (ε). In normal brains, these findings are highly accurate and reproducible landmarks for the motor hand region.

References:

Caulo M, Briganti C, Mattei PA, et al. New morphologic variants of the hand motor cortex as seen with MR imaging in a large study population. *AJNR Am J Neuroradiol*. 2007;28(8):1480-1485.

Yousry TA, Schmid UD, Alkadhi H, et al. Localization of the motor hand area to a knob on the precentral gyrus: a new landmark. *Brain*. 1997;120(pt 1):141-157.

DURAL/PACHYMENINGEAL ENHANCEMENT

Modalities:
CT, MR

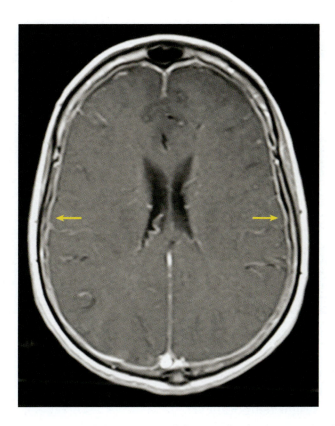

FINDINGS:

Axial contrast-enhanced T1-weighted MR shows diffuse enhancement of the dura mater (arrows).

DIFFERENTIAL DIAGNOSIS:

- Intracranial hypotension
- Inflammation/infection
- Malignancy
- Idiopathic hypertrophic pachymeningitis

DISCUSSION:

The dura mater (pachymeninges) include the periosteum of the inner table of the skull and its meningeal reflections (falx cerebri, tentorium cerebelli, and cavernous sinuses). Normally, the dura enhances mildly and discontinuously. Thick linear pachymeningeal enhancement can be seen in Intracranial hypotension (CSF hypovolemia), which leads to secondary vasocongestion and interstitial edema in the dura mater. This condition may be idiopathic (spontaneous intracranial hypotension) or secondary to lumbar puncture or trauma. Noncontrast FLAIR MR sequences are also effective for identifying pachymeningeal thickening and subdural effusions/hematomas in CSF hypotension. Thin linear dural enhancement is a common finding in postoperative patients. Focal or diffuse dural enhancement has been described in various other inflammatory, autoimmune, infectious, and neoplastic conditions. When no primary cause is identified, the condition is known as idiopathic hypertrophic pachymeningitis.

References:

Smirniotopoulos JG, Murphy FM, Rushing EJ, et al. Patterns of contrast enhancement in the brain and meninges. *Radiographics.* 2007;27(2):525-551.

Tosaka M, Sato N, Fujimaki H, et al. Diffuse pachymeningeal hyperintensity and subdural effusion/hematoma detected by fluid-attenuated inversion recovery MR imaging in patients with spontaneous intracranial hypotension. *AJNR Am J Neuroradiol.* 2008;29(6):1164-1170.

DURAL TAIL, FLARE, MENINGEAL

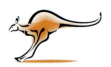

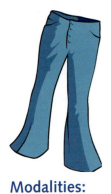

Modalities:
CT, MR

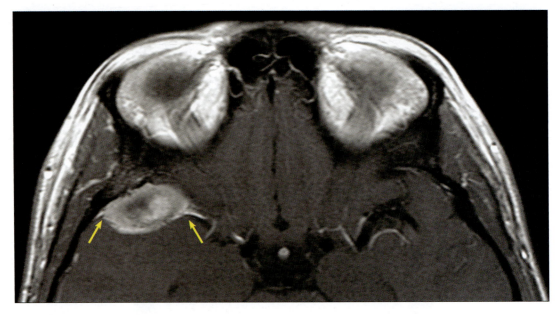

FINDINGS:

Axial contrast-enhanced T1-weighted MR shows a right middle cranial fossa mass with dural thickening along the greater sphenoid wing (arrows). There is posterior displacement of the right temporal gyri.

DIFFERENTIAL DIAGNOSIS:

- Meningioma
- Other dural masses

DISCUSSION:

The presence of a "dural tail" (dural thickening and enhancement contiguous with an intracranial mass) is classic for meningioma. This finding is most apparent on contrast-enhanced T1-weighted MR, and seen in about 60% of cases. The pathophysiology is not completely understood, but may relate to microscopic tumor invasion and/or reactive meningeal changes. Occasionally, other extra-axial and peripherally located intra-axial lesions can also involve the dura. The possibilities are wide and include metastasis, lymphoma, plasmacytoma, chloroma, glioma, nerve sheath tumors, pituitary lesions, inflammatory/granulomatous/histiocytic diseases, infection, primary bone tumors, and vascular abnormalities.

References:

Guermazi A, Lafitte F, Miaux Y, et al. The dural tail sign—beyond meningioma. *Clin Radiol.* 2005;60(2):171-188.

Wallace EW. The dural tail sign. *Radiology.* 2004;233(1):56-57.

EMPTY LIGHT BULB, HALO, HOLLOW SKULL, HOT NOSE

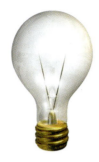

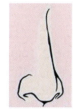

Modality:
NM

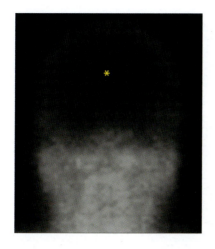

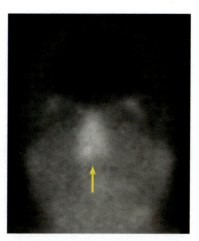

FINDINGS:

- Posterior planar ^{99m}Tc-HMPAO scan shows complete absence of tracer uptake in the brain (asterisk), with surrounding uptake in the scalp.
- Anterior planar image shows increased uptake in the nose (arrow) and facial soft tissues.

DIAGNOSIS:

Brain death

DISCUSSION:

Accurate diagnosis of brain death is critical prior to discontinuing life support in a comatose patient, particularly when organ donation is being considered. Clinical examination is only reliable in the absence of hypothermia, barbiturates, sedatives, and hypnotics. If the diagnosis is unclear, a nuclear medicine brain scan can be performed with technetium-99m ethyl cysteinate dimer (^{99m}Tc-ECD), hexamethylpropylene amine oxime (^{99m}Tc-HMPAO), or diethylene triamine pentaacetic acid (^{99m}Tc-DTPA). HMPAO and ECD are preferred, being lipophilic agents that selectively cross the blood-brain barrier and are taken up by the brain parenchyma. Initial dynamic flow images are acquired in the anterior projection, followed by delayed static blood pool images in anterior, posterior, and lateral projections. Brain death is diagnosed when there is complete absence of tracer uptake within the cranium on all images. Care must be taken to distinguish no flow from very slow flow within the cerebral arteries and/or veins. Occlusion of the ICAs prevents blood inflow to the brain, with increased collateral flow to the ECAs. This results in increased uptake of the nasopharyngeal soft tissues and scalp, producing the "hot nose" and "hollow skull" signs. In adults, a scalp band or tourniquet can be used to decrease scalp activity that might be confused for intracranial uptake. If the patient's head is resting on a firm surface, focal scalp compression may produce a photopenic defect known as the "halo" sign.

References:

Abdel-Dayem HM, Bahar RH, Sigurdsson GH, et al. The hollow skull: a sign of brain death in Tc-99m HM-PAO brain scintigraphy. *Clin Nucl Med.* 1989;14(12):912-916.

Huang AH. The hot nose sign. *Radiology.* 2005;235(1):216-217.

ENGULFED CALCIFICATION

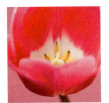

Modalities:
CT, MR

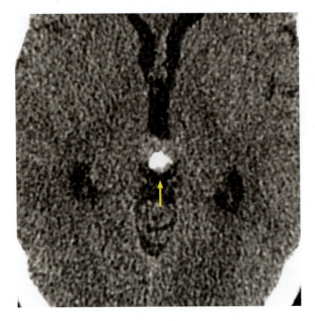

FINDINGS:

Axial CT shows a rounded hyperdense pineal mass with central calcification (arrow).

DIAGNOSIS:

Pineal germ cell tumor

DISCUSSION:

The differential for pineal region solid masses is wide and includes pineal parenchymal tumor, germ cell tumor, metastasis, glioma, lymphoma, neuroendocrine tumor, meningioma, and vascular lesions. Clinical symptoms include Parinaud syndrome (upward gaze palsy), headache, and ataxia. To determine whether a lesion is pineal or parapineal in origin, images should be reviewed to identify the pineal gland (if visible) and surrounding structures: internal cerebral veins (superior), midbrain tectum (anterior), cerebellar vermis (inferior), and tentorial incisura (posterior). In adults, physiologic calcification aids in identification of the pineal gland. For true pineal masses, the pattern of calcification is helpful: germ cell tumors tend to grow around and "engulf" preexisting pineal calcifications, whereas pineal parenchymal tumors disrupt and peripherally disperse ("explode") calcifications. Types of germ cell tumors include germinoma, teratoma, embryonal carcinoma, endodermal sinus (yolk sac) tumor, and choriocarcinoma. Germinomas, which are characteristically seen in young males, appear hyperdense on CT with avid homogeneous enhancement. They can be multifocal with additional lesions in the suprasellar region ("bifocal germinoma"), basal ganglia, and thalami. Tumors are exquisitely sensitive to radiation and/or chemotherapy, often resolving completely after treatment. When a pineal malignancy is diagnosed, the entire neuraxis should be imaged to assess for leptomeningeal spread of disease.

Reference:

Smith AB, Rushing EJ, Smirniotopoulos JG. From the archives of the AFIP: lesions of the pineal region: radiologic-pathologic correlation. *Radiographics*. 2010;30(7):2001-2020.

ENTRAPMENT, TRAPPED VENTRICLE

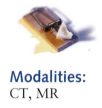

Modalities:
CT, MR

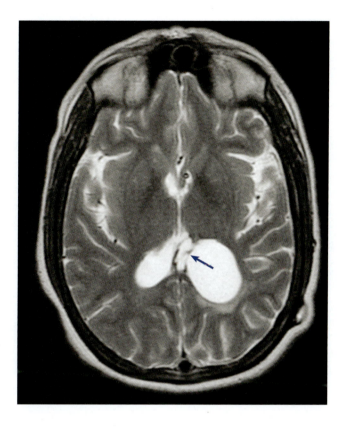

FINDINGS:

Axial T2-weighted MR shows a cystic mass in the left atrium (arrow), with asymmetric dilation of the left occipital horn.

DIFFERENTIAL DIAGNOSIS:

- Intraventricular mass
- Intraventricular adhesions
- Extraventricular mass

DISCUSSION:

"Trapped" ventricle refers to isolated ventricular dilation caused by blockage of cerebrospinal fluid outflow, and represents a focal form of obstructive hydrocephalus. Causes include prior surgery, trauma, or infection with residual adhesions; intraventricular neoplasms or cysts; and extraventricular lesions causing asymmetric mass effect. The lateral ventricles are most commonly affected, but rare entrapment of the third or fourth ventricles can also occur.

References:

Kuiper EJ, Vandertop WP. Trapped third ventricle. *Acta Neurochir (Wien)*. 2001;143(11):1169-1172.

Maurice Williams RS, Chokesy M. Entrapment of the temporal horn: a form of focal obstructive hydrocephalus. *J Neurol Neurosurg Psychiatry*. 1986;49:238-242.

EPENDYMAL DOT-DASH

Modality:
MR

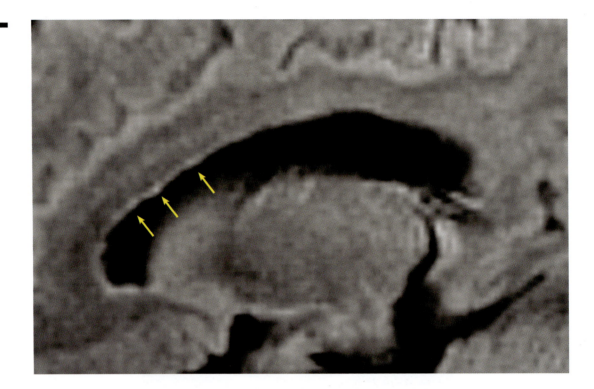

FINDINGS:

Sagittal FLAIR MR shows subcallosal hyperintense foci (arrows) separated by normal ependyma.

DIAGNOSIS:

Multiple sclerosis

DISCUSSION:

Multiple sclerosis (MS) is a chronic demyelinating disorder characterized by spatial and temporal heterogeneity. On thin-section sagittal FLAIR MR, there is irregularity of the ependymal stripe on the undersurface of the corpus callosum. Two or more rounded hyperintense "dots" are seen, with intervening normal ependymal "dashes." Lesions are not oriented perpendicular to the ependyma, in contrast to subcallosal striations and Dawson fingers. This finding has been shown to be highly sensitive and specific for detection of early MS, particularly in younger patients.

Reference:

Lisanti CJ, Asbach P, Bradley WG Jr. The ependymal "Dot-Dash" sign: an MR imaging finding of early multiple sclerosis. *AJNR Am J Neuroradiol.* 2005;26(8):2033-2036.

ÉTAT CRIBLÉ, HONEYCOMB, SWISS CHEESE

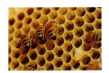

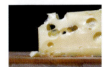

Modalities:
CT, MR

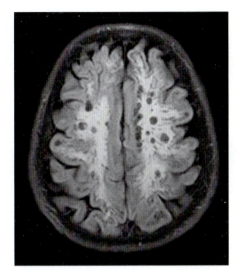

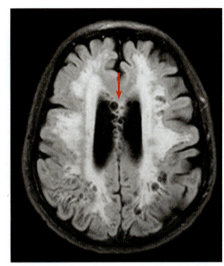

FINDINGS:

Axial FLAIR MR shows numerous cystic spaces throughout the brain, particularly the high convexity white matter and corpus callosum (arrow).

DIFFERENTIAL DIAGNOSIS:

- Dilated Virchow-Robin spaces
- Mucopolysaccharidosis
- Multiple sclerosis
- Lacunar infarcts

DISCUSSION:

Virchow-Robin (VR) spaces are interstitial fluid-containing spaces that surround vessels as they course from the subarachnoid space into the brain parenchyma. Small VR spaces are normally seen at imaging, and increase in size and number with advancing age. Dilated VR spaces are seen in three typical locations: type I, basal ganglia (lenticulostriate arteries); type II, high convexities (perforating medullary arteries); and type III, midbrain (collicular arteries). Diffusely enlarged VR spaces yield the "état criblé" appearance (French for "tissue riddled with holes" or "sievelike state"). This may be seen with the mucopolysaccharidoses, in which enzyme deficiencies disable breakdown of glycosaminoglycans (GAG). The VR spaces are dilated by accumulated GAG, producing a "cribriform" appearance of the white matter, corpus callosum, and basal ganglia. Toxic intracellular substrates also lead to cerebral atrophy and gliosis. Multiple sclerosis can show diffuse punctate (<2 mm) VR spaces, described as a "sandlike" appearance. Lacunar infarcts are usually larger (>5 mm), fewer, and less symmetric in distribution.

References:

Achiron A, Faibel M. Sandlike appearance of Virchow-Robin spaces in early multiple sclerosis: a novel neuroradiologic marker. *AJNR Am J Neuroradiol*. 2002;23(3):376-380.

Kwee RM, Kwee TC. Virchow-Robin spaces at MR imaging. *Radiographics*. 2007;27(4):1071-1086.

EXPLODED CALCIFICATION

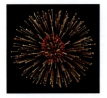

Modalities:
CT, MR

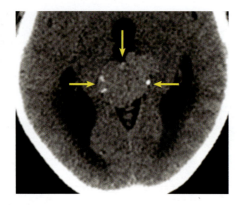

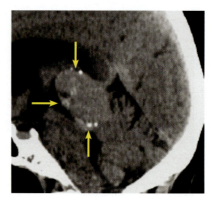

FINDINGS:

Axial and sagittal CT show a large irregular pineal mass with peripheral calcifications (arrows).

DIAGNOSIS:

Pineal cell tumor

DISCUSSION:

The differential for pineal region solid masses is wide and includes pineal parenchymal tumor, germ cell tumor, metastasis, glioma, lymphoma, neuroendocrine tumor, meningioma, and vascular lesions. Clinical symptoms include Parinaud syndrome (upward gaze palsy), headache, and ataxia. To determine whether a lesion is pineal or parapineal in origin, images should be reviewed to identify the pineal gland (if visible) and surrounding structures: internal cerebral veins (superior), midbrain tectum (anterior), cerebellar vermis (inferior), and tentorial incisura (posterior). In adults, physiologic calcification aids in identification of the pineal gland. For true pineal masses, the pattern of calcification is helpful: germ cell tumors tend to grow around and "engulf" preexisting pineal calcifications, whereas pineal parenchymal tumors disrupt and peripherally disperse ("explode") calcifications. Pineal parenchymal tumors are derived from pinealocytes with varying degrees of differentiation. Histologically, they are classified as pineocytoma [WHO grade I], pineal parenchymal tumor of intermediate differentiation (PPTID) [WHO grade II-III], papillary tumor of the pineal region (PPTR) [WHO grade II-III], and pineoblastoma (primitive neuroectodermal tumor of pineal gland) [WHO grade IV]. Lower-grade tumors are smaller, well-defined, and slowly growing, while higher-grade tumors appear larger, heterogeneous, and locally invasive. Pineoblastoma can be seen in patients with ocular retinoblastoma ("trilateral" retinoblastoma), along with suprasellar PNET ("quadrilateral" retinoblastoma). When a pineal malignancy is diagnosed, the entire neuraxis should be imaged to assess for leptomeningeal spread of disease.

Reference:

Smith AB, Rushing EJ, Smirniotopoulos JG. From the archives of the AFIP: lesions of the pineal region: radiologic-pathologic correlation. *Radiographics*. 2010;30(7):2001-2020.

EYE OF THE TIGER

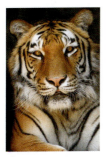

Modality:
MR

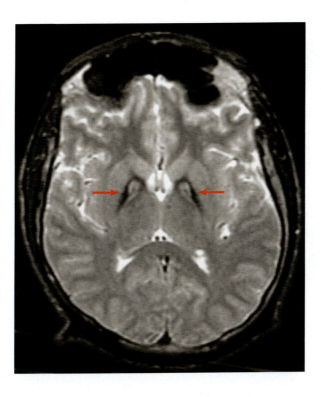

FINDINGS:

Axial T2-weighted MR shows hyperintense globus pallidi with hypointense rims (arrows).

DIFFERENTIAL DIAGNOSIS:

- Pantothenate kinase–associated neurodegeneration
- Other extrapyramidal parkinsonian disorders

DISCUSSION:

Neurodegeneration with brain iron accumulation (NBIA), previously known as Hallevorden-Spatz syndrome, refers to a spectrum of pediatric neurodegenerative disorders characterized by abnormal iron deposition in the basal ganglia. Symptoms begin in childhood with progressive extrapyramidal dysfunction causing rigidity, dystonia, impaired postural reflexes, and progressive dementia. Pantothenate kinase–associated neurodegeneration (PKAN) is the most common subtype of NBIA (NBIA1), and is caused by mutations in the pantothenate kinase 2 (*PANK2*) gene. On T2-weighted and SWI MR, the globus pallidi demonstrate high signal intensity with a hypointense rim ("eye of the tiger" sign). Histologically, this corresponds to central gliosis and vacuolization with surrounding iron deposition. This imaging finding is highly effective for distinguishing NBIA patients with the *PANK2* mutation from mutation-negative patients. However, other extrapyramidal parkinsonian disorders such as corticobasal degeneration, early-onset levodopa-responsive parkinsonism, and progressive supranuclear palsy can have similar imaging findings, and clinical correlation is crucial for diagnosis.

References:

Guillerman RP. The eye-of-the-tiger sign. *Radiology.* 2000;217(3):895-896.

Savoiardo M, Halliday WC, Nardocci N, et al. Hallervorden-Spatz disease: MR and pathologic findings. *AJNR Am J Neuroradiol.* 1993;14(1):155-162.

FACE OF THE GIANT PANDA, PANDA MIDBRAIN

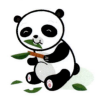

Modality:
MR

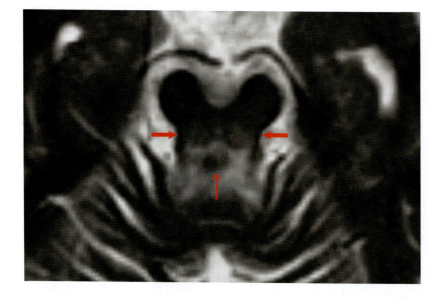

FINDINGS:

Axial T2-weighted MR of the midbrain shows high signal throughout the tegmentum, sparing the red nuclei (thick arrows) and periaqueductal gray (thin arrow). Low signal is seen in the substantia nigra and cerebral peduncles.

DIFFERENTIAL DIAGNOSIS:

- Wilson disease
- Leigh disease
- Glutaric aciduria type 1

DISCUSSION:

Wilson disease, or hepatolenticular degeneration, is an autosomal recessive disorder caused by mutations in the Wilson disease protein (*ATP7B*) gene on chromosome 13. This interferes with normal copper metabolism, resulting in pathologic accumulation of copper and other heavy metals in the central nervous system, liver, kidneys, and heart. On T2-weighted MR, the "face of the giant panda" refers to abnormal high signal in the midbrain tegmentum; preserved normal signal in the red nuclei ("eyes"), lateral pars reticulata of the substantia nigra ("ears"), and periaqueductal gray ("nose"); and hypointensity of the superior colliculi ("mouth"). Diffuse symmetric T2 hyperintensities in the subcortical white matter, internal and external capsules ("bright claustrum" sign), basal ganglia, and thalami can also be seen and are thought to represent edema or gliosis. The differential diagnosis includes other metabolic disorders, such as Leigh disease and glutaric aciduria type 1.

References:

Prashanth LK, Sinha S, Taly AB, et al. Do MRI features distinguish Wilson's disease from other early onset extrapyramidal disorders? An analysis of 100 cases. *Mov Disord.* 2010;25(6):672-678.

Schott JM. A neurological MRI menagerie. *Pract Neurol.* 2007;7:186-190.

FACE OF THE MINIATURE PANDA, PANDA CUB

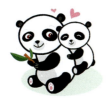

Modality:
MR

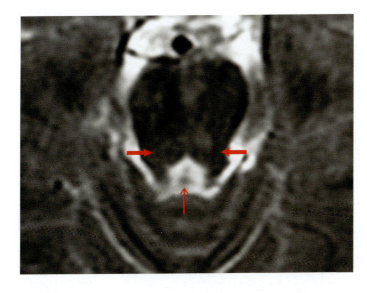

FINDINGS:

Axial T2-weighted MR of the pons shows hypointensity of the central tegmental tracts (thick arrows) and brachia conjunctivum. The fourth ventricle appears normally hyperintense with a central flow void (thin arrow).

DIAGNOSIS:

Wilson disease

DISCUSSION:

Wilson disease, or hepatolenticular degeneration, is an autosomal recessive disorder caused by mutations in the Wilson disease protein (*ATP7B*) gene on chromosome 13. This interferes with normal copper metabolism, resulting in pathologic accumulation of copper and other heavy metals in the central nervous system, liver, kidneys, and heart. On T2-weighted MR, the "face of the miniature panda" sign refers to abnormal high signal within the pontine tegmentum; normal signal in the cerebral peduncles ("ears"), hypointensity of the medial longitudinal fasciculi, central tegmental tracts ("eyes"), and superior cerebellar peduncles ("cheeks"); and hyperintense fluid signal within the aqueduct of Sylvius and fourth ventricle ("nose and mouth"). The combination of this sign with the "face of the giant panda" sign is termed the "double panda" sign, and is virtually pathognomonic for Wilson disease. Diffuse symmetric T2 hyperintensities in the subcortical white matter, internal and external capsules ("bright claustrum" sign), basal ganglia, and thalami can also be seen, and are thought to represent edema or gliosis.

References:

Jacobs DA, Markowitz CE, Liebeskind DS, et al. The "double panda sign" in Wilson's disease. *Neurology.* 2003;61(7):969.

Prashanth LK, Sinha S, Taly AB, et al. Do MRI features distinguish Wilson's disease from other early onset extrapyramidal disorders? An analysis of 100 cases. *Mov Disord.* 2010;25(6):672-678.

FAT/SAGGING/SWELLING MIDBRAIN

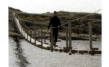

Modalities:
CT, MR

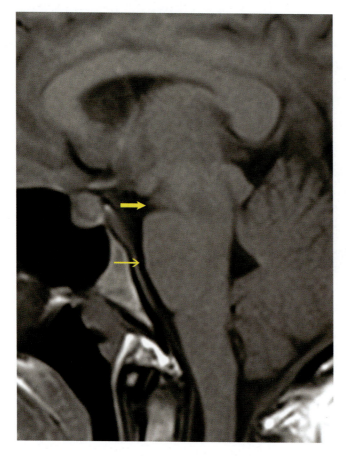

FINDINGS:

Sagittal T1-weighted MR shows distended midbrain (thick arrow) and inferior migration of the brainstem with flattening of the pons against the clivus (thin arrow). The pituitary gland is also distended.

DIAGNOSIS:

Intracranial hypotension

DISCUSSION:

Intracranial hypotension can be caused by idiopathic, degenerative, traumatic, and iatrogenic etiologies. Dural tears in the brain or spine cause continuous loss of fluid, resulting in cerebrospinal fluid hypovolemia. The Monro-Kellie doctrine states that in a closed compartment, the total volume of brain, blood, and CSF must remain constant. As a result, the high-capacitance venous system becomes engorged with blood. The deep cerebral structures and brainstem become swollen ("fat midbrain"), reflecting mild diffuse vasogenic edema. There is flattening of the pons against the clivus with effacement of the prepontine and interpeduncular cisterns. The entire brain migrates inferiorly with low-lying brainstem, cerebellar tonsils, third ventricle, optic chiasm, mammillary bodies, and splenium. Patients may present with orthostatic headaches, cranial neuropathies, nausea/vomiting, and fatigue. Strategies for identifying the site of leakage include radionuclide cisternography and conventional, CT, or MR myelography. Once identified, the leak can be repaired by epidural blood patch, percutaneous fibrin glue injection, or surgery.

References:

Hadizadeh DR, Kovács A, Tschampa H, et al. Postsurgical intracranial hypotension: diagnostic and prognostic imaging findings. *AJNR Am J Neuroradiol.* 2010;31(1):100-105.

Savoiardo M, Minati L, Farina L, et al. Spontaneous intracranial hypotension with deep brain swelling. *Brain.* 2007;130(pt 7):1884-1893.

FEATHERY, SOAP BUBBLE, SPREADING WAVEFRONT, SWISS CHEESE

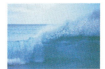

Modalities:
CT, MR

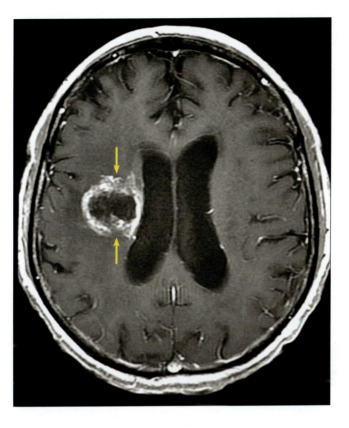

FINDINGS:

Axial contrast-enhanced T1-weighted MR shows a ring-enhancing lesion in the right corona radiata with ill-defined peripheral enhancement (arrows).

DIAGNOSIS:

Radiation necrosis

DISCUSSION:

Radiation necrosis refers to degradation of brain tissue following therapeutic irradiation for intracranial tumors (especially high-grade gliomas and metastases), arteriovenous malformations, and head and neck cancers. There is characteristic "soap bubble" or "Swiss cheese" enhancement, reflecting internal necrosis. The enhancing margins gradually blend in with surrounding brain, producing a "feathery" or "spreading wavefront" appearance. In the setting of treated tumor (particularly high-grade glioma), local recurrence and radiation necrosis are notoriously difficult to distinguish. Useful imaging studies include MR diffusion (reduced in recurrence, normal or increased in necrosis), CT/MR perfusion (increased in recurrence, decreased in radiation necrosis), MR spectroscopy (elevated choline-to-creatine and choline-to-NAA ratios in recurrence, reduced major metabolites and lactate peak in radiation necrosis), thallium-201 SPECT (increased uptake in recurrence, decreased in radiation necrosis), and 18F-FDG PET (increased metabolism in recurrence, decreased in radiation necrosis).

References:

Caroline I, Rosenthal MA. Imaging modalities in high-grade gliomas: pseudoprogression, recurrence, or necrosis? *J Clin Neurosci.* 2012;19(5):633-637.

Mullins ME, Barest GD, Schaefer PW, et al. Radiation necrosis versus glioma recurrence: conventional MR imaging clues to diagnosis. *AJNR Am J Neuroradiol.* 2005;26(8):1967-1972.

Shah R, Vattoth S, Jacob R, et al. Radiation necrosis in the brain: imaging features and differentiation from tumor recurrence. *Radiographics.* 2012;32(5):1343-1359.

FLECKED, MOTTLED, SALT AND PEPPER

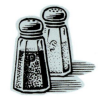

Modality:
CT

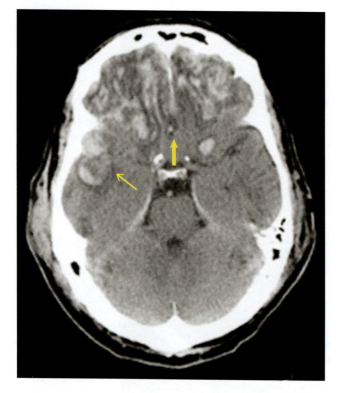

FINDINGS:

Axial CT shows mixed edema and hemorrhage in the bilateral inferior frontal (thick arrow) and right anterior temporal (thin arrow) lobes.

DIAGNOSIS:

Hemorrhagic contusions

DISCUSSION:

Cerebral contusions are caused by low-velocity direct head trauma. Coup injuries occur at the site of impact, whereas contrecoup injuries are caused by inertial force transmission to the opposite side. Confluent areas of edema in the inferior frontal and anterior temporal lobes are the result of impaction against the cribriform plate and sphenoid wings. Petechial hemorrhages reflect traumatic shearing of small vessels and may be seen at the gray-white junction, deep gray matter, brainstem, and periventricular regions. On CT, the combination of hypodense edema and hyperdense hemorrhage produces a "salt and pepper" appearance. Small simple contusions may normalize on follow-up imaging, whereas large and severe contusions progress to encephalomalacia. Late complications include attention, emotion, and memory deficits.

Reference:

Kurland D, Hong C, Aarabi B, et al. Hemorrhagic progression of a contusion after traumatic brain injury: a review. *J Neurotrauma.* 2012;29(1):19-31.

GELATINOUS PSEUDOCYSTS, SOAP BUBBLE

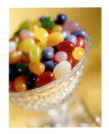

Modalities:
CT, MR

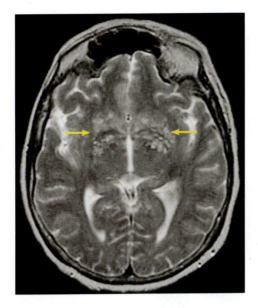

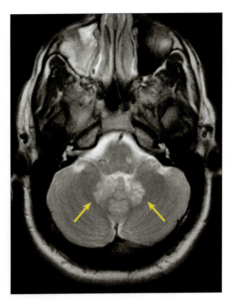

FINDINGS:

Axial T2-weighted MR shows clustered cystic lesions in the bilateral basal ganglia and cerebellar dentate nuclei (arrows).

DIAGNOSIS:

Cryptococcosis

DISCUSSION:

Cryptococcus neoformans is an encapsulated fungus found in soil contaminated by bird excreta. It is the most common fungal infection of the CNS, and the third most common in AIDS patients. In immunocompromised individuals, hematogenous spread from the lungs to the central nervous system results in CNS cryptococcosis (torulosis). Three patterns of disease have been identified: parenchymal granulomas (cryptococcomas or torulomas), gelatinous pseudocysts, and meningitis. Gelatinous pseudocysts represent dilated perivascular (Virchow-Robin) spaces filled with inflammatory cells and mucoid material produced by fungal capsules. These predominate in the basal ganglia, thalami, midbrain, cerebellum, and periventricular regions. There is high T2 and variable T1 signal, depending on the mucin content of cysts. Depending on the degree of immune competency, associated edema and enhancement may be present. Early treatment with intravenous antifungals is crucial to minimize morbidity and mortality.

References:

Andreula CF, Burdi N, Carella A. CNS cryptococcosis in AIDS: spectrum of MR findings. *J Comput Assist Tomogr.* 1993;17(3):438-441.

Smith AB, Smirniotopoulos JG, Rushing EJ. From the archives of the AFIP: central nervous system infections associated with human immunodeficiency virus infection: radiologic-pathologic correlation. *Radiographics.* 2008;28(7):2033-2058.

GYRIFORM, LEPTOMENINGEAL ENHANCEMENT, SERPENTINE

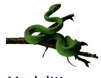

Modalities:
CT, MR

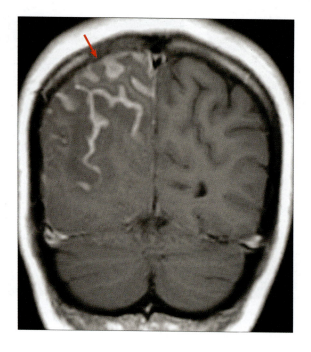

FINDINGS:

Coronal contrast-enhanced T1-weighted MR shows leptomeningeal enhancement in the right parietal lobe (arrow).

DIFFERENTIAL DIAGNOSIS:

- Infectious/inflammatory meningitis
- Vascular conditions
- Leptomeningeal carcinomatosis

DISCUSSION:

Enhancement of the arachnoid and pia mater reflects breakdown of the blood-brain barrier, with subsequent contrast leakage from vessels into cerebrospinal fluid. Common etiologies include infectious or inflammatory meningitis, vascular conditions, and leptomeningeal carcinomatosis. Bacterial (pyogenic) and viral (aseptic) meningitis demonstrate smooth linear leptomeningeal enhancement. Fungal, tuberculous, and other granulomatous (chronic) meningitides demonstrate more nodular enhancement with a predilection for the basilar cisterns. Vascular etiologies include acutely reperfused or subacute arterial infarction, posterior reversible leukoencephalopathy, vasculitis, and vasodilation associated with migraine or seizures. Typically, the subjacent cortex is also involved. Metastases from CNS primaries, breast, lung, melanoma, and lymphoma can diffusely involve the meninges. Inflammation secondary to prior surgery or subarachnoid hemorrhage can occasionally produce leptomeningeal enhancement.

Reference:

Smirniotopoulos JG, Murphy FM, Rushing EJ, et al. Patterns of contrast enhancement in the brain and meninges. *Radiographics*. 2007;27(2):525-551.

HOCKEY STICK, PULVINAR

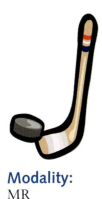

Modality:
MR

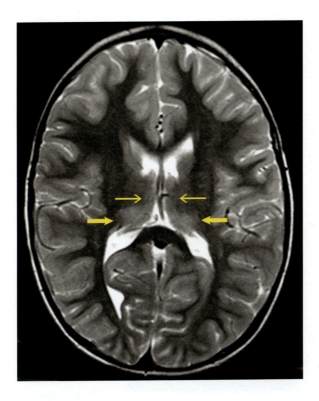

FINDINGS:

Axial T2-weighted MR shows symmetric increased signal in the dorsomedial (thin arrows) and pulvinar nuclei (thick arrows) of both thalami.

DIAGNOSIS:

Creutzfeldt-Jakob disease

DISCUSSION:

Creutzfeldt-Jakob disease (CJD) is a rapidly progressing and fatal dementia caused by prions, which are misfolded proteins that cannot be broken down by the body and subsequently convert their correctly folded counterparts. Subtypes of CJD include classical/sporadic (sCJD), inherited/familial (fCJD), variant (vCJD), and iatrogenic/acquired. vCJD, or "mad cow disease," was first described in the 1990s and linked to eating beef contaminated with bovine spongiform encephalopathy (BSE). Most cases have occurred in the United Kingdom, with a younger age of onset and longer duration of disease than in sCJD. On MR, there is rapidly progressive signal abnormality of the basal ganglia, thalami, and cerebral cortex. Symmetric T2 hyperintensities and reduced diffusion can be seen in the pulvinar and dorsomedial nuclei of the thalamus ("hockey stick" appearance), caudate heads, putamina, globus pallidi, insulae, cingulate cortex, and periaqueductal gray matter. Occasionally, intrinsic T1 shortening may be present, which is thought to represent deposition of prion proteins. In the late stages, there is massive loss of brain tissue that produces a "spongiform" or "Swiss cheese" appearance.

References:

Collie DA, Summers DM, Sellar RJ, et al. Diagnosing variant Creutzfeldt-Jakob disease with the pulvinar sign: MR imaging findings in 86 neuropathologically confirmed cases. *AJNR Am J Neuroradiol.* 2003;24(8):1560-1569.

Young GS, Geschwind MD, Fischbein NJ, et al. Diffusion-weighted and fluid-attenuated inversion recovery imaging in Creutzfeldt-Jakob disease: high sensitivity and specificity for diagnosis. *AJNR Am J Neuroradiol.* 2005;26(6):1551-1562.

HUMMINGBIRD, PENGUIN

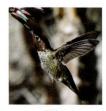

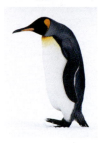

Modalities:
CT, MR

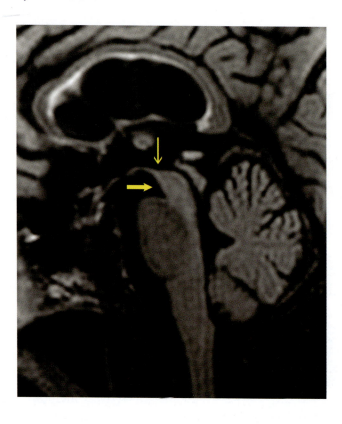

FINDINGS:

Sagittal FLAIR MR shows midbrain atrophy with concave superior margin (thin arrow) and deep interpeduncular fossa (thick arrow). The pons and medulla are normal in size.

DIAGNOSIS:

Progressive supranuclear palsy

DISCUSSION:

Progressive supranuclear palsy (Steele-Richardson-Olszewski syndrome), an adult-onset neurodegenerative disorder, is the most common cause of parkinsonism following Parkinson disease. Symptoms include dementia, postural instability, and vertical supranuclear gaze palsy. There is selective atrophy of the midbrain tectum and tegmentum, with flattened or concave margins and a deep interpeduncular fossa. On sagittal images, the "hummingbird" sign refers to midbrain atrophy juxtaposed with normal pons and medulla. On axial images, the "Mickey Mouse" or "morning glory" sign is produced by midbrain atrophy with preserved cerebral peduncles. Focal hypometabolism on PET gives rise to the "pimple" sign. Findings may be difficult to distinguish from age-related volume loss and other dementing disorders, and correlation with clinical symptoms is crucial for diagnosis.

References:

Botha H, Whitwell JL, Madhaven A, et al. The pimple sign of progressive supranuclear palsy syndrome. *Parkinsonism Relat Disord*. 2013 Nov 4. [Epub ahead of print]

Gröschel K, Kastrup A, Litvan I, et al. Penguins and hummingbirds: midbrain atrophy in progressive supranuclear palsy. *Neurology*. 2006;66(6):949-950.

HYPERDENSE FALX, HYPERDENSE TENTORIUM

Modality:
CT

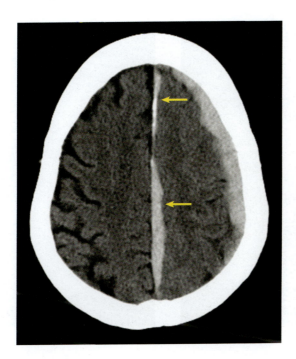 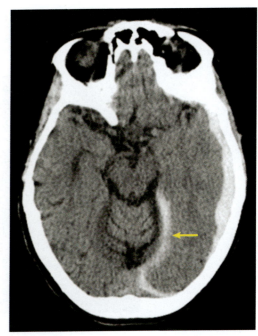

FINDINGS:

Axial CT shows a left holohemispheric subdural hematoma that extends superiorly along the falx cerebri and inferiorly along the tentorium cerebelli (arrows).

DIAGNOSIS:

Subdural hematoma

DISCUSSION:

Subdural hematomas (SDHs) are bleeds between the dura mater and arachnoid mater. These are caused by shear stress on bridging veins due to rotational and/or linear forces, resulting in low-pressure bleeding. In very young, elderly, and alcoholic patients, the presence of enlarged subdural spaces predisposes to SDH with minimal head trauma. Symptoms include gradually increasing headache and confusion. At imaging, SDH is typically crescentic in appearance, outlining the cerebral convexities and tracking along dural reflections (falx cerebri and tentorium cerebelli). A small SDH may present as subtle hyperdense thickening of the falx or tentorium, which can be easily missed. The differential for hyperdensity in the subdural space includes infectious (subdural empyema), inflammatory, and neoplastic etiologies, which can readily be distinguished on contrast-enhanced images.

Reference:

Brant WE, Helms C. *Fundamentals of Diagnostic Radiology*, 3rd ed. Baltimore: Lippincott Williams and Wilkins, 2012.

HYPERINTENSE RIM, PUTAMINAL HYPERINTENSITY, SLITLIKE

Modality:
MR

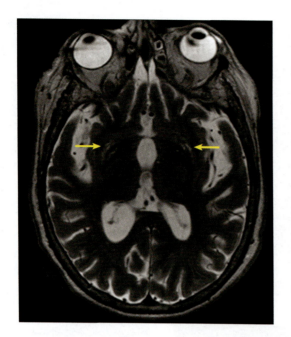
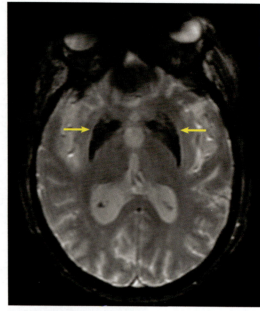

FINDINGS:

Axial T2-weighted and SWI MR show bilateral putaminal atrophy with T2-hypointense signal. There is linear hyperintensity along the lateral putaminal margins (arrows).

DIAGNOSIS:

Multiple system atrophy, parkinsonian subtype

DISCUSSION:

Multiple system atrophy (MSA) is an adult-onset neurodegenerative disease characterized by parkinsonism, autonomic failure, cerebellar ataxia, and pyramidal signs. Classification is based on the predominant clinical characteristics and includes MSA-P (parkinsonian) or striatonigral degeneration (SND), MSA-C (cerebellar) or olivopontocerebellar atrophy (OPCA), and MSA-A (autonomic) or Shy-Drager syndrome (SDS). MSA-P shows selective atrophy and mineralization of the putamina, with T2-hypointense and T1-hyperintense signal. On T2-weighted and FLAIR MR, the putamina appear abnormally hypointense with a residual hyperintense rim. There is linearization of the lateral margins, producing a "slitlike" appearance. Findings may be difficult to distinguish from age-related changes and other dementing disorders, and correlation with clinical symptoms is crucial for diagnosis.

References:

Ito S, Shirai W, Hattori T. Putaminal hyperintensity on T1-weighted MR imaging in patients with the Parkinson variant of multiple system atrophy. *AJNR Am J Neuroradiol.* 2009;30(4):689-692.

Lee JY, Yun JY, Shin CW, et al. Putaminal abnormality on 3-T magnetic resonance imaging in early parkinsonism-predominant multiple system atrophy. *J Neurol.* 2010;257(12):2065-2070.

KNIFE BLADE/EDGE

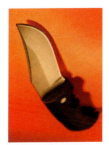

Modalities:
CT, MR

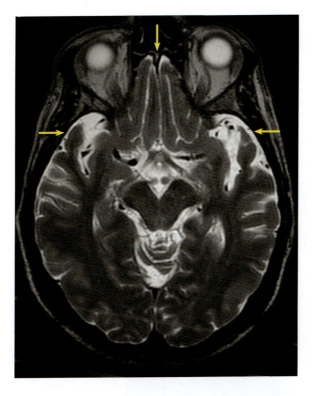

FINDINGS:

Axial T2-weighted MR shows selective atrophy of the frontal and temporal lobes, with enlargement of the Sylvian fissures and sharp pointed gyri (arrows).

DIAGNOSIS:

Frontotemporal lobar degeneration

DISCUSSION:

Frontotemporal lobar degeneration (FTLD) refers to a spectrum of neurodegenerative disorders characterized by selective, progressive atrophy of the frontal and temporal lobes. This has been linked to tissue deposition of abnormally aggregated proteins including phosphorylated tau protein, transactive response DNA-binding protein 43 (TDP-43), and fused in sarcoma (FUS) protein. 25-40% of cases are familial, with autosomal dominant inheritance in 10-20%. The three clinically defined subtypes of FTLD are frontotemporal dementia (Pick disease or behavioral variant, bvFTD), semantic dementia (SD), and progressive non-fluent aphasia (PNFA). Alternate presentations include extrapyramidal symptoms and motor neuron disease, producing clinical overlap with corticobasal degeneration (CBD) and progressive supranuclear palsy (PSP). At imaging, there is characteristic enlargement of the Sylvian fissures, widening of sulci, and pointed "knife-edge" gyri. Findings may be difficult to distinguish from age-related volume loss and other dementing disorders, and correlation with clinical symptoms is crucial for diagnosis.

References:

Lindberg O, Ostberg P, Zandbelt BB, et al. Cortical morphometric subclassification of frontotemporal lobar degeneration. *AJNR Am J Neuroradiol.* 2009;30(6):1233-1239.

Warren JD, Rohrer JD, Rossor MN. Clinical review. Frontotemporal dementia. *BMJ.* 2013 Aug 6; 347:f4827.

LAMB WOOL

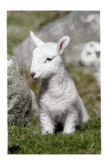

Modalities:
CT, MR

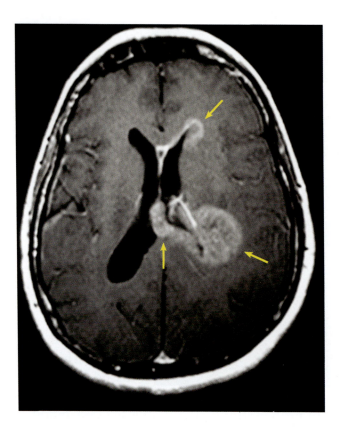

FINDINGS:

Axial contrast-enhanced T1-weighted MR shows multiple periventricular and subependymal masses involving the left frontal horn, atrium, septum pellucidum, and splenium with patchy contrast enhancement (arrows).

DIAGNOSIS:

Primary CNS lymphoma

DISCUSSION:

Primary central nervous system lymphoma (PCNSL) occurs in immunocompromised patients and immunocompetent individuals after the fifth decade. The most common type is non-Hodgkin B-cell lymphoma. Due to tumor hypercellularity, lesions are typically hyperdense on CT and hypointense on T2-weighted MR, with reduced diffusion. In immunocompetent patients, lymphoma demonstrates mild patchy enhancement with a "lamb's wool" appearance. Lesions can be multifocal and involve the brain parenchyma, vessels, ependyma, and meninges.

References:

Slone HW, Blake JJ, Shah R, et al. CT and MRI findings of intracranial lymphoma. *AJR Am J Roentgenol.* 2005;184(5):1679-1685.

Smirniotopoulos JG, Murphy FM, Rushing EJ, et al. Patterns of contrast enhancement in the brain and meninges. *Radiographics.* 2007;27(2):525-551.

LENTICULAR

Modalities:
CT, MR

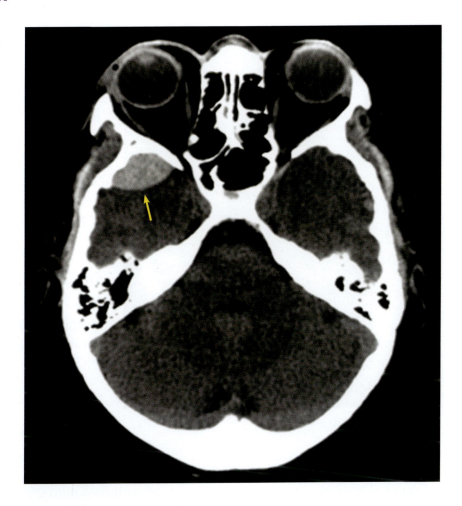

FINDINGS:

Axial CT shows a right temporal tip epidural hematoma (arrow).

DIAGNOSIS:

Epidural hematoma

DISCUSSION:

Epidural hematomas (EDHs) are bleeds located between the skull and dura mater. These are caused by major trauma with skull fractures producing lacerations of the meningeal arteries (usually MMA), or less commonly the dural venous sinuses. Classically, patients have a lucid interval, followed by rapid loss of consciousness as the high-pressure bleed begins to compress intracranial structures. At imaging, EDH has a "lenticular" appearance that is constrained by the cranial sutures. Prompt surgical intervention is critical for minimizing morbidity and mortality.

Reference:

Brant WE, Helms C. *Fundamentals of Diagnostic Radiology*, 3rd ed. Baltimore: Lippincott Williams and Wilkins, 2012.

LOW LYING TONSILS

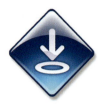

Modalities:
CT, MR

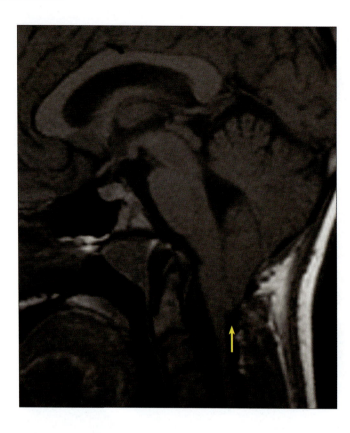

FINDINGS:

Sagittal T1-weighted MR shows the cerebellar tonsils extending below the foramen magnum (arrow).

DIFFERENTIAL DIAGNOSIS:

- Tonsillar ectopia
- Chiari I malformation
- Intracranial hypotension
- Tonsillar herniation

DISCUSSION:

The cerebellar tonsils are normally located above the foramen magnum, but may be at or slightly below this level. Tonsillar ectopia is a normal variant in which the tonsils are located within 5 mm of the foramen magnum, without other anatomic abnormalities. In Chiari I malformation, the tonsils have a peglike configuration and are displaced over 3 to 5 mm below the foramen magnum. There may be associated cervicomedullary kinking and obstruction of CSF outflow, which can result in syringohydromyelia. In intracranial hypotension (CSF hypovolemia), there is downward sagging of the entire brain, including the cerebellar tonsils. Associated findings include venous engorgement, brainstem and pituitary edema, and subdural effusions. Intracranial hypertension causes crowding of intracranial structures, which in severe cases can lead to tonsillar herniation.

Reference:

Barkovich AJ, Wippold FJ, Sherman JL, et al. Significance of cerebellar tonsillar position on MR. *AJNR Am J Neuroradiol.* 1986;7(5):795-799.

MICKEY MOUSE, MORNING GLORY

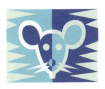

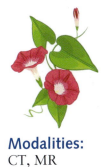

Modalities:
CT, MR

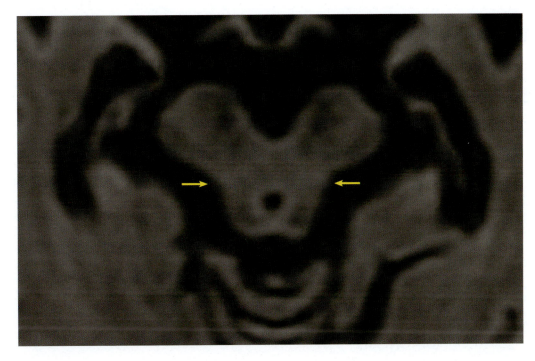

FINDINGS:

Axial FLAIR MR shows midbrain atrophy with concave lateral margins of the tegmentum (arrows). The cerebral peduncles are normal in size.

DIAGNOSIS:

Progressive supranuclear palsy

DISCUSSION:

Progressive supranuclear palsy (Steele-Richardson-Olszewski syndrome), an adult-onset neurodegenerative disorder, is the most common cause of parkinsonism following Parkinson disease. Symptoms include dementia, postural instability, and vertical supranuclear gaze palsy. There is selective atrophy of the midbrain tegmentum and tectum, with flattened or concave margins and a deep interpeduncular fossa. On axial images, the "Mickey Mouse" or "morning glory" sign is produced by midbrain atrophy with preserved cerebral peduncles. On sagittal images, the "hummingbird" sign refers to midbrain atrophy juxtaposed with normal pons and medulla. Focal hypometabolism on PET gives rise to the "pimple" sign. Findings may be difficult to distinguish from age-related volume loss and other dementing disorders, and correlation with clinical symptoms is crucial for diagnosis.

References:

Adachi M, Kawanami T, Ohshima H, et al. Morning glory sign: a particular MR finding in progressive supranuclear palsy. *Magn Reson Med Sci.* 2004;3(3):125-132.

Botha H, Whitwell JL, Madhaven A, et al. The pimple sign of progressive supranuclear palsy syndrome. *Parkinsonism Relat Disord.* 2013 Nov 4. [Epub ahead of print]

MICKEY MOUSE EARS

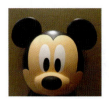

Modalities:
CT, MR

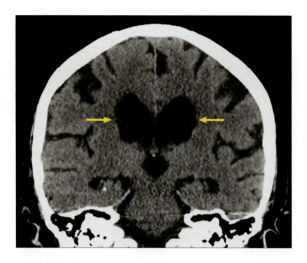

FINDINGS:

Coronal CT shows ballooning of the lateral (arrows) and third ventricles.

DIAGNOSIS:

Internal hydrocephalus

DISCUSSION:

Cerebrospinal fluid is produced in the choroid plexus of the ventricles, circulates continuously through the brain and spinal cord, and is reabsorbed by arachnoid granulations and/or lymphatic channels. Hydrocephalus refers to increased CSF accumulation in the brain, either internal (within ventricles) or external (within subarachnoid spaces). External hydrocephalus refers to enlarged subarachnoid spaces with normal-sized ventricles. This is a benign condition of infancy that resolves spontaneously by 2 years of age. Internal hydrocephalus may be produced by obstructive (noncommunicating) or nonobstructive (communicating) causes. In noncommunicating hydrocephalus, there is blockage of flow within the ventricular system, with continued upstream CSF production causing progressive dilation. In communicating hydrocephalus, the ventricular system is patent, but CSF overproduction or impaired absorption by arachnoid granulations results in increased CSF volume. Characteristic ballooning of the lateral ventricles creates a "Mickey Mouse ears" appearance. Clinical symptoms depend on the time course and severity of disease. Ventricular drainage or shunt placement can serve as a temporizing measure, but definitive treatment requires identification and correction of the underlying cause. True hydrocephalus should be distinguished from cerebral atrophy ("hydrocephalus ex vacuo"), in which parenchymal volume loss is responsible for diffuse enlargement of the CSF spaces.

Reference:

Brant WE, Helms C. *Fundamentals of Diagnostic Radiology*, 3rd ed. Baltimore: Lippincott Williams and Wilkins, 2012.

MOUNT FUJI, PEAKING

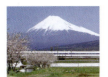

Modality:
CT

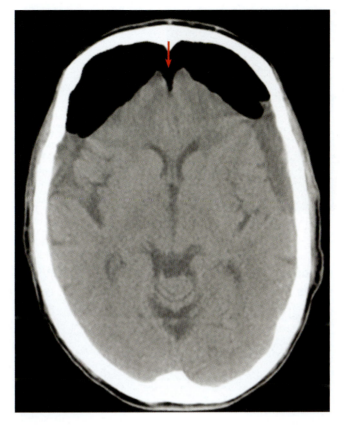

FINDINGS:

Axial CT shows bifrontal pneumocephalus and subdural fluid collections. There is compression of the frontal lobes and widening of the interhemispheric space (arrow).

DIFFERENTIAL DIAGNOSIS:

- Postsurgical pneumocephalus
- Tension pneumocephalus

DISCUSSION:

Pneumocephalus is a normal finding after surgery or trauma with violation of the dural space. Progressive air accumulation can develop because of a ball-valve mechanism, producing mass effect on adjacent brain. An important sign of tension pneumocephalus is compression and separation of the frontal lobes, resembling the double-peaked silhouette of Mount Fuji. The presence of gas within the interhemispheric space indicates that air pressure exceeds the surface tension of cerebrospinal fluid between the frontal lobes. Tension pneumocephalus is a neurosurgical emergency requiring immediate decompression.

Reference:

Michel SJ. The Mount Fuji sign. *Radiology.* 2004;232(2):449-450.

MUSHROOM, PANNUS

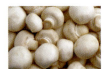

Modalities:
CT, MR

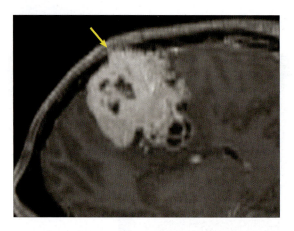

FINDINGS:

Sagittal contrast-enhanced T1-weighted MR shows a mixed solid and cystic mass with scalloping of the inner table of the calvarium (arrow), transdural invasion, and invagination into the frontal lobe.

DIFFERENTIAL DIAGNOSIS:

- Hemangiopericytoma
- Atypical meningioma
- Metastasis

DISCUSSION:

Hemangiopericytomas (formerly known as angioblastic meningiomas) are extraaxial tumors composed of pericytes of Zimmerman, the smooth muscle cells surrounding capillaries. The classic imaging appearance is a mixed solid/cystic mass with avid heterogeneous enhancement, flow voids reflecting hypervascularity, narrow dural attachment, and erosion of the overlying calvarium. When intraparenchymal invasion occurs through the relatively small dural attachment, it creates a "mushroom" appearance. In contrast, meningiomas appear more homogeneous, often calcify, have a broad dural base, and produce bony hyperostosis rather than erosion. Atypical meningiomas have a more irregular appearance, with the extradural variant involving the calvarium and subcutaneous tissues. Intra-axial invasion is rare and suggests malignant transformation; the broad dural attachment usually produces a "pannus" rather than "mushroom" appearance. Metastases may also behave aggressively with dural, calvarial and/or parenchymal invasion.

References:

Chiechi MV, Smirniotopoulos JG, Mena H. Intracranial hemangiopericytomas: MR and CT features. *AJNR Am J Neuroradiol.* 1996;17(7):1365-1371.

New PF, Hesselink JR, O'Carroll CP, Kleinman GM. Malignant meningiomas: CT and histologic criteria, including a new CT sign. *AJNR Am J Neuroradiol.* 1982;3(3):267-276.

Tokgoz N, Oner YA, Kaymaz M, et al. Primary intraosseous meningioma: CT and MRI appearance. *AJNR Am J Neuroradiol.* 2005;26(8):2053-2056.

(NEPTUNE) TRIDENT, TRIUMVIRATE

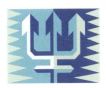

Modality:
NM

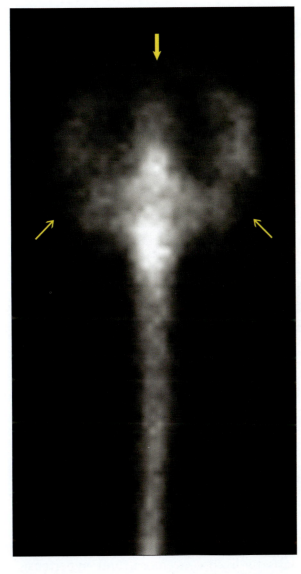

FINDINGS:

Anterior planar In-111 DTPA cisternogram shows expected ascent of radiopharmaceutical from the intrathecal injection site to the cerebral convexities, with no ventricular reflux. This results in normal tracer accumulation within the interhemispheric (thick arrow) and sylvian (thin arrows) cisterns.

DIAGNOSIS:

Normal cisternogram

DISCUSSION:

Radionuclide cisternography involves intrathecal injection of a radiolabeled pharmaceutical (usually indium-111 diethylene triamine pentaacetic acid) with sequential imaging to evaluate CSF flow. In a normal patient, tracer ascends up the spinal column to the level of the basal cisterns by 1 hour, the frontal poles and sylvian fissures by 2-6 hours, the cerebral convexities by 12 hours, and the sagittal sinus by 24 hours. Normal activity in the interhemispheric and sylvian cisterns creates the standard "trident" appearance. Tracer does not normally enter the ventricular system, because physiologic flow of CSF is in the opposite direction.

Reference:

Mettler FA, Guiberteau MJ. *Essentials of Nuclear Medicine Imaging*, 5th ed. St Louis, MO: Saunders, Elsevier, 2006.

NIBBLED CORTEX

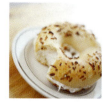

Modalities:
NM, CT, MR

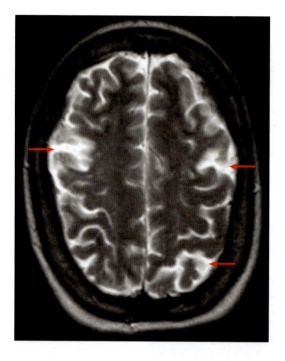

FINDINGS:

Axial T2-weighted MR shows multifocal encephalomalacia with cortical irregularity (arrows) and subcortical hyperintensities.

DIAGNOSIS:

Sneddon syndrome

DISCUSSION:

Sneddon syndrome is a noninflammatory arteriopathy causing cerebrovascular disease, livedo reticularis or livedo racemosa, and hypertension. Most cases are idiopathic, but a familial form of the disease exists with autosomal dominant inheritance. Antiphospholipid antibodies are positive in 50% of cases. Patients suffer from vasospastic episodes, transient ischemic attacks, strokes, and early-onset dementia. Small and medium-sized vessels are affected, with asymmetric multifocal cortical/subcortical infarcts. Nuclear medicine SPECT, CTP, or MRP studies may facilitate early diagnosis, identifying underperfused areas of brain prior to the development of irreversible infarcts. In late-stage disease, there is multifocal encephalomalacia with subcortical white matter signal abnormalities and irregular volume loss of the overlying cortex ("nibbled cortex").

References:

Karagülle AT, Karadağ D, Erden A, et al. Sneddon's syndrome: MR imaging findings. *Eur Radiol.* 2002;12(1):144-146.

Menzel C, Reinhold U, Grünwald F, et al. Cerebral blood flow in Sneddon syndrome. *J Nucl Med.* 1994;35(3):461-464.

NOTCH

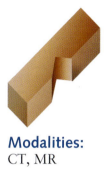

Modalities:
CT, MR

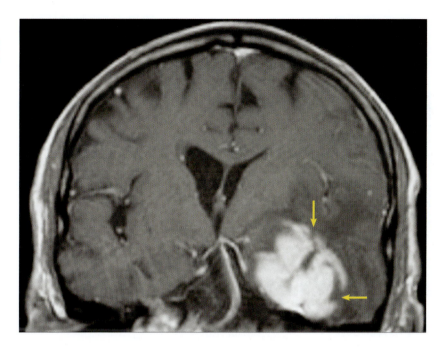

FINDINGS:

Coronal contrast-enhanced T1-weighted MR shows a left temporal enhancing mass with multiple peripheral indentations (arrows).

DIAGNOSIS:

CNS lymphoma

DISCUSSION:

Primary central nervous system lymphoma (PCNSL) occurs in immunocompromised patients and immunocompetent individuals after the fifth decade. The most common type is non-Hodgkin B-cell lymphoma. Due to tumor hypercellularity, lesions are typically hyperdense on CT and hypointense on T2-weighted MR, with reduced diffusion. The enhancement pattern is homogeneous and solid in immunocompetent patients, but more heterogeneous and ring-enhancing in immunocompromised patients. Lesions can be multifocal and involve the brain parenchyma, vessels, ependyma, and meninges. The "notch" sign has recently been described and refers to abnormally deep depressions of lesion margins. This is a rare but highly specific finding that effectively distinguishes PCNSL from other primary and metastatic brain tumors.

References:

Slone HW, Blake JJ, Shah R, et al. CT and MRI findings of intracranial lymphoma. *AJR Am J Roentgenol.* 2005;184(5):1679-1685.

Zhang D, Hu LB, Henning TD, et al. MRI findings of primary CNS lymphoma in 26 immunocompetent patients. *Korean J Radiol.* 2010;11(3):269-277.

OWL/SNAKE EYES

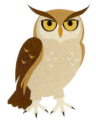

Modality:
MR

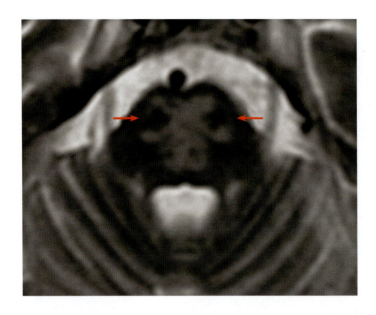

FINDINGS:

Axial T2-weighted MR shows hyperintense signal within the central pons, sparing the corticospinal tracts (arrows) and peripheral pons.

DIAGNOSIS:

Osmotic demyelination syndrome

DISCUSSION:

Osmotic demyelination syndrome (ODMS), formerly classified into central pontine myelinolysis (CPM) and extrapontine myelinolysis (EPM), refers to acute demyelination caused by rapid changes in serum osmolality. The classic presentation is an alcoholic, hyponatremic patient who undergoes rapid correction of serum sodium levels, resulting in massive fluid efflux from the brain into the serum. Symmetric T2-hyperintense signal and reduced diffusion are seen in the central pons, basal ganglia, and/or cerebral white matter. Mild injury produces signal abnormality in the median raphe and basis pontis, with a bilobed ("bat wing") or triangular ("trident") morphology. More profound injury affects the entire pons with relative sparing of the tegmentum, corticobulbar, and corticospinal tracts ("owl/snake eyes" appearance). In the subacute period, signal changes improve or resolve completely. The differential for central pontine T2 hyperintensity includes infarction, neoplasm, demyelination, infection, metabolic disorders, and radiation. However, combined findings of CPM and EPM are essentially pathognomonic for ODMS.

References:

Chua GC, Sitoh YY, Lim CC, et al. MRI findings in osmotic myelinolysis. *Clin Radiol.* 2002;57(9): 800-806.

Ho VB, Fitz CR, Yoder CC, et al. Resolving MR features in osmotic myelinolysis (central pontine and extrapontine myelinolysis). *AJNR Am J Neuroradiol.* 1993;14(1):163-167.

PERIVENTRICULAR HYPERINTENSITY/HYPODENSITY

Modalities:
CT, MR

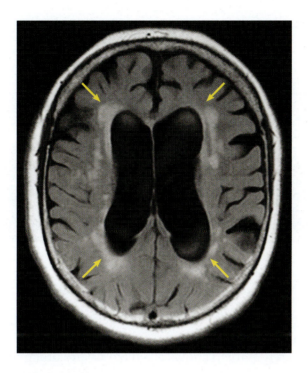

FINDINGS:

Axial FLAIR MR shows multiple T2-hyperintense foci in the periventricular white matter (arrows). There is diffuse enlargement of ventricles and sulci.

DIFFERENTIAL DIAGNOSIS:

- Normal aging
- Vasculopathy
- Demyelinating disease
- Dementia
- Hydrocephalus

DISCUSSION:

Foci of CT hypodensity/MR hyperintensity in the white matter are known as leukoaraiosis, and are common incidental findings at imaging. They increase proportionally with patient age, cerebral atrophy, and vascular risk factors. At pathology, these foci are found to consist of dilated perivascular spaces, myelin pallor, and/or gliosis. Periventricular signal abnormalities greater than expected for patient age should raise the question of other pathologies such as vasculopathy, demyelinating disease, dementia, and hydrocephalus with transependymal flow of CSF.

References:

Debette S, Markus HS. The clinical importance of white matter hyperintensities on brain magnetic resonance imaging: systematic review and meta-analysis. *BMJ*. 2010;341:c3666.

Matsusue E, Sugihara S, Fujii S, et al. White matter changes in elderly people: MR-pathologic correlations. *Magn Reson Med Sci*. 2006;5(2):99-104.

PNEUMOSINUS DILATANS

Modalities:
XR, MR

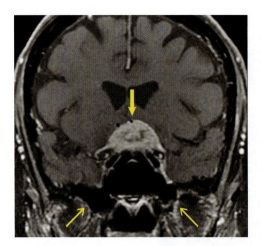
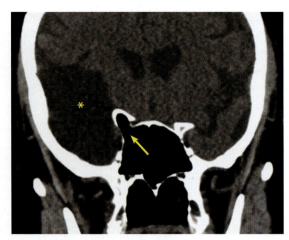

FINDINGS:

- Coronal contrast-enhanced T1-weighted MR shows an enhancing planum sphenoidale mass (thick arrow). There is enlargement and hyperaeration of the sphenoid sinuses (thin arrows).
- Coronal CT in a different patient shows a sylvian fissure arachnoid cyst (asterisk). There is hyperaeration of the sphenoid sinuses and right anterior clinoid process (arrow).

DIFFERENTIAL DIAGNOSIS:

- Meningioma
- Arachnoid cyst

DISCUSSION:

Pneumosinus dilatans refers to abnormal dilatation of one or more paranasal sinuses without bone destruction, hyperostosis, or mucosal thickening. This most commonly affects the frontal sinus, followed by the sphenoid, ethmoid, and maxillary sinuses. The mechanism is unknown, but proposed etiologies include ball-valve obstruction, dural tethering, aerobic infection, mucocele discharge, and hormonal dysregulation. Pneumosinus dilatans has been described in conjunction with meningioma, arachnoid cyst, meningocele, nerve sheath tumors, sinonasal polyposis, Dyke-Davidoff-Masson syndrome, fibro-osseous dysplasia, hydrocephalus, and trauma. Diffuse involvement of the paranasal sinuses and mastoid air cells is known as pneumosinus dilatans multiplex, and is associated with mental retardation and craniofacial malformations. Spontaneous pneumocephalus can occur after minimal trauma. Other types of sinus air cysts include hypersinus, sinus enlargement contained within normal boundaries; pneumocele, sinus enlargement with bone thinning/erosion; and pneumatocele, subperiosteal air along the sinus wall.

Reference:

Teh BM, Hall C, Chan SW. Pneumosinus dilatans, pneumocoele or air cyst? A case report and literature review. *J Laryngol Otol.* 2012;126(1):88-93.

PSEUDO-SUBARACHNOID HEMORRHAGE

Modality:
CT

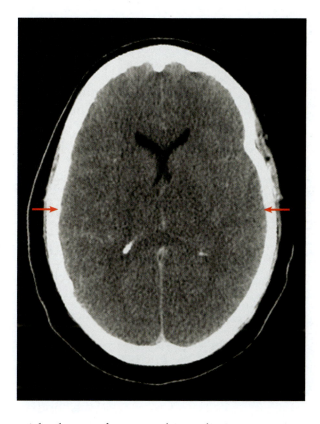

FINDINGS:

Axial noncontrast CT shows diffuse cerebral edema with apparent hyperdensity throughout the subarachnoid space (arrows).

DIFFERENTIAL DIAGNOSIS:

- Cerebral edema
- Meningitis
- Leptomeningeal carcinomatosis
- Intracranial hypotension
- Prior contrast administration

DISCUSSION:

Increased attenuation in the subarachnoid spaces and basal cisterns does not always represent subarachnoid hemorrhage. In diffuse cerebral edema, the brain parenchyma is diffusely hypodense with loss of gray-white distinction. Increased intracranial pressure causes displacement of cerebrospinal fluid from the subarachnoid spaces, as well as engorgement of superficial veins, yielding a dense appearance of the leptomeninges ("pseudo-subarachnoid hemorrhage" sign). The MR correlate of this finding is known as the "FLAIR hyperintensity" sign. Other processes that affect the subarachnoid space include meningitis (proteinaceous fluid), leptomeningeal carcinomatosis (tumor cells), and prior contrast administration (intrathecal or intravascular). Intracranial hypotension can produce superficial venous engorgement in the pachymeninges and/or leptomeninges.

References:

Given CA 2nd, Burdette JH, Elster AD, et al. Pseudo-subarachnoid hemorrhage: a potential imaging pitfall associated with diffuse cerebral edema. *AJNR Am J Neuroradiol.* 2003;24(2):254-256.

Lang JL, Leach PL, Emelifeonwu JA, et al. Meningitis presenting as spontaneous subarachnoid haemorrhage (pseudo-subarachnoid haemorrhage). *Eur J Emerg Med.* 2013;20(2):140-141

Schievink WI, Maya MM, Tourje J, Moser FG. Pseudo-subarachnoid hemorrhage: a CT-finding in spontaneous intracranial hypotension. *Neurology.* 2005;65(1):135-137.

SANDWICH

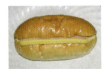

Modality:
MR

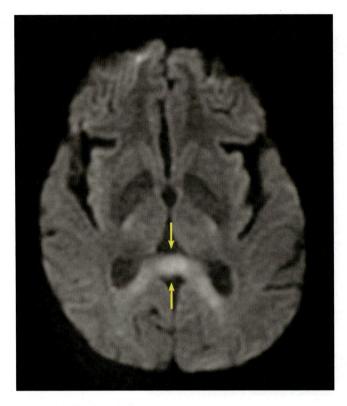

FINDINGS:

Axial DWI MR shows reduced diffusion in the central (arrows) and lateral splenium. The ventral and dorsal layers of the corpus callosum are relatively preserved.

DIAGNOSIS:

Marchiafava-Bignami disease

DISCUSSION:

Marchiafava-Bignami disease typically occurs in chronic alcoholics with severe malnutrition. Deficiency of the vitamin B complex results in degeneration of the corpus callosum. This first involves the body, followed by the genu and splenium. Other affected areas include the anterior/posterior commissures, corticospinal tracts, brachia pontis, and hemispheric white matter. On MR, the corpus callosum appears T2-hyperintense and T1-hypointense. Preferential involvement of the central layer, with relative sparing of the dorsal and ventral layers, creates a "sandwich" appearance. In the acute phase, there may be reduced diffusion and peripheral enhancement. In the chronic phase, lesions necrose and cavitate. Other processes that can affect the corpus callosum include infarction, demyelination, and trauma (diffuse axonal injury). However, these entities have disparate clinical presentations and do not typically produce a "layered" appearance.

References:

Arbelaez A, Pajon A, Castillo M. Acute Marchiafava-Bignami disease: MR findings in two patients. *AJNR Am J Neuroradiol.* 2003;24(10):1955-1957.

Ménégon P, Sibon I, Pachai C, et al. Marchiafava-Bignami disease: diffusion-weighted MRI in corpus callosum and cortical lesions. *Neurology.* 2005;65(3):475-477.

SATELLITE

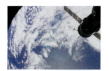

Modalities:
CT, MR

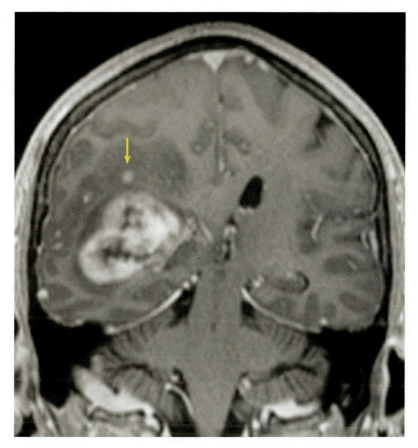

FINDINGS:

Coronal contrast-enhanced T1-weighted MR shows a heterogeneously enhancing right subinsular mass. There is a second focus of enhancement (arrow) superior to and separate from the dominant lesion.

DIFFERENTIAL DIAGNOSIS:

- Glioblastoma multiforme
- Metastases
- Abscesses

DISCUSSION:

"Satellite" foci refer to smaller lesions adjacent to, but separate from, a primary mass. Glioblastoma multiforme, which shows an aggressive and infiltrative growth pattern, is the most common primary brain tumor with this appearance. Metastases can present as multiple discrete masses throughout the brain. Daughter abscesses may develop adjacent to a parent abscess, but are usually contiguous and evolve rapidly over time with progressive organization and rim enhancement.

Reference:

Dobelbower MC, Burnett OL III, Nordal RA, et al. Patterns of failure for glioblastoma multiforme following concurrent radiation and temozolomide. *J Med Imaging Radiat Oncol.* 2011;55(1):77-81.

SCALLOPED

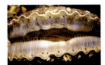

Modalities:
CT, MR

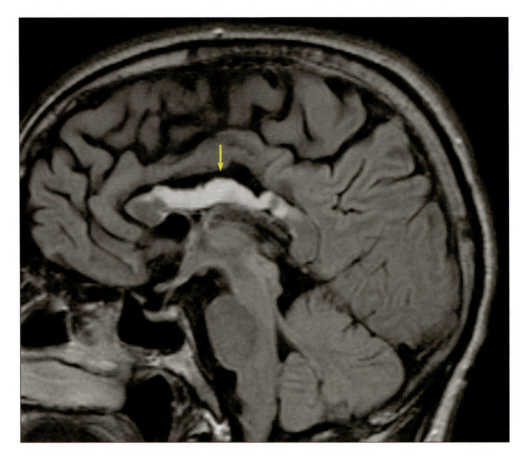

FINDINGS:

Sagittal FLAIR MR shows hyperintense signal and scalloped morphology (arrow) of the corpus callosum.

DIAGNOSIS:

Decompressed chronic hydrocephalus

DISCUSSION:

Chronic hydrocephalus produces ventriculomegaly with elevation of the corpus callosum. Following CSF drain or shunt placement, the corpus callosum rapidly descends away from the rigid falx cerebri. The dorsal body of the corpus callosum can develop a "scalloped" appearance, reflecting tethering by pericallosal artery branches to the overlying cingulate cortex. T2-hyperintense, T1-hypointense MR signal changes have been suggested to represent biomechanical compression, edema, ischemia, and/or demyelination.

References:

Lane JI, Luetmer PH, Atkinson JL. Corpus callosal signal changes in patients with obstructive hydrocephalus after ventriculoperitoneal shunting. *AJNR Am J Neuroradiol.* 2001;22(1):158-162.

Numaguchi Y, Kristt DA, Joy C, et al. Scalloping deformity of the corpus callosum following ventricular shunting. *AJNR Am J Neuroradiol.* 1993;14(2):355-362.

SLIT VENTRICLES

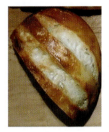

Modalities:
CT, MR

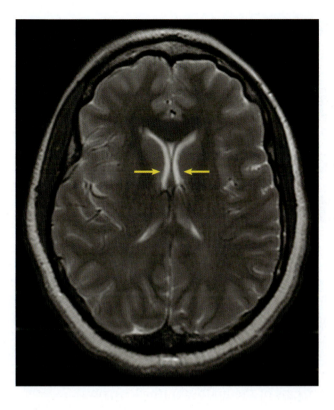

FINDINGS:

Axial T2-weighted MR shows diminutive lateral ventricles (arrows). There is effacement of the subarachnoid spaces with gyral remodeling of the inner table, indicating chronically increased intracranial pressure.

DIFFERENTIAL DIAGNOSIS:

- Increased intracranial pressure
- Excessive CSF removal

DISCUSSION:

The Monro-Kellie doctrine states that the brain, CSF, and blood are in volume equilibrium within the fixed cranial compartment. Causes of increased intracranial pressure including pseudotumor cerebri (idiopathic intracranial hypertension), supratentorial masses, and cerebral edema can force out CSF from the ventricles, producing a "slitlike" appearance. Other imaging features of increased intracranial pressure include effacement of the subarachnoid spaces, empty sella, papilledema, venous pseudostenosis, and calvarial remodeling. The cavernous sinuses, Meckel caves, and cranial nerve meati may be narrowed in the acute phase, but can expand in the chronic phase due to transmitted CSF pulsations. In patients who undergo lumbar puncture, ventricular drainage, or shunting, the cranial compartment is no longer isolated from the external environment. Excessive CSF removal can also cause a slit ventricle appearance in these cases. In patients with indwelling ventricular shunts, the combination of new-onset mental status changes, slit ventricles on imaging, and abnormally low CSF pressures is diagnostic of shunt malfunction.

References:

Bruce DA, Weprin B. The slit ventricle syndrome. *Neurosurg Clin N Am*. 2001;12(1).709-717, viii.

Degnan AJ, Levy LM. Narrowing of Meckel's cave and cavernous sinus and enlargement of the optic nerve sheath in pseudotumor cerebri. *J Comput Assist Tomogr*. 2011;35(2):308-312.

SPINNING TOP, SQUARE, TRIANGLE

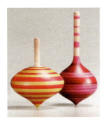

Modalities:
CT, MR

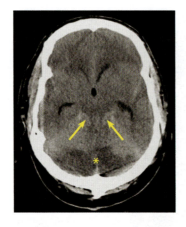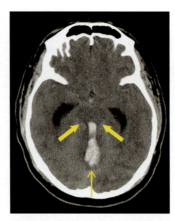

FINDINGS:

- Axial CT shows diffuse cerebral and cerebellar edema (asterisk) with upward transtentorial herniation. There is a triangular appearance of the quadrigeminal plate cistern with compression of the posterolateral margins of the midbrain (arrows).
- Axial CT in a different patient shows hemorrhage and edema within the cerebellar vermis (thin arrow). Upward transtentorial herniation compresses the posterolateral margins of the midbrain (thick arrows).

DIAGNOSIS:

Ascending transtentorial herniation

DISCUSSION:

Cerebral herniation is a response to increased intracranial pressure caused by hemorrhage, edema, and/or mass lesions. The Monro-Kellie doctrine states that in a closed compartment, the total volume of brain, blood, and CSF must remain constant. Types of cerebral herniation include subfalcine (cingulate); transalar (sphenoid); transtentorial (uncal, central); cerebellar (tonsillar, foramen magnum); and external (transcalvarial, extracranial). Transtentorial herniation refers to herniation across the tentorium cerebelli. Descending (downward) transtentorial herniation occurs in the setting of supratentorial mass effect, and is more common. Upward (ascending) transtentorial herniation occurs secondary to posterior fossa mass effect. There is effacement of the quadrigeminal plate cistern ("triangle" or "square" appearance), compression of the posterolateral midbrain ("spinning top" appearance), and flattening of the third ventricle. Cerebral herniation is an urgent imaging finding that should be addressed with prompt correction of the underlying cause. Additional strategies for lowering intracranial pressure include mannitol diuresis, ventriculostomy placement, and decompressive craniectomy.

References:

Laine FJ, Shedden AI, Dunn MM, et al. Acquired intracranial herniations: MR imaging findings. *AJR Am J Roentgenol.* 1995;165(4):967-973.

Osborn AG, Heaston DK, Wing SD. Diagnosis of ascending transtentorial herniation by cranial computed tomography. *AJR Am J Roentgenol.* 1978;130(4):755-760.

STAR

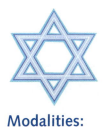

Modalities:
CT, MR

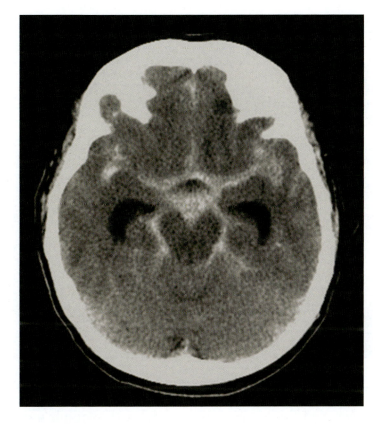

FINDINGS:

Axial CT shows hyperdense material within the suprasellar cistern.

DIAGNOSIS:

Subarachnoid hemorrhage

DISCUSSION:

The suprasellar cistern is a CSF–filled space located inferior to the hypothalamus and superior to the sella turcica. It contains the optic chiasm, pituitary infundibulum, and circle of Willis. The boundaries of the suprasellar cistern include the interhemispheric fissure anteriorly; the unci laterally; and the pons and cerebral peduncles posteriorly. It is shaped like a five-pointed star at the level of the pons, and a six-pointed star at the level of the cerebral peduncles. Apparent hyperdensity in the suprasellar cistern indicates subarachnoid hemorrhage or its mimics (diffuse cerebral edema, basilar meningitis, leptomeningeal carcinomatosis, prior contrast administration). Loss of the normal star appearance can occur with transtentorial herniation.

Reference:

Chen R, Zhang S, Zhang W, et al. A comparative study of thin-layer cross-sectional anatomic morphology and CT images of the basal cistern and its application in acute craniocerebral traumas. *Surg Radiol Anat.* 2009;31(2):129-138.

STIPPLED

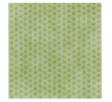

Modality:
CT

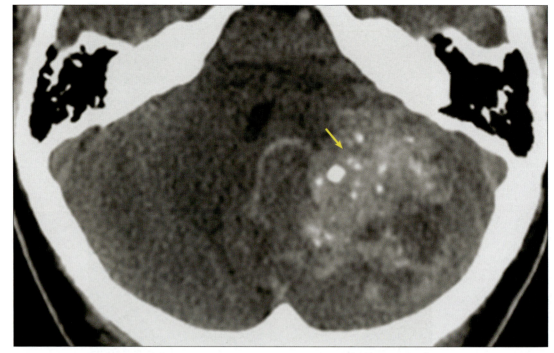

FINDINGS:

Axial CT shows a mixed-density mass (arrow) with multiple punctate calcifications in the left cerebellar hemisphere and vermis.

DIFFERENTIAL DIAGNOSIS:

- Dermoid/epidermoid
- Vascular malformation

DISCUSSION:

Punctate "stippled" calcifications are seen in a variety of benign and malignant brain lesions, most classically dermoid/epidermoid cysts. These are congenital ectodermal inclusion cysts lined by squamous epithelium (epidermoid) and varying amounts of hair, sebaceous, and sweat glands (dermoid). Calcification is also common in vascular lesions, including cavernomas and arteriovenous malformations. Primary and metastatic brain tumors (breast, lung, thyroid, osteosarcoma, chondrosarcoma) can also calcify, but the calcifications are usually coarser and more confluent.

References:

Smirniotopoulos JG, Chiechi MV. Teratomas, dermoids, and epidermoids of the head and neck. *Radiographics*. 1995;15(6):1437-1455.

Vilanova JC, Barceló J, Smirniotopoulos JG, et al. Hemangioma from head to toe: MR imaging with pathologic correlation. *Radiographics*. 2004;24(2):367-385.

SUBDURAL EFFUSIONS

Modalities:
CT, MR

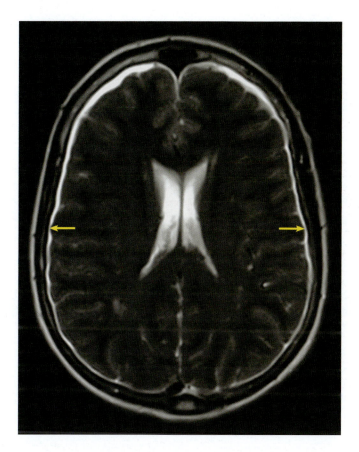

FINDINGS:

Axial T2-weighted MR shows bilateral holohemispheric subdural fluid collections (arrows).

DIFFERENTIAL DIAGNOSIS:

- Intracranial hypotension
- Subdural empyemas
- Subdural hygromas
- Subdural hematomas

DISCUSSION:

Intracranial hypotension can be caused by idiopathic, degenerative, traumatic, and iatrogenic etiologies. Dural tears in the brain or spine cause continuous loss of fluid, resulting in CSF hypovolemia. The Monro-Kellie doctrine states that in a closed compartment, the total volume of brain, blood, and CSF must remain constant. As the pressure within the intracranial compartment decreases, the brain migrates inferiorly, with distension of veins and CSF spaces overlying the cerebral convexities. Other types of subdural collections include subdural empyemas (infection), subdural hygromas (CSF), and subdural hematomas (blood). Clinical presentation and correlation with other MR sequences (FLAIR, SWI, contrast-enhanced T1) should enable distinction of these various etiologies.

References:

Tosaka M, Sato N, Fujimaki H, et al. Diffuse pachymeningeal hyperintensity and subdural effusion/hematoma detected by fluid-attenuated inversion recovery MR imaging in patients with spontaneous intracranial hypotension. *AJNR Am J Neuroradiol.* 2008;29(6):1164-1170.

Wetterling T, Rama B. Differential diagnosis of subdural effusions. *Rontgenblatter.* 1989;42(12):508-514.

SUPERNORMAL, SUPERSCAN, WHITE CEREBRUM

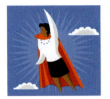

Modality:
MR

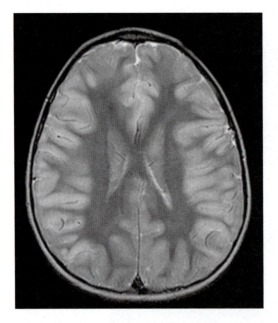 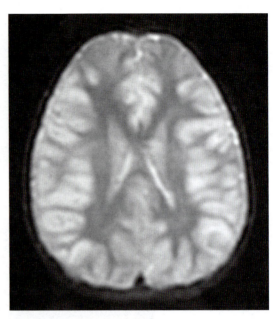

FINDINGS:

Axial T2-weighted and DWI MR show T2 hyperintensity and reduced diffusion throughout the cortex and subcortical white matter, exaggerating the normal gray-white distinction.

DIAGNOSIS:

Hypoxic-ischemic encephalopathy

DISCUSSION:

Severe hypoxic-ischemic encephalopathy results in globally reduced diffusion throughout the cortex and subcortical white matter. The gray matter, which is eight times more metabolically active than the white matter, is more susceptible to injury and undergoes diffuse cortical laminar necrosis. On other MR sequences, the gray-white matter distinction is preserved or may even be accentuated. In the subacute period, worsening edema becomes more apparent on T2/FLAIR images, with pseudonormalization on DWI.

References:

McKinney AM, Teksam M, Felice R, et al. Diffusion-weighted imaging in the setting of diffuse cortical laminar necrosis and hypoxic-ischemic encephalopathy. *AJNR Am J Neuroradiol.* 2004;25(10):1659-1665.

Wijdicks EF, Campeau NG, Miller GM. MR imaging in comatose survivors of cardiac resuscitation. *AJNR Am J Neuroradiol.* 2001;22(8):1561-1565.

TADPOLE

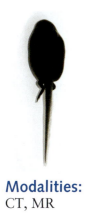

Modalities:
CT, MR

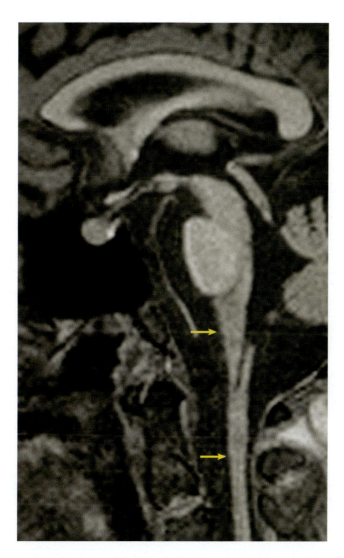

FINDINGS:

Sagittal T1-weighted MR shows severe cervicomedullary atrophy (arrows) with normal midbrain and pons.

DIAGNOSIS:

Adult-onset Alexander disease

DISCUSSION:

Alexander disease is a fatal, autosomal dominant neurodegenerative disorder caused by mutations in the *GFAP* gene on chromosome 17q21. This results in pathologic formation of Rosenthal fibers, astrocytic inclusions of long-chain fatty acids that lead to myelin destruction. Infantile (less than 2 years), juvenile (4 to 10 years), and adult-onset (over 12 years) forms have been described, with later presentations demonstrating less severe and slower progression of disease. At imaging, the infantile form usually shows frontal lobe white matter abnormalities with macrocephaly. The juvenile form typically has nodular brainstem lesions and periventricular "garlands." The adult form is characterized by a "tadpole" brainstem with selective atrophy of the medulla oblongata and cervical cord.

References:

Namekawa M, Takiyama Y, Honda J, et al. Adult-onset Alexander disease with typical "tadpole" brainstem atrophy and unusual bilateral basal ganglia involvement: a case report and review of the literature. *BMC Neurol.* 2010;10:21.

van der Knaap MS, Naidu S, Breiter SN, et al. Alexander disease: diagnosis with MR imaging. *AJNR Am J Neuroradiol.* 2001;22(3):541-552.

THICK CORTEX

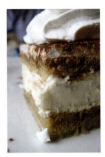

Modality:
CT

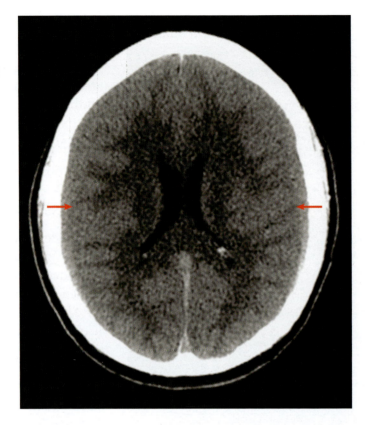

FINDINGS:

Axial CT shows bilateral subdural fluid collections isodense to gray matter (arrows), obscuring the normal sulci and gyri.

DIAGNOSIS:

Isodense subdural hematomas

DISCUSSION:

Subdural hematomas (SDHs) are bleeds between the dura mater and arachnoid mater. These are caused by shear stress on bridging veins due to rotational and/or linear forces, with low-pressure bleeding. At imaging, SDH is typically crescentic in appearance, tracking along the cerebral convexities. Acute bleeds (< 3 days) appear hyperdense because of clotted blood, whereas chronic bleeds (> 3 weeks) liquefy and become hypodense to gray matter. In the subacute stage, hemorrhage may be isodense and difficult to distinguish from gray matter. Acute bleeds in patients with anemia can also appear iso- to hypodense. On CT, this results in nonvisualization of the normal sulci/gyri with displacement from the inner table. With MR, subdural hematomas are readily distinguished from subjacent brain.

Reference:

Brant WE, Helms C. *Fundamentals of Diagnostic Radiology*, 3rd ed. Baltimore: Lippincott Williams and Wilkins, 2012.

ZEBRA

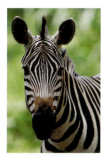

Modalities:
CT, MR

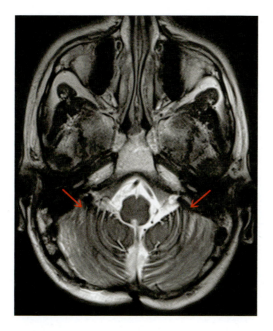 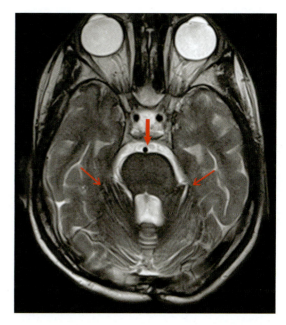

FINDINGS:

Axial T2-weighted MR shows hypointense hemosiderin outlining the pons (thick arrow), temporal tips, and cerebellar folia (thin arrows).

DIFFERENTIAL DIAGNOSIS:

- Posterior fossa hemorrhage
- Superficial siderosis

DISCUSSION:

In the adult, posterior fossa hemorrhage can be caused by traumatic, iatrogenic, ischemic, vascular, and neoplastic (particularly metastases and hemangioblastoma) etiologies. This produces a characteristic streaky appearance of blood outlining the cerebellar folia ("zebra" sign), which is hyperintense on CT in the acute phase, and hypointense on T2-weighted and SWI MR in the chronic phase. Subarachnoid hemorrhage anywhere along the neuraxis leads to superficial siderosis, in which hemosiderin is deposited along the surface of the brain, spinal cord, and nerves. On T2-weighted MR, linear hypointense signal outlines the brain and spinal cord, often with associated demyelination and gliosis.

References:

Figueiredo EG, de Amorim RL, Teixeira MJ. Remote cerebellar hemorrhage (zebra sign) in vascular neurosurgery: pathophysiological insights. *Neurol Med Chir (Tokyo).* 2009;49(6):229-233; discussion 233-234.

Kumar N, Cohen-Gadol AA, Wright RA, et al. Superficial siderosis. *Neurology.* 2006;66(8):1144-1152.

CHAPTER TWO

PEDIATRIC BRAIN

ABSENT BUTTERFLY, MONOVENTRICLE

Modalities:
US, CT, MR

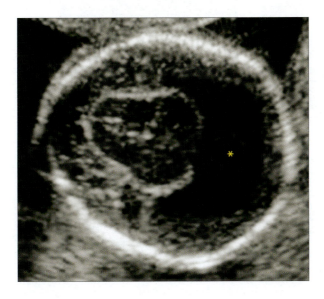

FINDINGS:

Fetal US, axial plane, shows a large monoventricle (asterisk) with absence of normal choroid plexus. The thalami are also fused.

DIAGNOSIS:

Alobar holoprosencephaly

DISCUSSION:

Holoprosencephaly refers to a spectrum of congenital malformations in which the embryonic forebrain (prosencephalon) fails to separate completely. Based on the degree of midline fusion, these are classified as alobar, semilobar, lobar, and middle interhemispheric variant (syntelencephaly). The alobar variant is the most severe, with holospheric cortical fusion; absent corpus callosum, septum pellucidum, and falx cerebri; single monoventricle; and fusion of the basal ganglia and thalami. On prenatal US, failure to identify the normal "butterfly" appearance of hyperechoic choroid plexus within the paired lateral ventricles is an early harbinger of holoprosencephaly.

References:

Hahn JS, Barnes PD. Neuroimaging advances in holoprosencephaly: refining the spectrum of the midline malformation. *Am J Med Genet C Semin Med Genet*. 2010;154C(1):120-132.

Sepulveda W, Dezerega V, Be C. First-trimester sonographic diagnosis of holoprosencephaly: value of the "butterfly" sign. *J Ultrasound Med*. 2004;23(6):761-765; quiz 766-767.

ABSENT POSTERIOR LIMB, 1-2-3-4

Modality:
MR

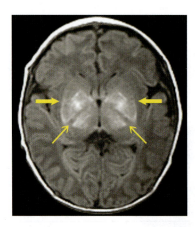 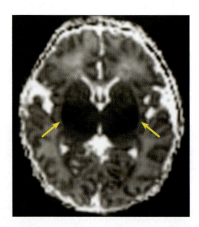

FINDINGS:

- Axial T1-weighted MR shows markedly increased signal in the bilateral basal ganglia (thick arrows) and thalami. There is loss of the normal T1-hyperintense signal in the posterior limbs of the internal capsules (thin arrows).
- Axial ADC MR shows reduced diffusion in the basal ganglia and thalami (arrows).

DIAGNOSIS:

Hypoxic-ischemic encephalopathy, term infant

DISCUSSION:

In the term infant, hypoxic-ischemic encephalopathy (HIE) manifests differently than in older children and adults. Although US and CT can be used for screening, MR is the modality of choice for diagnosing HIE. After 37 weeks of gestational age, normal myelination involves the dorsal portion of the posterior limb of the internal capsule (PLIC) and ventrolateral nucleus of the thalamus, which appear T1-hyperintense and T2-hypointense. Severe HIE is caused by sudden total loss of oxygenation, which injures metabolically active structures including the putamina, globus pallidi, thalami, hippocampi, corticospinal tracts, lateral geniculate nuclei, and sensorimotor cortex. The constellation of findings has been termed the "1-2-3-4" sign and includes T1-hyperintense signal in the basal ganglia and thalami, loss of T1 signal in the PLIC ("absent posterior limb" sign), and reduced diffusion. ADC data should always be reviewed because the high T2 values of unmyelinated tissue can mask diffusion changes on DWI. On MR spectroscopy, an elevated choline-to-creatine ratio, decreased NAA, and lactate peak may be present. More profound hypoxia can cause diffuse gray and white matter injury. Partial HIE occurs with prolonged incomplete loss of oxygenation and results in parasagittal cortical/subcortical watershed injury.

References:

Heinz ER, Provenzale JM. Imaging findings in neonatal hypoxia: a practical review. *AJR Am J Roentgenol*. 2009;192(1):41-47.

Huang BY, Castillo M. Hypoxic-ischemic brain injury: imaging findings from birth to adulthood. *Radiographics*. 2008;28(2):417-439.

ANGEL WING, TRIPLE PEAK

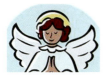

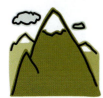

Modalities:
CT, MR

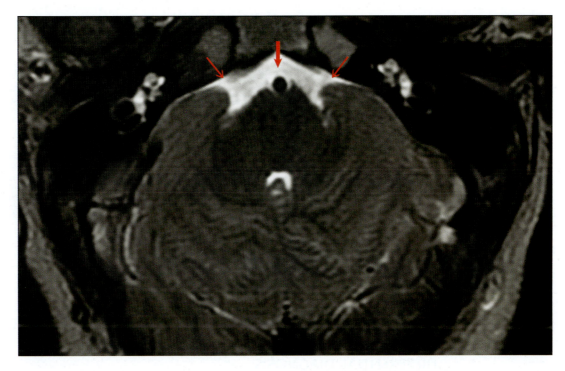

FINDINGS:

Axial T2-weighted MR shows inferior herniation of the cerebellar hemispheres (thin arrows), wrapping laterally around the pons (thick arrow).

DIAGNOSIS:

Chiari II malformation

DISCUSSION:

The Chiari II malformation is a complex congenital anomaly consisting of small posterior fossa, inferior displacement of the cerebellum and brainstem, and lumbosacral myelomeningocele. The cerebellar hemispheres wrap laterally around the pons and extend into the cerebellopontine angles, forming a "triple peak" appearance. Other characteristic imaging signs of Chiari II malformation include beaked tectum, cervicomedullary kink, wide incisura with towering cerebellum, and fenestrated falx with interdigitating gyri. In the Chiari III malformation, there is also an occipital or high cervical encephalocele.

Reference:

Naidich TP, Pudlowski RM, Naidich JB. Computed tomographic signs of Chiari II malformation, II: midbrain and cerebellum. *Radiology.* 1980;134(2):391-398.

ANGULAR, POINT, SQUARE, TRIANGLE

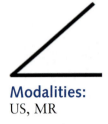

Modalities:
US, MR

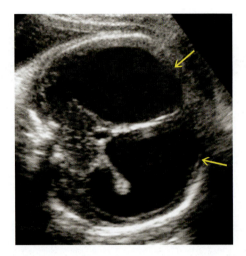

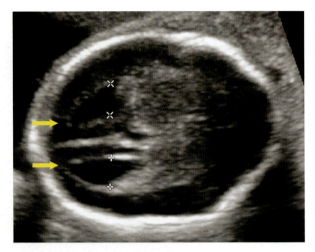

FINDINGS:

Fetal US, coronal and axial planes, show dilated lateral ventricles with an angular morphology (thin arrows) and pointed occipital horns (thick arrows).

DIFFERENTIAL DIAGNOSIS:

- Fetal Chiari malformation
- Spinal dysraphism

DISCUSSION:

Accurate diagnosis of fetal neural tube defects is crucial for guiding further imaging evaluation, genetic workup, and prenatal counseling. The Chiari II malformation is a complex congenital deformity involving small posterior fossa and lumbosacral myelomeningocele. Infratentorial abnormalities can be difficult to detect in early pregnancy. Before 24 weeks of gestational age, there is characteristic pointing and posterior displacement of the occipital horn ("too-far-back" ventricle). After 24 weeks, the occipital horns become increasingly dilated and angular, with various geometric appearances depending on the severity of the malformation. Fetal MR may help to further characterize the spectrum of anatomic abnormalities.

References:

Callen AL, Filly RA. Supratentorial abnormalities in the Chiari II malformation, I: the ventricular "point." *J Ultrasound Med.* 2008;27(1):33-38.

Fujisawa H, Kitawaki J, Iwasa K, et al. New ultrasonographic criteria for the prenatal diagnosis of Chiari type 2 malformation. *Acta Obstet Gynecol Scand.* 2006;85(12):1426-1429.

ANGULAR, FAN, SCALLOPED, TRIANGLE

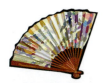

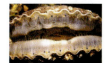

Modalities:
US, CT, MR

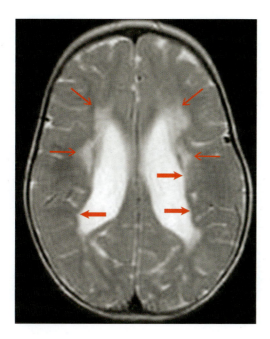

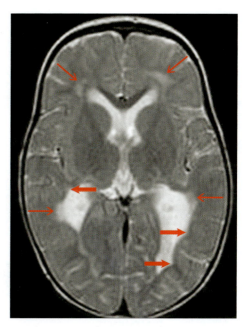

FINDINGS:

Axial T2-weighted MR shows multifocal periventricular hyperintensities (thin arrows). There is ex vacuo dilation of the lateral ventricles, with irregular contours (thick arrows).

DIAGNOSIS:

Periventricular leukomalacia

DISCUSSION:

In premature infants, the periventricular white matter is most susceptible to hypoxic injury because it is supplied by ventriculopetal penetrating arteries from the cortical surface. Periventricular leukomalacia (PVL) is the most common preterm brain injury, manifesting with periventricular white matter changes that appear echogenic on US, hypodense on CT, and hyperintense on T2-weighted MR. Localized venous infarctions produce "fan" or "triangle"-shaped abnormalities, reflecting the vascular borderzones in this age group. After 2-6 weeks, the white matter begins to involute, causing ex vacuo dilation of the ventricles with an "angular" or "scalloped" morphology. End-stage PVL is characterized by cystic encephalomalacia ("Swiss cheese" brain) with severe white matter loss and ventriculomegaly.

References:

Chao CP, Zaleski CG, Patton AC. Neonatal hypoxic-ischemic encephalopathy: multimodality imaging findings. *Radiographics*. 2006;26(Suppl 1):S159-S172.

Nakamura Y, Okudera T, Hashimoto T. Vascular architecture in white matter of neonates: its relationship to periventricular leukomalacia. *J Neuropathol Exp Neurol*. 1994;53(6):582-589.

BALL, BOOMERANG, CRESCENT, CUP, HORSESHOE, PANCAKE

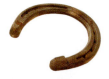

Modalities:
US, CT, MR

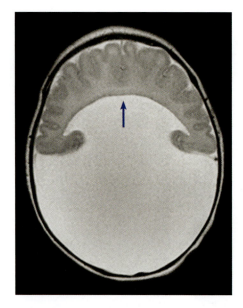

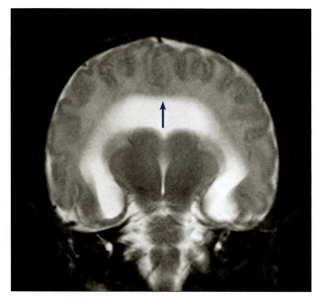

FINDINGS:

Axial and coronal T2-weighted MR show fusion of the cerebral cortex (arrows) and thalami across the midline. There is a monoventricular cavity that communicates widely with a dorsal cyst.

DIAGNOSIS:

Alobar holoprosencephaly

DISCUSSION:

Holoprosencephaly refers to a spectrum of congenital malformations in which the embryonic forebrain (prosencephalon) fails to separate completely. Based on the degree of midline fusion, these are classified as alobar, semilobar, lobar, and middle interhemispheric variant (syntelencephaly). The alobar variant is the most severe, with holospheric cortical fusion; absent corpus callosum, septum pellucidum, and falx cerebri; and fusion of the basal ganglia and thalami. There is a single "crescent"-shaped monoventricle that communicates widely with a dorsal cyst. The surrounding dysmorphic brain parenchyma has an appearance that is variably described as "ball," "boomerang," "cup," "horseshoe," or "pancake"-shaped. Holoprosencephaly should be distinguished from hydranencephaly caused by bilateral ICA occlusion in utero. In this condition, diffuse cortical destruction is present, but the posterior fossa and thalami are normal.

Reference:

Hahn JS, Barnes PD. Neuroimaging advances in holoprosencephaly: refining the spectrum of the midline malformation. *Am J Med Genet C Semin Med Genet.* 2010;154C(1):120-132.

BANANA, TIGHT POSTERIOR FOSSA

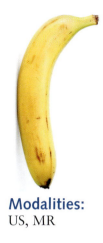

Modalities:
US, MR

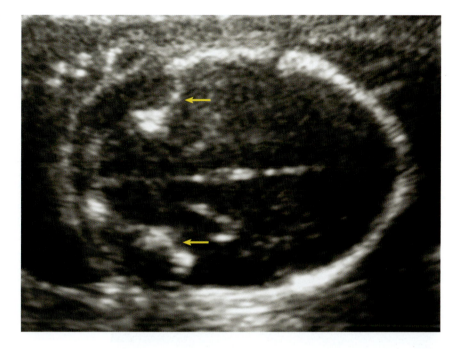

FINDINGS:

Fetal US, axial plane, shows hypoplastic posterior fossa with cerebellar hemispheres (arrows) wrapping around the brainstem.

DIFFERENTIAL DIAGNOSIS:

- Fetal Chiari malformation
- Spinal dysraphism

DISCUSSION:

Accurate diagnosis of fetal neural tube defects is crucial for guiding further imaging evaluation, genetic workup, and prenatal counseling. The Chiari II malformation is a complex congenital deformity involving small posterior fossa and lumbosacral myelomeningocele. Before 24 weeks of gestational age, the posterior fossa shows a "banana" configuration with cerebellar hemispheres wrapping around the posterior brainstem, due to downward traction on the spinal cord. After 24 weeks, the cerebellum descends further below the foramen magnum and is not well seen at US ("vanishing cerebellum"). Fetal MR may help to further characterize the spectrum of anatomic abnormalities.

References:

Ando K, Ishikura R, Ogawa M, et al. MRI tight posterior fossa sign for prenatal diagnosis of Chiari type II malformation. *Neuroradiology.* 2007;49(12):1033-1039.

Boltshauser E, Schneider J, Kollias S, et al. Vanishing cerebellum in myelomeningocoele. *Eur J Paediatr Neurol.* 2002;6(2):109-113.

Nicolaides KH, Campbell S, Gabbe SG, et al. Ultrasound screening for spina bifida: cranial and cerebellar signs. *Lancet.* 1986;2(8498):72-74.

BAT WING, BEAK, DOUBLE POINT

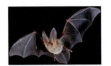

Modalities:
CT, MR

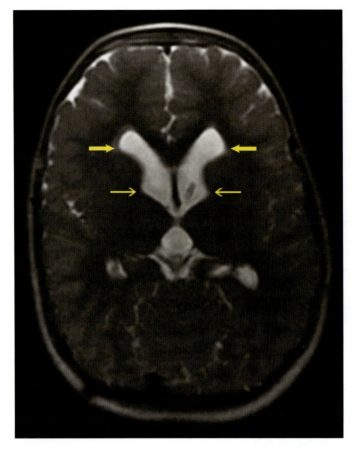

FINDINGS:

Axial T2-weighted MR shows dilated frontal horns with notching along the lateral walls (thick and thin arrows), due to prominent caudate heads.

DIAGNOSIS:

Chiari II malformation

DISCUSSION:

The Chiari II malformation is a complex congenital anomaly consisting of small posterior fossa, inferior displacement of the cerebellum and brainstem, and lumbosacral myelomeningocele. The frontal horns of the lateral ventricles are dilated and assume a "double pointed" or "bat wing" appearance, reflecting indentation of the lateral walls by prominent caudate nuclei. Other characteristic imaging signs of Chiari II malformation include beaked tectum, cervicomedullary kink, wide incisura with towering cerebellum, and fenestrated falx with interdigitating gyri. In the Chiari III malformation, there is also an occipital or high cervical encephalocele.

Reference:

Naidich TP, Pudlowski RM, Naidich JB. Computed tomographic signs of the Chiari II malformation, III: ventricles and cisterns. *Radiology.* 1980;134(3):657-663.

BAT WING, BULL/RAM/STEER HORN, CANDELABRA, CRESCENT, MOOSE HEAD, TRIDENT, VIKING HELMET

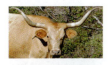

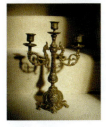

Modalities:
US, CT, MR

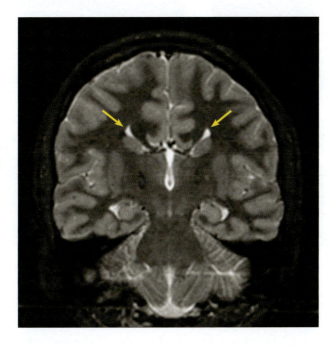

FINDINGS:

Coronal T2-weighted MR shows absent corpus callosum with widely separated and curvilinear frontal horns (arrows).

DIAGNOSIS:

Callosal agenesis

DISCUSSION:

Dysgenesis of the corpus callosum is caused by abnormalities in neural development between 12 and 18 weeks of gestation. The sequence of formation is largely ventral to dorsal, beginning with the genu and progressing through the anterior body, posterior body, splenium, and rostrum. In callosal agenesis, there is complete absence of the normal crossing white matter tracts. Instead, nondecussating white matter fibers known as Probst bundles course anteroposteriorly along the medial edges of the lateral ventricles. The lateral ventricles assume a parallel orientation, with narrow curvilinear frontal horns that are widely separated ("bull horn" configuration) and dilated occipital horns (colpocephaly). Without crossing fibers to displace and invert them, the cingulate gyri remain everted and the cingulate sulcus is unformed. Other imaging signs of callosal agenesis include high-riding third ventricle, radiating gyri, and "keyhole" temporal horns.

References:

Atlas SW. *Magnetic Resonance Imaging of the Brain and Spine*. 4th ed, vol. 1. Philadelphia: Wolters Kluwer; 2008.

Barkovich AJ, Raybaud C. *Pediatric Neuroimaging*. 5th ed. Philadelphia: Wolters Kluwer; 2011.

BAT WING, RECTANGLE, UMBRELLA

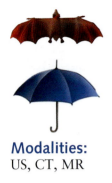

Modalities:
US, CT, MR

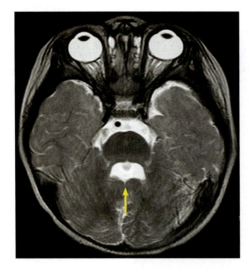

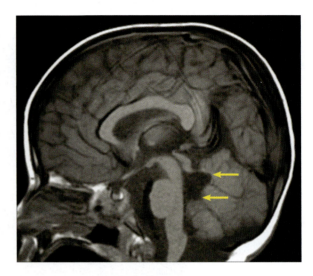

FINDINGS:

- Axial T2-weighted MR shows absent cerebellar vermis with apposition of the cerebellar hemispheres and pointed roof of the fourth ventricle (arrow).
- Sagittal T1-weighted MR shows angular bulging of the roof of the fourth ventricle (arrows) in the region of the absent vermis.

DIAGNOSIS:

Joubert syndrome-related disorders

DISCUSSION:

Joubert syndrome–related disorders (JSRD), or cerebello-oculo-renal disorders, are autosomal recessive disruptions of midbrain-hindbrain development with associated ocular, facial, hepatic, renal, and digital anomalies. Hypoplasia of the cerebellar vermis results in dilation of the fourth ventricle and bulging of its roof, creating a "rectangular" appearance on sagittal images. Just below the pontomesencephalic junction, there is notching of the fourth ventricular roof between the cerebellar hemispheres. This is best appreciated on axial images, and yields the "bat wing" or "umbrella" appearance. Other imaging signs of JSRD include the "molar tooth" appearance of the midbrain and "bullet" third ventricle.

References:

Alorainy IA, Sabir S, Seidahmed MZ, et al. Brain stem and cerebellar findings in Joubert syndrome. *J Comput Assist Tomogr.* 2006;30(1):116-121.

Brancati F, Dallapiccola B, Valente EM. Joubert syndrome and related disorders. *Orphanet J Rare Dis.* 2010;5:20.

BOXCAR VENTRICLES

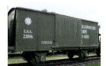

Modalities:
US, CT, MR

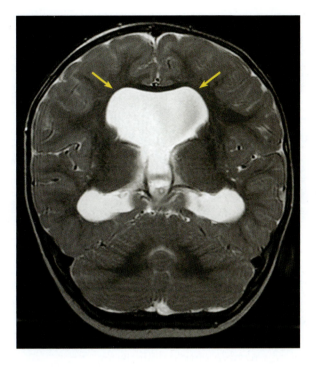

FINDINGS:

Coronal T2-weighted MR shows absent septum pellucidum and squared lateral ventricles (arrows).

DIFFERENTIAL DIAGNOSIS:

- Septo-optic dysplasia
- Holoprosencephaly

DISCUSSION:

Septo-optic dysplasia, also known as de Morsier syndrome, is a congenital anomaly that may represent a forme fruste of lobar holoprosencephaly. Classic findings are optic nerve hypoplasia, absent septum pellucidum, and hypothalamic-pituitary dysfunction. Midline defects result in closely apposed lateral ventricles with a squared ("boxcar") appearance. Two subsets of disease have been identified, based on the presence or absence of schizencephaly. Patients with schizencephaly ("septo-optic dysplasia plus") tend to have less severe midline defects. Patients without schizencephaly exhibit diffuse white matter hypoplasia, resulting in ventriculomegaly with squaring of the frontal horns. The olfactory bulbs may also be absent (Kallmann syndrome). In true holoprosencephaly, incomplete separation of forebrain structures can also yield a "boxcar" appearance of the frontal horns, with more severe midline and facial abnormalities.

Reference:

Barkovich AJ, Fram EK, Norman D. Septo-optic dysplasia: MR imaging. *Radiology*. 1989;171(1): 189-192.

BRACKET

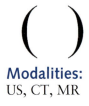

Modalities:
US, CT, MR

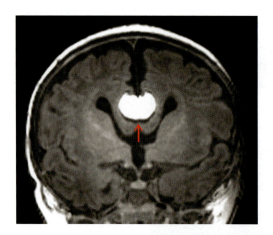
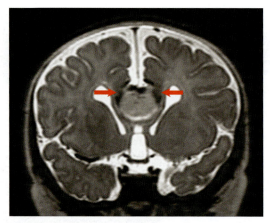

FINDINGS:

- Coronal T1-weighted MR shows a hyperintense mass (thin arrow) in the anterior interhemispheric fissure with chemical shift artifact along the inferior margin. There is associated callosal dysgenesis with abnormal configuration of the frontal horns.
- Coronal T2-weighted MR shows susceptibility along the lateral margins of the mass (thick arrows), compatible with calcification.

DIAGNOSIS:

Pericallosal lipoma, tubulonodular subtype

DISCUSSION:

Intracranial lipoma is thought to result from abnormal persistence of the meninx primitiva, the mesenchymal precursor to the meninges. Normally, the inner meninx is resorbed between weeks 8 and 10 of gestation and gives rise to the subarachnoid cisterns. When residual meninx is present, it differentiates into lipomatous tissue and can interfere with normal growth. Pericallosal lipomas are the most common, and may be tubulonodular or curvilinear in morphology. Tubulonodular lipomas are large round or cylindrical masses, usually greater than 1-2 cm in diameter. They arise earlier in development and are usually located along the genu, with peripheral calcifications producing a "bracket" sign on coronal images. There is a high rate of associated malformations including callosal dysgenesis, sincipital encephaloceles, and migration/gyration anomalies. Curvilinear lipomas are thin ribbonlike masses that typically curve around the splenium. They arise later in development, with no or mild associated anomalies. Lipomas appear echogenic on US, hypodense on CT, hyperintense on T1-weighted MR, and variably hyperintense on T2-weighted MR. Identification of chemical shift artifact and signal dropout on fat-suppressed sequences is diagnostic.

References:

Tart RP, Quisling RG. Curvilinear and tubulonodular varieties of lipoma of the corpus callosum: an MR and CT study. *J Comput Assist Tomogr.* 1991;15(5):805-810.

Truwit CL, Barkovich AJ. Pathogenesis of intracranial lipoma: an MR study in 42 patients. *AJR Am J Roentgenol.* 1990;155(4):855-864; discussion 865.

BRIGHT RIM, HYPERINTENSE RING

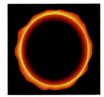

Modality:
MR

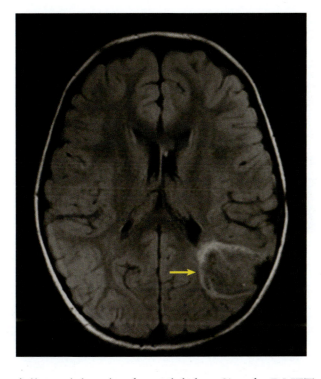

FINDINGS:

Axial FLAIR MR shows a peripheral left temporo-occipital mass with hyperintense rim (arrow).

DIAGNOSIS:

Dysembryoplastic neuroepithelial tumor

DISCUSSION:

Dysembryoplastic neuroepithelial tumors (DNETs) are benign, slow-growing neuroepithelial tumors arising from cortical or deep gray matter. Patients are typically male and under age 20. The temporal lobe is the most common location, followed by the frontal lobe. Simple DNETs are T2-hyperintense multiseptated "bubbly" masses with little vasogenic edema, enhancement, or mass effect. On FLAIR MR, there is nulling of the cystic components of tumor with a characteristic "bright rim," which may be complete or incomplete. Pathologically, this corresponds to peripheral loose neuroglial elements, and suggests residual or recurrent tumor in the postoperative setting. Complex DNETs have varying amounts of solid tissue and low-level enhancement. Lesions typically have a wedge-shaped morphology, in which the apex points toward the ventricle, and the outer surface extends to cortex with remodeling of the inner table. Associated cortical dysplasia is common. Other pediatric cystic tumors include ganglioglioma (GGL), pleomorphic xanthoastrocytoma (PXA), and juvenile pilocytic astrocytoma (JPA), which tend to be associated with mural nodules. In GGLs, edema is rare and calcification is common. PXAs tend to be larger and produce dural tails without skull erosion. When supratentorial, JPAs are usually adjacent to the third ventricle.

References:

Koeller KK, Henry JM. From the archives of the AFIP: superficial gliomas: radiologic pathologic correlation. Armed Forces Institute of Pathology. *Radiographics*. 2001;21(6):1533-1556.

Parmar HA, Hawkins C, Ozelame R, et al. Fluid-attenuated inversion recovery ring sign as a marker of dysembryoplastic neuroepithelial tumors. *J Comput Assist Tomogr*. 2007;31(3):348-353.

BRIGHT SPOTS, UNIDENTIFIED BRIGHT OBJECTS

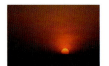

Modality:
MR

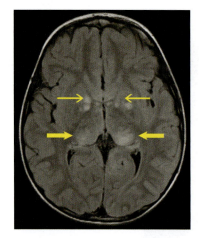
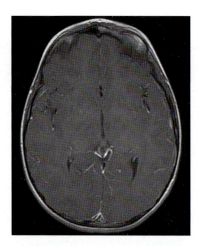

FINDINGS:

- Axial FLAIR MR shows multiple hyperintense, mildly expansile lesions in the bilateral basal ganglia (thin arrows) and thalami (thick arrows).
- Axial contrast-enhanced T1-weighted MR shows no appreciable enhancement.

DIAGNOSIS:

Neurofibromatosis type I

DISCUSSION:

Neurofibromatosis type I (NF1), also known as von Recklinghausen disease, is the most common phakomatosis. Caused by a mutation in the *NF1* gene on the long arm of chromosome 17, it is transmitted with autosomal dominant inheritance. At least two of the following diagnostic criteria must be present to make the diagnosis: café-au-lait spots, multiple or plexiform neurofibromas, axillary or inguinal freckling, optic gliomas, Lisch nodules (iris hamartomas), osseous abnormalities (sphenoid dysplasia, long bone thinning and pseudoarthrosis), and a first-degree relative with NF1. On MR, 30% to 60% of patients demonstrate T2-hyperintense foci with predilection for the basal ganglia, cerebellum, and brainstem. Known as unidentified bright objects (UBOs), these are considered benign hamartomas and correlate histologically with spongiform myelinopathy (myelin vacuolization with edema). Higher UBO burden is associated with cognitive dysfunction, though most lesions regress with age. Children with large numbers and volumes of UBOs should undergo regular imaging surveillance, given the increased risk of both benign and malignant CNS tumors. Lesion enlargement and/or contrast enhancement are suspicious imaging features that raise concern for neoplastic transformation.

References:

Gutmann DH, Aylsworth A, Carey JC, et al. The diagnostic evaluation and multidisciplinary management of neurofibromatosis 1 and neurofibromatosis 2. *JAMA*. 1997;278(1):51-57.

Mentzel HJ, Seidel J, Fitzek C, et al. Pediatric brain MRI in neurofibromatosis type I. *Eur Radiol*. 2005;15(4):814-822.

BUBBLY, FEATHERY, SOAP BUBBLE, SWISS CHEESE

Modalities:
CT, MR

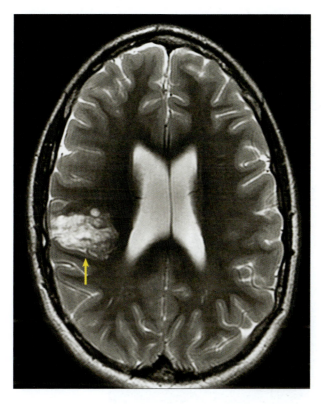

FINDINGS:

Axial T2-weighted MR shows a multiloculated hyperintense mass in the right perirolandic region (arrow).

DIAGNOSIS:

Dysembryoplastic neuroepithelial tumor

DISCUSSION:

Dysembryoplastic neuroepithelial tumors (DNETs) are benign, slow-growing neuroepithelial tumors arising from cortical or deep gray matter. Patients are typically male and under age 20. The temporal lobe is the most common location, followed by the frontal lobe. Simple DNETs are T2-hyperintense multiseptated "bubbly" masses with little vasogenic edema, enhancement, or mass effect. On FLAIR MR, there is nulling of the cystic components of tumor with a characteristic "bright rim," which may be complete or incomplete. Pathologically, this corresponds to peripheral loose neuroglial elements, and suggests residual or recurrent tumor in the postoperative setting. Complex DNETs have varying amounts of solid tissue and low-level enhancement. Lesions typically have a wedge-shaped morphology, in which the apex points toward the ventricle, and the outer surface extends to cortex with remodeling of the inner table. Associated cortical dysplasia is common. Other pediatric cystic tumors include ganglioglioma (GGL), pleomorphic xanthoastrocytoma (PXA), and juvenile pilocytic astrocytoma (JPA), which tend to be associated with enhancing mural nodules. In GGLs, edema is rare and calcification is common. PXAs tend to be larger and produce dural tails rather than skull erosion. When supratentorial, JPAs are usually adjacent to the third ventricle.

References:

Fernandez C, Girard N, Paz Paredes A, et al. The usefulness of MR imaging in the diagnosis of dysembryoplastic neuroepithelial tumor in children: a study of 14 cases. *AJNR Am J Neuroradiol.* 2003;24:829-834.

Koeller KK, Henry JM. From the archives of the AFIP: superficial gliomas: radiologic-pathologic correlation. Armed Forces Institute of Pathology. *Radiographics.* 2001;21(6):1533-1556.

BULLET

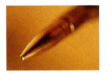

Modalities:
CT, MR

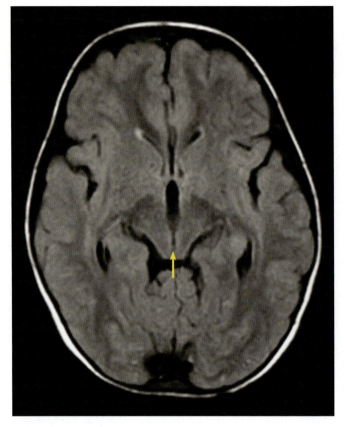

FINDINGS:

Axial FLAIR MR shows a deep interpeduncular fossa with dorsal pointing of the third ventricle (arrow).

DIAGNOSIS:

Joubert syndrome–related disorders

DISCUSSION:

Joubert syndrome–related disorders (JSRD), or cerebello-oculo-renal disorders, are autosomal recessive disruptions of midbrain-hindbrain development with associated ocular, facial, hepatic, renal, and digital anomalies. Lack of decussation of the superior cerebellar peduncles within the midbrain results in deepening of the interpeduncular fossa, with elongation of the third ventricle posteriorly ("bullet" appearance). Other imaging signs of JSRD include the "molar tooth" appearance of the midbrain, "bat-wing" fourth ventricle, and vermian dysplasia.

References:

Alorainy IA, Sabir S, Seidahmed MZ, et al. Brain stem and cerebellar findings in Joubert syndrome. *J Comput Assist Tomogr.* 2006;30(1):116-121.

Brancati F, Dallapiccola B, Valente EM. Joubert syndrome and related disorders. *Orphanet J Rare Dis.* 2010;5:20.

BULLET/HEART/TOWERING CEREBELLUM, TENTORIAL PSEUDOTUMOR

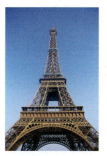

Modalities:
CT, MR

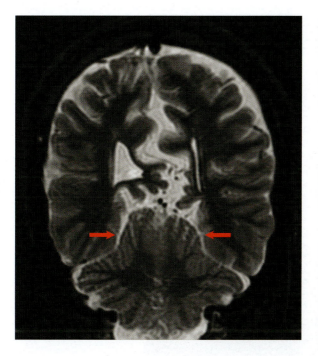

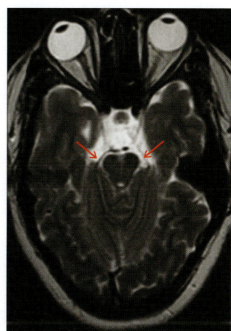

FINDINGS:

Axial and coronal T2-weighted MR show a widened incisura, with the cerebellum herniating superiorly (thick arrows) above the tentorium and wrapping laterally around the midbrain (thin arrows).

DIAGNOSIS:

Chiari II malformation

DISCUSSION:

The Chiari II malformation is a complex congenital anomaly consisting of small posterior fossa and lumbosacral myelomeningocele. Hypoplasia of the tentorium cerebelli produces a wide incisura, through which the cerebellum can herniate superiorly ("towering cerebellum"). Other characteristic imaging signs of Chiari II malformation include beaked tectum, cervicomedullary kink, and fenestrated falx with interdigitating gyri. In the Chiari III malformation, there is also an occipital or high cervical encephalocele.

References:

el Gammal T, Mark EK, Brooks BS. MR imaging of Chiari II malformation. *AJR Am J Roentgenol.* 1988;150(1):163-170.

Naidich TP, Pudlowski RM, Naidich JB. Computed tomographic signs of Chiari II malformation, II: midbrain and cerebellum. *Radiology.* 1980;134(2):391-398.

BUMPY, COBBLESTONE, NODULAR, PEBBLE, VERRUCOUS

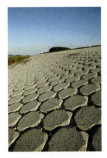

Modalities:
US, CT, MR

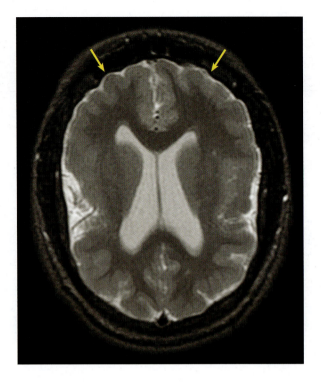

FINDINGS:

Axial T2-weighted MR shows dysplastic gyri and sulci with a micronodular appearance of the cortex, most pronounced in the frontal lobes (arrows).

DIAGNOSIS:

Lissencephaly, type II

DISCUSSION:

Congenital brain malformations with incomplete cortical sulcation include agyria (no gyri), pachygyria (broad gyri), and lissencephaly (underdeveloped gyri). Lissencephaly can be divided into type I (classic) and type II (cobblestone) types. Type I lissencephaly results from undermigration, while type II lissencephaly results from overmigration of neuroblasts and glial cells into the subarachnoid space during development. In type II lissencephaly, a thinned multinodular cortex ("cobblestone" appearance) and thickened meninges are seen, often in an anterior distribution. There is an association with muscular dystrophy–like syndromes. From most to least severe, these are Walker-Warburg syndrome (WWS), muscle-eye-brain disease (MEB), and Fukuyama congenital muscular dystrophy (FCMD). Associated ocular hypoplasia, midline anomalies, and hydrocephalus may be present.

References:

Abdel Razek AA, Kandell AY, Elsorogy LG, et al. Disorders of cortical formation: MR imaging features. *AJNR Am J Neuroradiol.* 2009;30(1):4-11.

Pilz DT, Quarrell OW. Syndromes with lissencephaly. *J Med Genet.* 1996;33(4):319-323.

BUTTERFLY

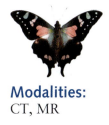

Modalities:
CT, MR

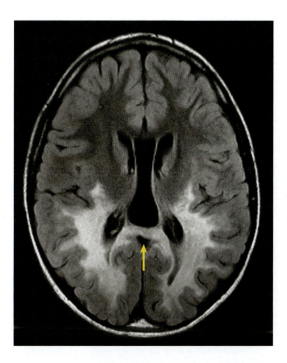
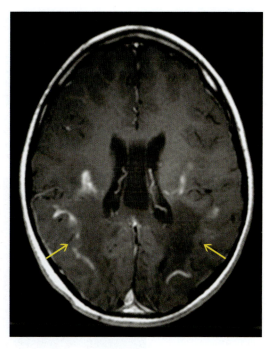

FINDINGS:

- Axial FLAIR MR shows symmetric hyperintensity within the periatrial white matter and splenium (arrow).
- Axial contrast-enhanced T1-weighted MR shows peripheral enhancement along the areas of FLAIR signal abnormality (arrows).

DIAGNOSIS:

Adrenoleukodystrophy

DISCUSSION:

Adrenoleukodystrophy (ALD) is an X-linked hereditary leukoencephalopathy caused by mutations in the ABCD1 peroxisomal protein, which is responsible for β-oxidation of very long chain fatty acids (VLCFAs). Most patients are young males, but there are additional subtypes of disease that affect neonates, adolescents, and adults. Accumulation of VLCFAs is toxic to the brain and causes symmetric demyelination of the splenium and periatrial white matter, producing a "butterfly" appearance. Demyelination progresses from central to peripheral, with characteristic enhancement along the leading edges. Less commonly, disease involves the frontal lobes, genu, cerebellum, and/or brainstem. There is also dysfunction of the adrenal cortex and testicular Leydig cells, yielding Addison disease and gonadal insufficiency.

References:

Cheon JE, Kim IO, Hwang YS, et al. Leukodystrophy in children: a pictorial review of MR imaging features. *Radiographics.* 2002;22(3):461-476.

Kim JH, Kim HJ. Childhood X-linked adrenoleukodystrophy: clinical-pathologic overview and MR imaging manifestations at initial evaluation and follow-up. *Radiographics.* 2005;25(3):619-631.

BUTTOCK

Modalities:
US, CT, MR

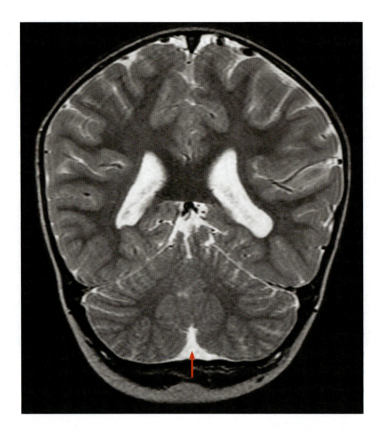

FINDINGS:

Coronal T2-weighted MR shows absent cerebellar vermis with apposition of the cerebellar hemispheres, separated by a thin CSF cleft (arrow).

DIAGNOSIS:

Joubert syndrome–related disorders

DISCUSSION:

Joubert syndrome–related disorders (JSRD), or cerebello-oculo-renal disorders, are autosomal recessive disruptions of midbrain-hindbrain development with associated ocular, facial, hepatic, renal, and digital anomalies. There is vermian hypoplasia with enlarged cisterna magna, creating a CSF-filled notch between the apposed cerebellar hemispheres ("buttock" sign). Other imaging signs of JSRD include the "molar tooth" appearance of the midbrain and "bat-wing" fourth ventricle. Another condition involving vermian aplasia is rhombencephalosynapsis, in which the cerebellar hemispheres and deep nuclei are fused across midline with no intervening cleft.

References:

Alorainy IA, Sabir S, Seidahmed MZ, et al. Brain stem and cerebellar findings in Joubert syndrome. *J Comput Assist Tomogr.* 2006;30(1):116-121.

Brancati F, Dallapiccola B, Valente EM. Joubert syndrome and related disorders. *Orphanet J Rare Dis.* 2010;5:20.

CANDLE GUTTERING/WAX

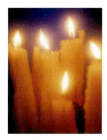

Modalities:
US, CT, MR

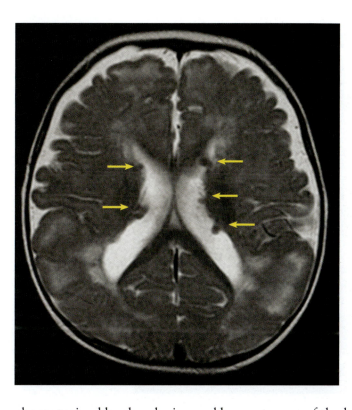

FINDINGS:

Axial T2-weighted MR shows ovoid subependymal nodules (arrows) along the lateral ventricular walls. Several cortical/subcortical hyperintense lesions are also present.

DIFFERENTIAL DIAGNOSIS:

- Tuberous sclerosis
- CNS lymphoma
- Metastases
- Gray matter heterotopia

DISCUSSION:

Tuberous sclerosis complex (TSC) is a phakomatosis or neuroectodermal syndrome characterized by dysplasias and hamartomas of the brain, retinae, skin, heart, lungs, kidneys, and bones. Histologically, there is abnormal neuronal/glial formation and migration, with disorganized myelination and gliosis. Neuroimaging manifestations include cortical/subcortical hamartomas, white matter abnormalities, and subependymal nodules or giant cell astrocytomas (SEGAs). Subependymal nodules of TSC are elongated and irregular ("candle guttering" appearance), frequently with calcification. In infants younger than 3 months, MR signal is T1-hyperintense and T2-hypointense. As myelination progresses with age, nodules become T2-hyperintense with variable T1 signal. There should not be associated diffusion abnormalities or contrast enhancement. Large enhancing nodules near the foramen of Monro suggest SEGAs—benign tumors that are typically resected because of their propensity for hemorrhage and ventricular obstruction. Other causes of ependymal nodularity include primary CNS lymphoma and ependymal metastases. These are typically larger and more enhancing, with reduced diffusion. The imaging differential also includes subependymal gray matter heterotopia, in which nodules have a smoother and more regular appearance. Signal is isointense to gray matter on all sequences, and there is no contrast enhancement.

References:

Baron Y, Barkovich AJ. MR imaging of tuberous sclerosis in neonates and young infants. *AJNR Am J Neuroradiol.* 1999;20(5):907-916.

Pinto Gama HP, da Rocha AJ, Braga FT, et al. Comparative analysis of MR sequences to detect structural brain lesions in tuberous sclerosis. *Pediatr Radiol.* 2006;36(2):119-125.

CAULIFLOWER

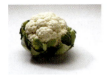

Modalities:
US, CT, MR

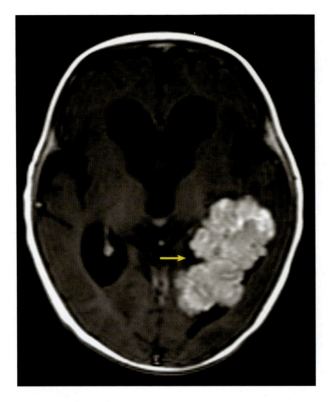

FINDINGS:

Axial contrast-enhanced T1-weighted MR shows a lobulated hyperenhancing mass in the left trigone (arrow), with associated hydrocephalus.

DIAGNOSIS:

Choroid plexus tumor

DISCUSSION:

The choroid plexus is the most vascular structure within the ventricular system and continuously produces cerebrospinal fluid. As a result, choroid plexus tumors are markedly hypervascular and associated with hydrocephalus. Benign choroid plexus papilloma (CPP) classically has a well-circumscribed, frondlike "cauliflower" appearance and is contained within the ventricle. Malignant choroid plexus carcinoma (CPC) tends to be larger and more irregular, with local invasion and metastasis. However, there is a great deal of overlap in imaging appearances. Choroid plexus tumors most commonly occur in the trigones in children and the fourth ventricle in adults. There is an association with von Hippel-Lindau disease.

References:

Anderson DR, Falcone S, Bruce JH, et al. Radiologic-pathologic correlation. Congenital choroid plexus papillomas. *AJNR Am J Neuroradiol.* 1995;16(10):2072-2076.

Koeller KK, Sandberg GD. From the archives of the AFIP. Cerebral intraventricular neoplasms: radiologic-pathologic correlation. *Radiographics.* 2002;22(6):1473-1505.

(CERVICO)MEDULLARY BUCKLE/KINK/SPUR, TRUMPET

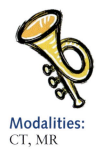

Modalities:
CT, MR

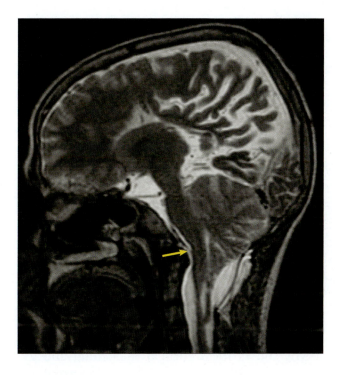

FINDINGS:

Sagittal T2-weighted MR shows acute angulation at the cervicomedullary junction (arrow), with edema in the medulla and atrophy of the cervical cord. The cerebellar tonsils are peglike and displaced far below the foramen magnum.

DIAGNOSIS:

Chiari malformation

DISCUSSION:

Chiari malformations involve a spectrum of complex congenital anomalies, all with inferior displacement of the cerebellum and brainstem through the foramen magnum. In Chiari I, tonsillar displacement may cause syringohydromyelia due to obstruction of cerebrospinal fluid (CSF) flow. With Chiari II, a lumbosacral myelomeningocele produces additional traction on the spinal cord, resulting in a hypoplastic posterior fossa. Inferior migration of the cerebellar tonsils causes crowding of the foramen magnum, with brainstem elongation and kinking at the level of the cervicomedullary junction. Edema of the medulla and atrophy of the cervical cord yields a flared ("trumpet") appearance. In Chiari III, there is also an occipital or high cervical encephalocele.

References:

Geerdink N, van der Vliet T, Rotteveel JJ, et al. Essential features of Chiari II malformation in MR imaging: an interobserver reliability study—part 1. *Childs Nerv Syst.* 2012;28(7):977-985.

Naidich TP, McLone DG, Fulling KH. The Chiari II malformation: Part IV. The hindbrain deformity. *Neuroradiology.* 1983;25(4):179-197.

CLEFT-DIMPLE

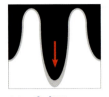

Modalities:
CT, MR

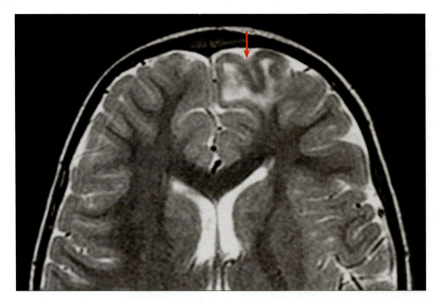

FINDINGS:

Axial T2-weighted MR shows focal cortical thickening and gyral enlargement in the left frontal lobe, with dilated overlying CSF space (arrow) and subcortical white matter hyperintensity.

DIAGNOSIS:

Cortical dysgenesis

DISCUSSION:

Cortical dysgenesis represents a spectrum of congenital cortical malformations resulting from abnormal cellular proliferation, migration, or postmigrational development. Abnormalities of neuronal and glial proliferation include focal cortical dysplasia type II (Taylor dysplasia), microcephaly, and megalencephaly. Abnormalities of neuronal migration include lissencephaly and gray matter heterotopia. Abnormalities of postmigrational development include polymicrogyria, schizencephaly, and non-Taylor cortical dysplasias. Imaging features of cortical dysgenesis include cortical thickening, undersulcation, macrogyria, loss of gray-white distinction, and abnormal white matter signal. The "cleft-dimple" complex refers to inward buckling of the cortex (cortical "dimple") with a prominent CSF space ("cleft") overlying the area of dysgenesis. This feature is particularly helpful in detecting subtle cortical malformations and distinguishing them from true atrophy (with volume loss and cortical thinning) or mass lesions (expanding into and effacing the overlying CSF space).

References:

Barkovich AJ, Guerrini R, Kuzniecky RI, et al. A developmental and genetic classification for malformations of cortical development: update 2012. *Brain*. 2012;135(Pt 5):1348-1369.

Bronen RA, Spencer DD, Fulbright RK. Cerebrospinal fluid cleft with cortical dimple: MR imaging marker for focal cortical dysgenesis. *Radiology*. 2000;214(3):657-663.

CLOSED LIP

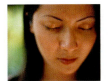

Modalities:
US, CT, MR

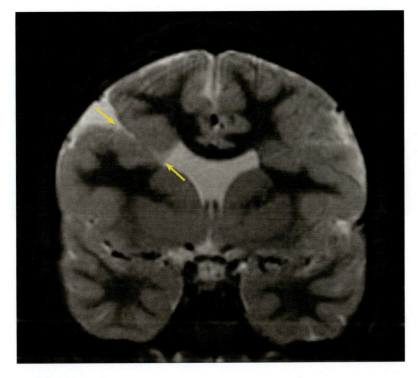

FINDINGS:

Coronal T2-weighted MR shows a right frontal transcortical defect (arrows) lined by gray matter, without intervening CSF.

DIAGNOSIS:

Closed-lip schizencephaly

DISCUSSION:

Schizencephaly is caused by a full-thickness insult to the cerebral cortex during cortical organization, which produces a gray matter-lined cleft extending from the ventricular system to the subarachnoid space. Clefts may be small or large, unilateral or bilateral, and classified as type I (closed-lip) or type II (open-lip). In closed-lip schizencephaly, the lips are in contact with each other; in open-lip schizencephaly, the lips are separated by intervening CSF. The gray matter lining the cleft is frequently polymicrogyric (multiple tiny gyri) and can extend into the ventricle, forming subependymal gray matter heterotopia. Schizencephaly should not be confused with porencephaly, in which an acquired insult results in a white matter-lined cavity adjacent to the ventricular system and/or subarachnoid space.

References:

Abdel Razek AA, Kandell AY, Elsorogy LG, et al. Disorders of cortical formation: MR imaging features. *AJNR Am J Neuroradiol.* 2009;30(1):4-11.

Barkovich AJ, Norman D. MR imaging of schizencephaly. *AJR Am J Roentgenol.* 1988;150(6): 1391-1396.

CONVOLUTED, CURVILINEAR, GYRIFORM, SERPENTINE, TRAM LINE/TRACK

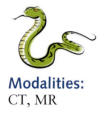

Modalities:
CT, MR

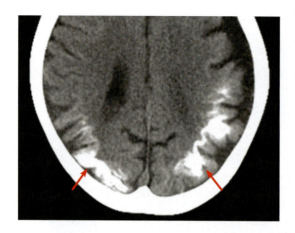 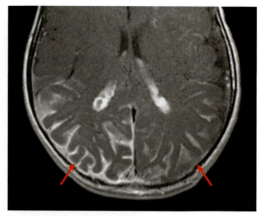

FINDINGS:

- Axial CT shows cortical calcifications in both parietal lobes (arrows).
- Axial contrast-enhanced T1-weighted MR shows leptomeningeal (arrows) and choroid plexus hyperenhancement, right greater than left.

DIFFERENTIAL DIAGNOSIS:

- Sturge-Weber syndrome
- Cortical laminar necrosis
- Meningitis
- Radiation

DISCUSSION:

Sturge-Weber syndrome (encephalotrigeminal angiomatosis) is a neurocutaneous syndrome consisting of facial port-wine stain and leptomeningeal angiomatosis. During development, subarachnoid vascular malformations between the arachnoid and pia mater prevent development of cortical bridging veins that normally connect the superficial and deep venous systems. Cerebral venous outflow is impaired and causes enlargement of cortical, medullary, and subependymal veins and choroid plexus ("choroidal angiomatosis"). Chronic venous hypertension causes white matter damage and cortical calcifications, particularly in the parietal and occipital lobes. Calcifications in apposing gyri form the classic "tram track" appearance. An associated condition is Dyke-Davidoff-Masson syndrome, or cerebral hemiatrophy with ipsilateral enlargement of the sinuses, mastoid air cells, and diploic space. Other causes of gyriform calcification include infarcts with cortical laminar necrosis, meningitis, radiation, anticonvulsant therapy, folic acid deficiency, leukemia treated with intrathecal methotrexate, gliomas, and calcifying hamartomas in tuberous sclerosis. Correlation with other radiologic and clinical findings is crucial for diagnosis.

References:

Akpinar E. The tram-track sign: cortical calcifications. *Radiology.* 2004;231(2):515-516.

Juhász C, Haacke EM, Hu J, et al. Multimodality imaging of cortical and white matter abnormalities in Sturge-Weber syndrome. *AJNR Am J Neuroradiol.* 2007;28(5):900-906.

CORTICAL/SUBCORTICAL ISLANDS, TUBERS

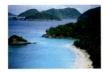

Modalities:
CT, MR

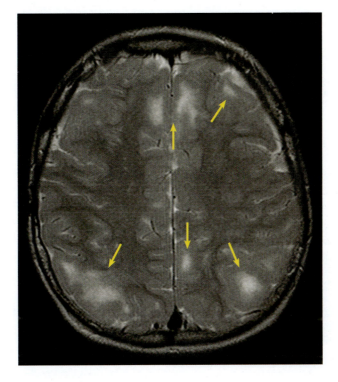

FINDINGS:

Axial T2-weighted MR shows multiple hyperintense lesions (arrows) in the cortex and subcortical white matter.

DIAGNOSIS:

Tuberous sclerosis

DISCUSSION:

Tuberous sclerosis complex (TSC) is a phakomatosis or neuroectodermal syndrome characterized by dysplasias and hamartomas of the brain, retinae, skin, heart, lungs, kidneys, and bones. Histologically, there is abnormal neuronal/glial formation and migration, with disorganized myelination and gliosis. Neuroimaging manifestations include cortical/subcortical hamartomas ("islands"), white matter abnormalities, and subependymal nodules or giant cell astrocytomas (SEGAs). Tubers are focal protrusions of gyri in the cerebrum and/or cerebellum, which expand the cortex and obscure the gray-white junction. In infants younger than 3 months, MR signal is T1-hyperintense and T2-hypointense. As myelination progresses with age, tubers become T2-hyperintense with variable T1 signal and central cystic changes.

References:

Inoue Y, Nemoto Y, Murata R, et al. CT and MR imaging of cerebral tuberous sclerosis. *Brain Dev.* 1998;20(4):209-221.

Pinto Gama HP, da Rocha AJ, Braga FT, et al. Comparative analysis of MR sequences to detect structural brain lesions in tuberous sclerosis. *Pediatr Radiol.* 2006;36(2):119-125.

CYST WITH NODULE, MURAL NODULE

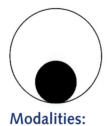

Modalities:
CT, MR

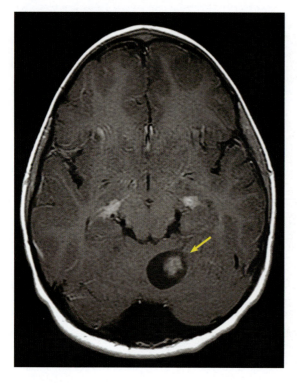

FINDINGS:

Axial contrast-enhanced T1-weighted MR shows a left cerebellar cystic lesion with enhancing mural nodule (arrow).

DIFFERENTIAL DIAGNOSIS:

- Juvenile pilocytic astrocytoma
- Pleomorphic xanthoastrocytoma
- Ganglioglioma
- Dysembryoplastic neuroepithelial tumor

DISCUSSION:

Pediatric mixed solid/cystic tumors include juvenile pilocystic astrocytoma (JPA), ganglioglioma (GGL), pleomorphic xanthoastrocytoma (PXA), and dysembryoplastic neuroepithelial tumor (DNET). The enhancing "mural nodule" corresponds to tumor, while the cystic component represents secreted fluid. JPAs are typically infratentorial in the posterior fossa, but when supratentorial are usually adjacent to the third ventricle. GGL, PXA, and DNET favor the superficial temporal lobes. GGLs are typically well circumscribed with a small mural nodule. Classic DNETs are multilobulated nonenhancing masses with calvarial scalloping. PXAs tend to be larger and produce dural tails without skull erosion.

Reference:

Koeller KK, Henry JM. From the archives of the AFIP: superficial gliomas: radiologic-pathologic correlation. Armed Forces Institute of Pathology. *Radiographics.* 2001;21(6):1533-1556.

DANGLING CHOROID

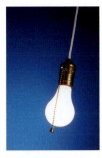

Modalities:
US, MR

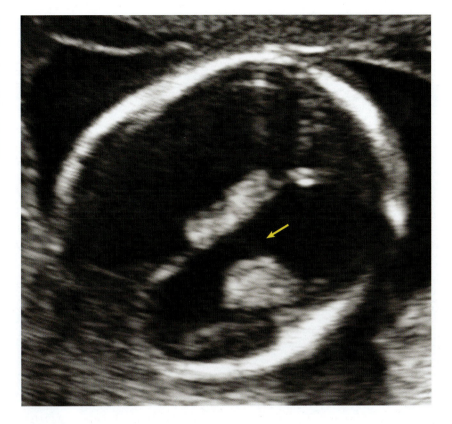

FINDINGS:

Fetal US, axial plane, shows enlarged lateral ventricles with dependent choroid plexi. The choroid plexus farther from the transducer is abnormally angulated and "dangles" from its attachment at the foramen of Monro (arrow).

DIFFERENTIAL DIAGNOSIS:

- Fetal ventriculomegaly
- Fetal hydrocephalus

DISCUSSION:

Fetal ventriculomegaly is defined as enlargement of the lateral ventricles, with atrial diameter greater than 10 mm or choroid plexus ventricular wall separation greater than 3 to 4 mm. Normally, the choroid plexi course parallel to the ventricles and contact both ventricular walls. In severe ventriculomegaly or hydrocephalus (>15 mm), the choroid angles increase and the free-hanging choroid "dangles" from its attachment at the foramen of Monro.

References:

Cardoza JD, Filly RA, Podrasky AE. The dangling choroid plexus: a sonographic observation of value in excluding ventriculomegaly. *AJR Am J Roentgenol.* 1988;151(4):767-770.

Nyberg DA, McGahan JP, Pretorius DH, et al. *Diagnostic Imaging of Fetal Anomalies.* 2nd ed. Philadelphia: Lippincott Williams & Wilkins; 2002.

DARK CEREBELLUM

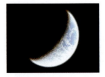

Modality:
CT

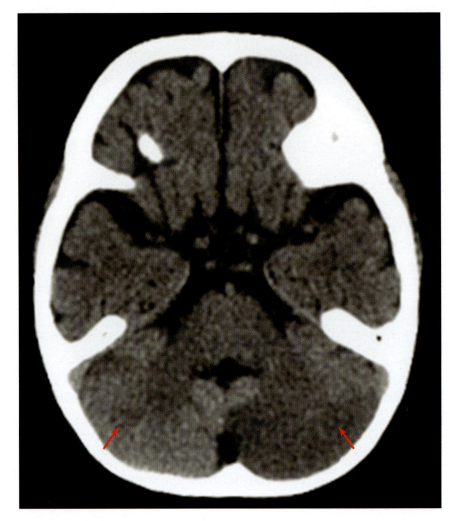

FINDINGS:

Axial CT shows prominent hypodensities in the cerebellar hemispheres, left greater than right. Involvement of both gray and white matter indicates cytotoxic edema.

DIAGNOSIS:

Cerebellar infarcts

DISCUSSION:

Diffuse hypodensity of the cerebellum on CT ("dark cerebellum") is a rare finding that raises concern for ischemia, particularly when both gray and white matter are involved. Isolated cerebellar infarction is occasionally seen in premature neonates, or in children and adolescents following an overdose of tricyclic antidepressants (TCA). In the acute setting, MR can be ordered to confirm the presence of reduced diffusion.

Reference:

Huisman TA, Kubat SH, Eckhardt BP. The "dark cerebellar sign." *Neuropediatrics*. 2007;38(3):160-163.

DIAMOND, KEYHOLE, TRAPEZOID

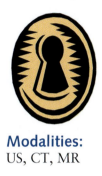

Modalities:
US, CT, MR

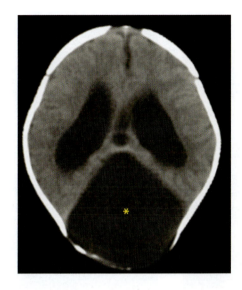

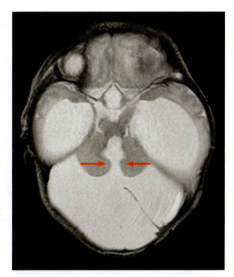

FINDINGS:

- Axial CT shows a gaping posterior fossa with diamond-shaped CSF space (asterisk).
- Axial T2-weighted MR shows a dilated fourth ventricle communicating (arrows) with an enlarged cisterna magna.

DIFFERENTIAL DIAGNOSIS:

- Dandy-Walker complex
- Rhombencephalosynapsis
- Communicating hydrocephalus
- Arachnoid cyst

DISCUSSION:

Dandy-Walker complex represents a continuum of posterior fossa anomalies, which from most to least severe are Dandy-Walker malformation, Dandy-Walker variant, and mega cisterna magna. The posterior fossa is small with varying degrees of vermian hypoplasia, torcular-lambdoid inversion (torcular herophili elevated above the lambdoid suture), and cisterna magna enlargement. There is dilation of the fourth ventricle, which communicates with the cisterna magna through a CSF space between the cerebellar hemispheres, creating a "keyhole" or "diamond" appearance. Rhombencephalosynapsis is a severe malformation that involves vermian hypoplasia, dorsal fusion of the cerebellar hemispheres, and apposition or fusion of the dentate nuclei and cerebellar peduncles. Other mimics include communicating hydrocephalus, posterior fossa arachnoid cyst, and the normal rhombencephalic cavity before 18 weeks of gestational age.

Reference:

Wolfson BJ, Faerber EN, Truex RC Jr. The "keyhole": a sign of herniation of a trapped fourth ventricle and other posterior fossa cysts. *AJNR Am J Neuroradiol.* 1987;8(3):473-477.

DIAMOND, STAR

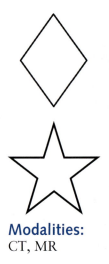

Modalities:
CT, MR

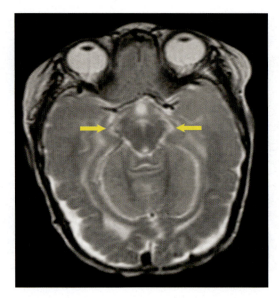

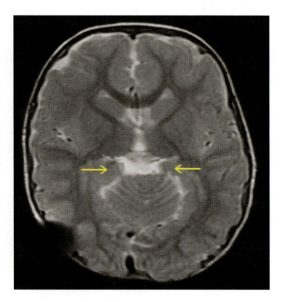

FINDINGS:

Axial T2-weighted MR of different patients show diamond- (thick arrows) and star-shaped (thin arrows) basilar cisterns. Also seen are wide incisurae, superior herniation of the cerebellum, and interdigitation of occipital gyri.

DIAGNOSIS:

Chiari II malformation

DISCUSSION:

The Chiari II malformation is a complex congenital anomaly consisting of small posterior fossa and lumbosacral myelomeningocele. The basilar cisterns assume a "diamond"- or "star"-shaped morphology formed by the cistern of velum interpositum, superior vermian cistern, and ambient cisterns. Other characteristic imaging signs of Chiari II malformation include beaked tectum, cervicomedullary kink, wide incisura with towering cerebellum, and fenestrated falx with interdigitating gyri. In the Chiari III malformation, there is also an occipital or high cervical encephalocele.

Reference:

Naidich TP, Pudlowski RM, Naidich JB. Computed tomographic signs of the Chiari II malformation, III: ventricles and cisterns. *Radiology*. 1980;134(3):657-663.

DIMPLE, NIPPLE

Modalities:
US, CT, MR

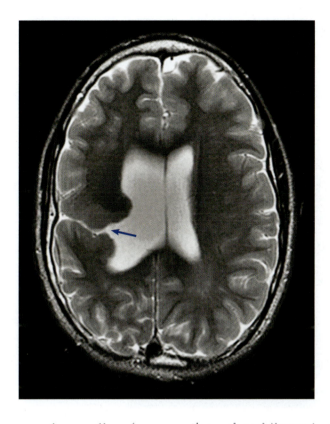

FINDINGS:

Axial T2-weighted MR shows a right perirolandic transcortical defect lined by dysmorphic gray matter, with a thin intervening CSF cleft. There is associated contour irregularity of the lateral ventricle (arrow).

DIAGNOSIS:

Schizencephaly

DISCUSSION:

Schizencephaly is caused by a full-thickness insult to the cerebral cortex during cortical organization, producing a gray matter-lined cleft that extends from the ventricular system to the subarachnoid space. Clefts may be small or large, unilateral or bilateral, and classified as type I (closed-lip) or type II (open-lip). In closed-lip schizencephaly, the lips are in contact with each other; in open-lip schizencephaly, the lips are separated by intervening CSF. The pia mater and ependyma meet within the cleft to form the pial-ependymal seam, which is visible as a "dimple" along the superficial wall of the ventricle. The gray matter lining the cleft is frequently polymicrogyric (multiple tiny gyri) and can extend into the ventricle, forming subependymal gray matter heterotopia. Schizencephaly should not be confused with porencephaly, in which an acquired insult results in a white matter-lined cavity adjacent to the ventricular system and/ or subarachnoid space.

References:

Abdel Razek AA, Kandell AY, Elsorogy LG, et al. Disorders of cortical formation: MR imaging features. *AJNR Am J Neuroradiol.* 2009;30(1):4-11.

Barkovich AJ, Norman D. MR imaging of schizencephaly. *AJR Am J Roentgenol.* 1988;150(6): 1391-1396.

DOUBLE CORTEX, THREE LAYER CAKE

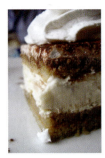

Modalities:
CT, MR

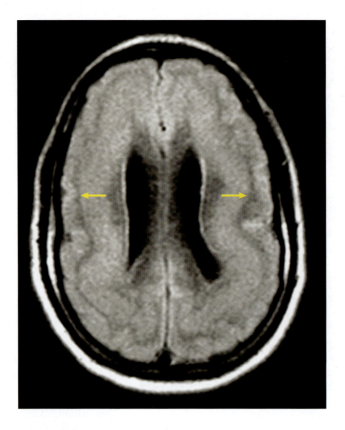

FINDINGS:

Axial FLAIR MR shows cortical undersulcation and a continuous band of heterotopic gray matter (arrows) that is separated from the cortex by intervening white matter.

DIAGNOSIS:

Band heterotopia

DISCUSSION:

Gray matter heterotopia is caused by abnormal neuronal migration, and can occur anywhere between the subependymal region and cerebral cortex. The major types are band, subcortical, and periventricular (subependymal). Band heterotopia is associated with type I lissencephaly. Females are predominantly affected, with an X-linked dominant pattern of inheritance. At imaging, symmetric bands of gray matter are seen coursing parallel to the cortex ("double cortex"), with an intervening layer of white matter ("three layer cake"). Bands may be partial, complete, or even duplicated. The overlying cortex can be normal or pachygyric.

References:

Abdel Razek AA, Kandell AY, Elsorogy LG, et al. Disorders of cortical formation: MR imaging features. *AJNR Am J Neuroradiol.* 2009;30(1):4-11.

Franzoni E, Bernardi B, Marchiani V, et al. Band brain heterotopia. Case report and literature review. *Neuropediatrics.* 1995;26(1):37-40.

ENLARGED MASSA INTERMEDIA

Modalities:
CT, MR

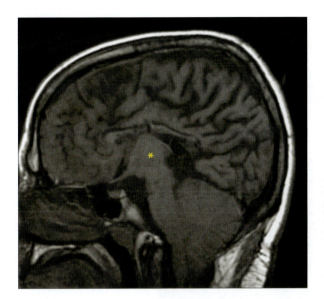
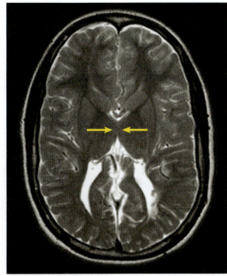

FINDINGS:

- Sagittal T1-weighted MR shows an enlarged massa intermedia (asterisk), hypoplastic posterior fossa with tonsillar descent, and callosal dysgenesis.
- Axial T2-weighted MR again shows the prominent massa intermedia (arrows).

DIAGNOSIS:

Chiari II malformation

DISCUSSION:

The Chiari II malformation is a complex congenital anomaly consisting of small posterior fossa, inferior displacement of the cerebellum and brainstem, and lumbosacral myelomeningocele. Thickening of the massa intermedia (interthalamic adhesion) is a classic finding. Other characteristic imaging signs of Chiari II malformation include beaked tectum, cervicomedullary kink, wide incisura with towering cerebellum, and fenestrated falx with interdigitating gyri. In the Chiari III malformation, there is also an occipital or high cervical encephalocele.

References:

Geerdink N, van der Vliet T, Rotteveel JJ, et al. Essential features of Chiari II malformation in MR imaging: an interobserver reliability study—part 1. *Childs Nerv Syst.* 2012;28(7):977-985.

Naidich TP, Pudlowski RM, Naidich JB. Computed tomographic signs of Chiari II malformation, II: midbrain and cerebellum. *Radiology.* 1980;134(2):391-398.

FENESTRATED FALX, INTERDIGITATING/INTERLOCKING GYRI

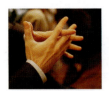

Modalities:
US, CT, MR

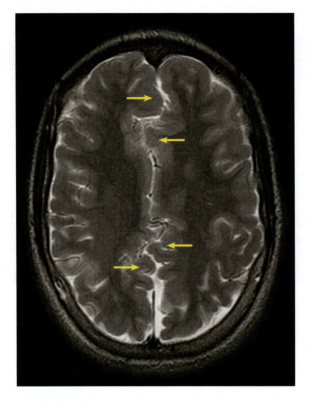

FINDINGS:

Axial T2-weighted MR shows absent falx cerebri, with gyri interdigitating across the midline (arrows).

DIAGNOSIS:

Chiari II malformation

DISCUSSION:

The Chiari II malformation is a complex congenital anomaly consisting of small posterior fossa, inferior displacement of the cerebellum and brainstem, and lumbosacral myelomeningocele. Midline anomalies are common, including partial absence of the falx cerebri ("fenestrated falx") with the cerebral gyri extending across the midline ("interdigitating gyri"). There may be associated stenogyria (packed shallow gyri and sulci with normal cortical organization). Other characteristic imaging signs of Chiari II malformation include beaked tectum, cervicomedullary kink, and wide incisura with towering cerebellum. In the Chiari III malformation, there is also an occipital or high cervical encephalocele.

References:

Geerdink N, van der Vliet T, Rotteveel JJ, et al. Essential features of Chiari II malformation in MR imaging: an interobserver reliability study—part 1. *Childs Nerv Syst.* 2012;28(7):977-985.

Naidich TP, Pudlowski RM, Naidich JB, et al. Computed tomographic signs of the Chiari II malformation. Part I: skull and dural partitions. *Radiology.* 1980;134(1):65-71.

FIGURE EIGHT, HOURGLASS, OVAL

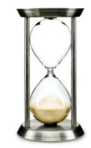

Modalities:
US, CT, MR

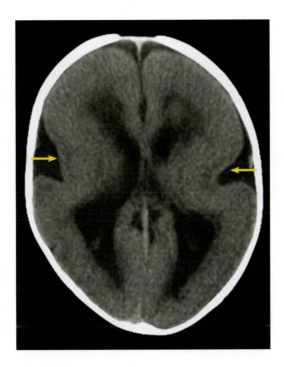
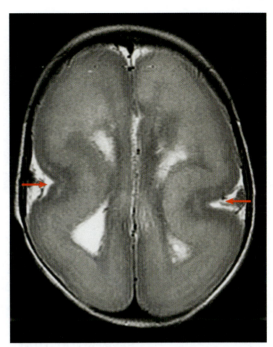

FINDINGS:

Axial CT and T2-weighted MR show poorly developed gyri with shallow sylvian fissures (arrows). The cerebral cortex is diffusely smooth and thickened.

DIAGNOSIS:

Lissencephaly, type I

DISCUSSION:

Congenital brain malformations with incomplete cortical sulcation include agyria (no gyri), pachygyria (broad gyri), and lissencephaly (underdeveloped gyri). Lissencephaly can be divided into type I (classic) and type II (cobblestone) types. Type I lissencephaly results from neuronal undermigration during development, with formation of four cortical layers rather than the normal six. At imaging, there is a diffusely thickened cortex (>3 mm) with poorly formed gyri, shallow sylvian fissures, and a smooth outer surface ("figure 8" or "hourglass" appearance). Subcortical band heterotopia is frequently associated. The anomaly can be isolated or seen as part of the Miller-Dieker syndrome with associated cardiac, pulmonary, gastrointestinal, genitourinary, and musculoskeletal anomalies. Type I lissencephaly should not be confused with polymicrogyria, in which multiple tiny gyri are present; or with the normal fetal brain between 18 and 22 weeks, when the primary fissures begin to develop.

References:

Abdel Razek AA, Kandell AY, Elsorogy LG, et al. Disorders of cortical formation: MR imaging features. *AJNR Am J Neuroradiol.* 2009;30(1):4-11.

Ghai S, Fong KW, Toi A, et al. Prenatal US and MR imaging findings of lissencephaly: review of fetal cerebral sulcal development. *Radiographics.* 2006;26(2):389-405.

FIGURE EIGHT, MENISCUS

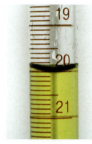

Modalities:
CT, MR

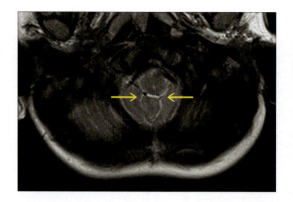 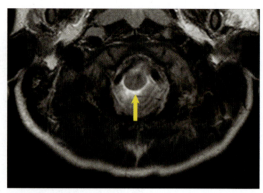

FINDINGS:

- Axial T2-weighted MR shows crowding of the foramen magnum with the inferior vermis (thin arrows) immediately dorsal to the medulla.
- Axial T2-weighted MR at a lower level shows a thin rim of CSF (thick arrow) surrounding the cervical cord.

DIFFERENTIAL DIAGNOSIS:

- Tonsillar ectopia
- Tonsillar herniation
- Chiari malformation

DISCUSSION:

Inferior displacement of the cerebellar tonsils through the foramen magnum can be seen as a normal variant, secondary to increased intracranial pressure, or as part of a Chiari malformation. Crowding of the spinal cord and cerebellum within the foramen magnum partially obliterates the CSF space, and in severe cases can lead to CSF flow obstruction with syringohydromyelia. The "figure 8" appearance is created by the abnormal juxtaposition of the medulla and inferior vermis, as well as the cervical cord and cerebellar tonsils. The "meniscus" sign refers to the thin rim of CSF surrounding the brainstem and cervical cord.

Reference:

Naidich TP, McLone DG, Fulling KH. The Chiari II malformation: Part IV. The hindbrain deformity. *Neuroradiology.* 1983;25(4):179-197.

FLAT FLOOR OF FOURTH VENTRICLE

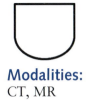

Modalities:
CT, MR

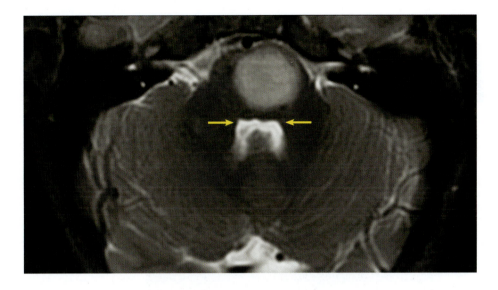

FINDINGS:

Axial T2-weighted MR shows a hyperintense pontine mass with effacement of the floor of the fourth ventricle (arrows). There is a left ventral exophytic component that partially encases the basilar artery.

DIFFERENTIAL DIAGNOSIS:

- Brainstem glioma
- Rhombencephalitis

DISCUSSION:

The floor (ventral surface) of the fourth ventricle normally slopes up toward midline, with indentations from the facial colliculi on each side. A flattened floor indicates pontine edema and/or mass effect, which can be seen in primary/metastatic tumors or infection (rhombencephalitis); and rarely in central pontine myelinolysis, demyelinating disease, and infarction. Brainstem gliomas are infiltrative, expansile primary tumors that can be focal or diffuse, and are most commonly centered in the pons. There is an association with neurofibromatosis type I (NF1). Lesions have hypodense CT attenuation and hyperintense signal on T2-weighted MR. Enhancement and reduced diffusion are rare, but indicate higher-grade tumor with a worse prognosis. Encasement of the basilar artery and compression of surrounding structures are highly specific imaging findings for neoplasia. Rhombencephalitis demonstrates signal abnormality with enhancement and/or reduced diffusion, and may extend to involve noncontiguous structures.

References:

Donaldson SS, Laningham F, Fisher PG. Advances toward an understanding of brainstem gliomas. *J Clin Oncol.* 2006;24(8):1266-1272.

Ueoka DI, Nogueira J, Campos JC, et al. Brainstem gliomas—retrospective analysis of 86 patients. *J Neurol Sci.* 2009;281(1-2):20-23.

FROG

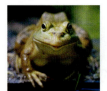

Modalities:
US, MR

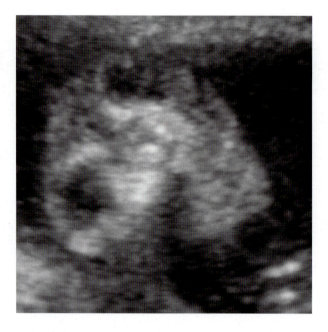

FINDINGS:

Fetal US, coronal plane, reveals bulging orbits and absence of supraorbital tissues.

DIAGNOSIS:

Anencephaly

DISCUSSION:

Anencephaly is the most severe neural tube defect, with absence of normal cortical tissue and calvarium above the level of the orbits. There may be a small amount of supraorbital angiomatous stroma or residual vascularized tissue. The orbits are prominent, and the facial features are preserved ("frog face"). The skull base, brainstem, and cerebellum are variably formed. Anencephaly is thought to represent the final stage of the acrania-exencephaly-anencephaly sequence. In acrania, there is absence of the calvarium but normally formed cerebral hemispheres and meninges. Without overlying bone, the brain and meninges are continually exposed to amniotic fluid and progressively disintegrate. Exencephaly refers to the stage in which some residual brain is present and the cerebral hemispheres can still be identified. Once the brain has completely degraded, the defect is termed anencephaly. This diagnosis should be made only after 14 weeks of gestation, once the skull has ossified. Anencephaly must be distinguished from amniotic band syndrome, in which the head and other structures are entrapped and lacerated by crossing fibrous bands.

References:

Goldstein RB, Filly RA. Prenatal diagnosis of anencephaly: spectrum of sonographic appearances and distinction from the amniotic band syndrome. *AJR Am J Roentgenol.* 1988;151(3):547-550.

Hidalgo H, Bowie J, Rosenberg ER, et al. Review. In utero sonographic diagnosis of fetal cerebral anomalies. *AJR Am J Roentgenol.* 1982;139(1):143-148.

FUSED THALAMI

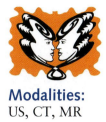

Modalities:
US, CT, MR

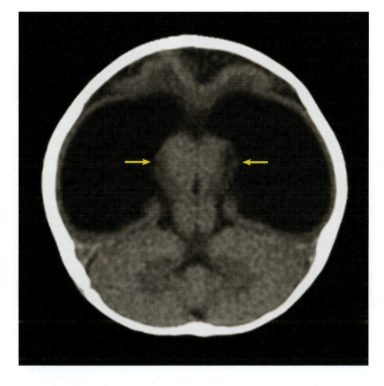

FINDINGS:

Axial CT shows partial fusion of midline structures including thalami (arrows), with dilated lateral ventricles.

DIAGNOSIS:

Holoprosencephaly

DISCUSSION:

Holoprosencephaly refers to a spectrum of congenital malformations in which the embryonic forebrain (prosencephalon) fails to separate completely. Based on the degree of midline fusion, these are classified as alobar, semilobar, lobar, and middle interhemispheric variant (syntelencephaly). The alobar variant is the most severe with holospheric cortical fusion; absent corpus callosum, septum pellucidum, and falx cerebri; single monoventricle; and fusion of the basal ganglia and thalami. Semilobar and middle interhemispheric variants are less severe and exhibit variable degrees of thalamic fusion. Lobar holoprosencephaly is the mildest form, in which the anterior corpus callosum and falx are hypoplastic, and the thalami are usually fully separate. Holoprosencephaly should be distinguished from hydranencephaly caused by bilateral ICA occlusion in utero. In this condition, diffuse cortical destruction is present, but the posterior fossa and thalami are normal.

Reference:

Hahn JS, Barnes PD. Neuroimaging advances in holoprosencephaly: Refining the spectrum of the midline malformation. *Am J Med Genet C Semin Med Genet.* 2010;154C(1):120-132.

GAPING/HEART/WIDE INCISURA

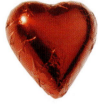

Modalities:
CT, MR

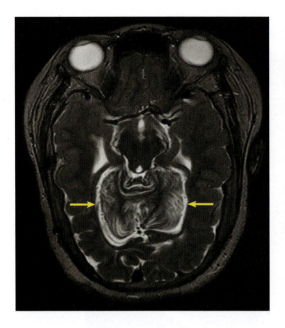

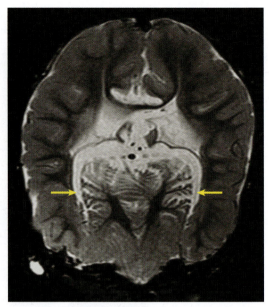

FINDINGS:

Axial and coronal T2-weighted MR show a hypoplastic tentorium with wide incisura (arrows), through which the cerebellum herniates superiorly.

DIAGNOSIS:

Chiari II malformation

DISCUSSION:

The Chiari II malformation is a complex congenital anomaly consisting of small posterior fossa and lumbosacral myelomeningocele. Hypoplasia of the tentorium results in a wide "heart"-shaped incisura, through which the cerebellum can herniate superiorly and laterally around the brainstem. Other characteristic imaging signs of Chiari II malformation include beaked tectum, cervicomedullary kink, and fenestrated falx with interdigitating gyri. In the Chiari III malformation, there is also an occipital or high cervical encephalocele.

References:

Geerdink N, van der Vliet T, Rotteveel JJ, et al. Essential features of Chiari II malformation in MR imaging: an interobserver reliability study—part 1. *Childs Nerv Syst.* 2012;28(7):977-985.

Naidich TP, Pudlowski RM, Naidich JB, et al. Computed tomographic signs of the Chiari II malformation, part I: skull and dural partitions. *Radiology.* 1980;134(1):65-71.

HOURGLASS, SHARK TOOTH

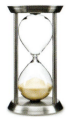

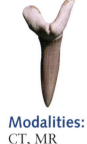

Modalities:
CT, MR

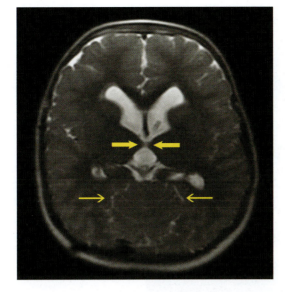

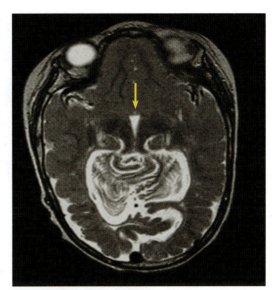

FINDINGS:

- Axial T2-weighted MR shows mild ventriculomegaly with an enlarged massa intermedia (thick arrows) that causes waisting of the third ventricle. There is also a wide incisura and superior herniation of the cerebellum (thin arrows).
- Axial T2-weighted MR in a different patient shows a triangular third ventricle (arrow) with pointed dorsal tip. There is also a wide incisura, superior herniation of the cerebellum, and interdigitating occipital gyri.

DIAGNOSIS:

Chiari II malformation

DISCUSSION:

The Chiari II malformation is a complex congenital anomaly consisting of small posterior fossa and lumbosacral myelomeningocele. Because of mass effect from an enlarged massa intermedia (interthalamic adhesion), the third ventricle can assume an "hourglass" or "shark tooth" appearance. Other characteristic imaging signs of Chiari II malformation include beaked tectum, cervicomedullary kink, wide incisura with towering cerebellum, and fenestrated falx with interdigitating gyri. In the Chiari III malformation, there is also an occipital or high cervical encephalocele.

Reference:

Naidich TP, Pudlowski RM, Naidich JB. Computed tomographic signs of the Chiari II malformation, III: ventricles and cisterns. *Radiology.* 1980;134(3):657-663.

INTERHEMISPHERIC CYST

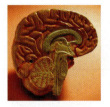

Modalities:
US, CT, MR

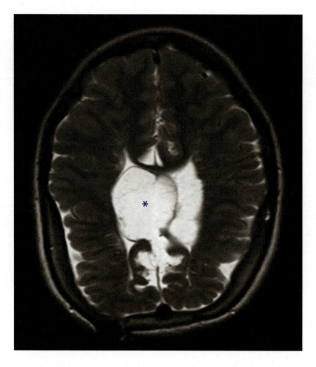

FINDINGS:

Axial T2-weighted MR shows an encapsulated midline cyst (asterisk) between the cerebral hemispheres and spanning the septum pellucidum.

DIFFERENTIAL DIAGNOSIS:

- Callosal dysgenesis
- Arachnoid cyst
- Normal variants

DISCUSSION:

Interhemispheric cysts are focal fluid collections that are located in the interhemispheric fissure and may communicate with the ventricular system. There is a strong association with callosal dysgenesis, in which the third ventricle is high-riding and forms a cyst at the level of the absent corpus callosum. Other congenital brain malformations, including Chiari II, Dandy-Walker, holoprosencephaly, and heterotopias, may also develop midline cysts. If there are no accompanying anatomic abnormalities, differential considerations include isolated arachnoid cyst and normal variants of midline structures (cavum septum pellucidum, cavum vergae, cavum velum interpositum).

References:

Epelman M, Daneman A, Blaser SI, et al. Differential diagnosis of intracranial cystic lesions at head US: correlation with CT and MR imaging. *Radiographics.* 2006;26(1):173-196.

Spennato P, Ruggiero C, Aliberti F, et al. Interhemispheric and quadrigeminal cysts. *World Neurosurg.* 2012;79(2 Suppl):S20.e1-e7.

KEYHOLE

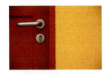

Modalities:
US, CT, MR

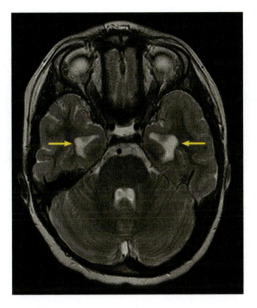 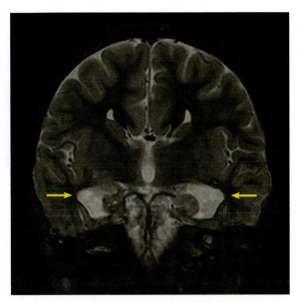

FINDINGS:

Axial and coronal T2-weighted MR show enlarged and curved temporal horns (arrows), with hypoplastic and vertically oriented hippocampi.

DIAGNOSIS:

Hippocampal hypoplasia

DISCUSSION:

The hippocampal neocortex is located along the lateral temporal lobe and grows more rapidly than the allocortex during development, resulting in medial displacement and inversion into the temporal horns. Hippocampal hypoplasia can occur with a variety of congenital brain malformations including callosal agenesis, lissencephaly, schizencephaly, polymicrogyria, holoprosencephaly, and heterotopia. Failure of hippocampal infolding produces vertically oriented and "globular" perihippocampal fissures, as well as a dilated "keyhole" appearance of the temporal horns.

Reference:

Sato N, Hatakeyama S, Shimizu N, et al. MR evaluation of the hippocampus in patients with congenital malformations of the brain. *AJNR Am J Neuroradiol.* 2001;22(2):389-393.

LACK OF CENTRAL RED DOT

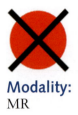

Modality:
MR

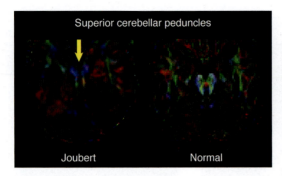

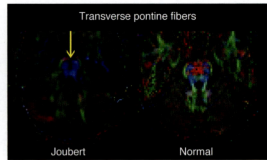

FINDINGS:

Axial DTI MR of Joubert syndrome versus normal patient. In Joubert syndrome, there is no central red dot at the level of the superior cerebellar peduncles (thick arrow) or transverse pontine fibers (thin arrow) in the middle cerebellar peduncles.

DIAGNOSIS:

Joubert syndrome-related disorders

DISCUSSION:

Joubert syndrome–related disorders (JSRD), or cerebello-oculo-renal disorders, are autosomal recessive disruptions of midbrain-hindbrain development with associated ocular, facial, hepatic, renal, and digital anomalies. Diffusion tensor imaging is an MR technique that measures the directional diffusion of water molecules in three dimensions. This can be used to map white matter fiber tracts using a variety of algorithms. DTI maps are color-coded according to the principal eigenvector (red, left to right; blue, cranial to caudal; green, anterior to posterior). In Joubert syndrome, there is lack of decussation of the pyramidal tracts within the superior cerebellar peduncles. Instead, the superior cerebellar peduncles become elongated and thickened, with a parallel orientation forming the roots of the "molar tooth." The transverse pontine fibers in the middle cerebellar peduncles also fail to decussate. This leads to "absence of the focal red dot" in the midbrain and pons, as compared to normal patients.

References:

Brancati F, Dallapiccola B, Valente EM. Joubert syndrome and related disorders. *Orphanet J Rare Dis.* 2010;5:20.

Poretti A, Boltshauser E, Loenneker T, et al. Diffusion tensor imaging in Joubert syndrome. *AJNR Am J Neuroradiol.* 2007;28(10):1929-1933.

LEOPARD SKIN, STRIPE, TIGROID

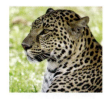

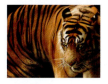

Modality:
MR

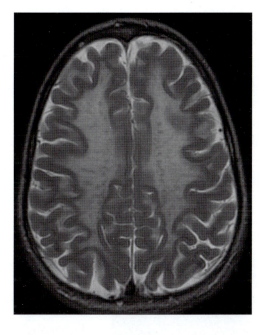 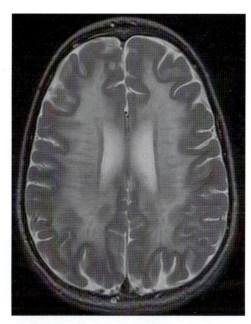

FINDINGS:

Axial T2-weighted MR shows widespread periventricular white matter hyperintensity, with internal linear radiating hypointensities.

DIFFERENTIAL DIAGNOSIS:

- Metachromatic leukodystrophy
- Pelizaeus-Merzbacher disease

DISCUSSION:

Metachromatic leukodystrophy (MLD), the most common hereditary leukodystrophy, is an autosomal recessive disorder caused by arylsulfatase A deficiency. Accumulation of sulfatides in multiple organ systems impairs myelination. This initially involves the periventricular white matter, with sparing of the subcortical U (arcuate) fibers and perivascular spaces. On T2-weighted MR, multiple hypointense lines within diffusely hyperintense white matter produces a "leopard skin" appearance. Other dysmyelinating diseases with a similar appearance include Pelizaeus-Merzbacher disease, Alexander disease, and other lysosomal storage disorders. Pelizaeus-Merzbacher disease (PMD) is a rare X-linked leukodystrophy caused by proteolipidprotein (PLP1) mutations, with arrested myelin development that involves the subcortical U fibers. Disease distribution may be diffuse or patchy with perivascular sparing.

References:

Cheon JE, Kim IO, Hwang YS, et al. Leukodystrophy in children: a pictorial review of MR imaging features. *Radiographics.* 2002;22(3):461-476.

Kim TS, Kim IO, Kim WS, et al. MR of childhood metachromatic leukodystrophy. *AJNR Am J Neuroradiol.* 1997;18(4):733-738.

LINEAR, MIGRATION TRACTS, RADIAL BANDS

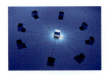

Modalities:
CT, MR

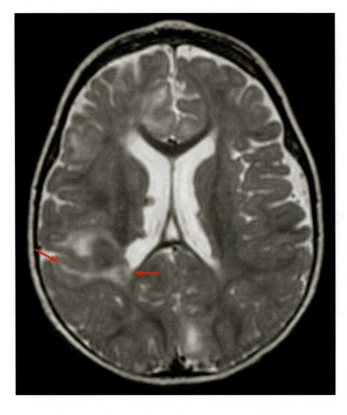

FINDINGS:

Axial T2-weighted MR shows linear hyperintensity radiating from the right atrium to parietal cortex (arrows). Multiple subcortical tubers and subependymal nodules are also present.

DIFFERENTIAL DIAGNOSIS:

- Tuberous sclerosis
- Other migrational abnormalities

DISCUSSION:

Tuberous sclerosis complex (TSC) is a phakomatosis or neuroectodermal syndrome characterized by dysplasias and hamartomas of the brain, retinae, skin, heart, lungs, kidneys, and bones. Neuroimaging manifestations include cortical/subcortical hamartomas, white matter abnormalities, and subependymal nodules or giant cell astrocytomas (SEGAs). Radial bands are straight or curvilinear areas of abnormal white matter signal. These are usually seen supratentorially, radiating from the periventricular to subcortical regions; but can occasionally be present in the cerebellum. Histologically, these correspond to heterotopic clusters of cells along the glial-neuronal migration unit. In infants younger than 3 months, MR signal is T1-hyperintense and T2-hypointense. As myelination progresses with age, bands become T2-hyperintense with variable T1 signal. Radial bands can be seen in association with cortical tubers and other migrational abnormalities, including cortical dysplasia.

References:

Abdel Razek AA, Kandell AY, Elsorogy LG, et al. Disorders of cortical formation: MR imaging features. *AJNR Am J Neuroradiol.* 2009;30(1):4-11.

Bernauer TA. The radial bands sign. *Radiology.* 1999;212(3):761-762.

MICKEY MOUSE

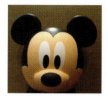

Modalities:
US, MR

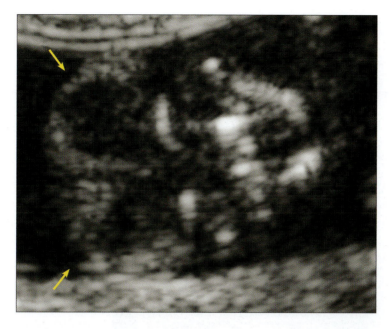

FINDINGS:

Fetal US, coronal plane, reveals absent cranium above the level of the orbits. The cerebral hemispheres (arrows) float freely in the amniotic fluid.

DIAGNOSIS:

Exencephaly

DISCUSSION:

Exencephaly is a lethal neural tube defect characterized by a poorly formed cranial vault. Some brain tissue is present, but it is not covered by meninges or bone. The cerebral hemispheres project from the head ("Mickey Mouse" sign), float freely in the amniotic fluid, and may attach to the amniotic membrane. Exencephaly is thought to represent the middle stage of the acrania-exencephaly-anencephaly sequence. In acrania, there is absence of the calvarium, but normally formed cerebral hemispheres and meninges. Without overlying bone, the brain and meninges are continually exposed to amniotic fluid and progressively disintegrate. Exencephaly refers to the stage in which some residual brain is present, and the cerebral hemispheres can still be identified. Once the brain has completely degraded, the defect is termed anencephaly. This diagnosis should be made only after 14 weeks of gestation, once the skull has ossified. Anencephaly must be distinguished from amniotic band syndrome, in which the head and other structures are entrapped and lacerated by crossing fibrous bands.

References:

Goldstein RB, Filly RA. Prenatal diagnosis of anencephaly: spectrum of sonographic appearances and distinction from the amniotic band syndrome. *AJR Am J Roentgenol.* 1988;151(3):547-550.

Hidalgo H, Bowie J, Rosenberg ER, et al. Review. In utero sonographic diagnosis of fetal cerebral anomalies. *AJR Am J Roentgenol.* 1982;139(1):143-148.

MOLAR TOOTH

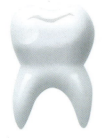

Modalities:
US, CT, MR

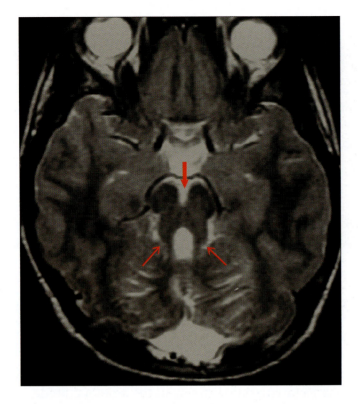

FINDINGS:

Axial T2-weighted MR shows a deep interpeduncular fossa (thick arrow), thin midbrain isthmus, and parallel enlarged superior cerebellar peduncles (thin arrows). There is also vermian hypoplasia and enlarged cisterna magna.

DIAGNOSIS:

Joubert syndrome–related disorders

DISCUSSION:

Joubert syndrome–related disorders (JSRD), or cerebello-oculo-renal disorders, are autosomal recessive disruptions of midbrain-hindbrain development with associated ocular, facial, hepatic, renal, and digital anomalies. Lack of decussation of the superior cerebellar peduncles across the midline results in thinning of the midbrain isthmus and deepening of the interpeduncular fossa ("crown" of the molar tooth). The nondecussating pyramidal tracts run parallel to each other within the superior cerebellar peduncles, which have a thickened and horizontal orientation ("root" of the molar tooth). Other imaging signs of JSRD include "bullet" third ventricle, "bat-wing" fourth ventricle, and vermian hypoplasia.

References:

Brancati F, Dallapiccola B, Valente EM. Joubert syndrome and related disorders. *Orphanet J Rare Dis.* 2010;5:20.

McGraw P. The molar tooth sign. *Radiology.* 2003;229(3):671-672.

MUSHROOM

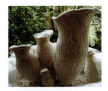

Modalities:
US, CT, MR

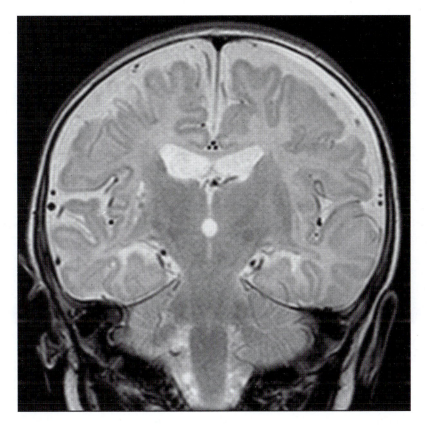

FINDINGS:

Coronal T2-weighted MR shows enlargement of deep sulci with sparing of surface gyri, particularly in the parasagittal cortex. There is abnormal hyperintense signal throughout the subcortical white matter.

DIAGNOSIS:

Ulegyria

DISCUSSION:

Ulegyria refers to cortical injury with preferential atrophy of the deep cortical layers (cortical laminar necrosis). The usual etiology is mild hypoxic-ischemic injury in full-term infants, preferentially affecting the parasagittal watershed areas. This results in atrophy of the deep sulci with sparing of surface gyri, creating a "mushroom" appearance. Associated subcortical white matter signal abnormalities are common. Clinical presentation includes mental retardation, cerebral palsy, and epilepsy.

References:

Nikas I, Dermentzoglou V, Theofanopoulou M, et al. Parasagittal lesions and ulegyria in hypoxic-ischemic encephalopathy: neuroimaging findings and review of the pathogenesis. *J Child Neurol.* 2008;23(1):51-58.

Villani F, D'Incerti L, Granata T, et al. Epileptic and imaging findings in perinatal hypoxic-ischemic encephalopathy with ulegyria. *Epilepsy Res.* 2003;55(3):235-243.

NODULAR, PEARLS ON A STRING

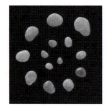

Modalities:
US, CT, MR

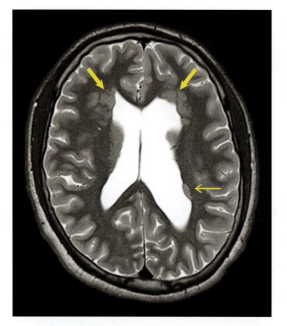

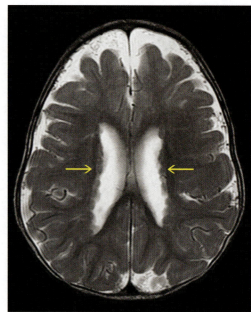

FINDINGS:

Axial T2-weighted MR in two different patients show multiple heterotopic nodules of gray matter in the deep periventricular white matter (thick arrows) and subependymal lateral ventricles (thin arrows).

DIFFERENTIAL DIAGNOSIS:

- Gray matter heterotopia
- Tuberous sclerosis

DISCUSSION:

Gray matter heterotopia is caused by abnormal neuronal migration and can occur anywhere between the subependymal region and cerebral cortex. The major types are band, subcortical, and periventricular (subependymal). Subcortical heterotopias are located within the subcortical or deep white matter, contiguous with the cortex or ventricular system. Morphology tends to be curvilinear when superficial, and nodular when deep. Periventricular heterotopias are located close to ventricular walls and project into the ventricular lumen or periventricular white matter. Location is frequently along the atria or occipital horns, and more common on the right due to later migration of right-sided neuroblasts. Lesions appear smooth and ovoid, with signal isointense to gray matter and absence of contrast enhancement. In tuberous sclerosis, the subependymal nodules have a more irregular morphology ("candle guttering"), signal distinct from gray matter, and often calcify. Primary CNS lymphoma and metastases are also enhancing and more irregular.

Reference:

Abdel Razek AA, Kandell AY, Elsorogy LG, et al. Disorders of cortical formation: MR imaging features. *AJNR Am J Neuroradiol.* 2009;30(1):4-11.

OPEN LIP

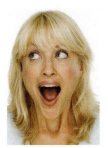

Modalities:
US, CT, MR

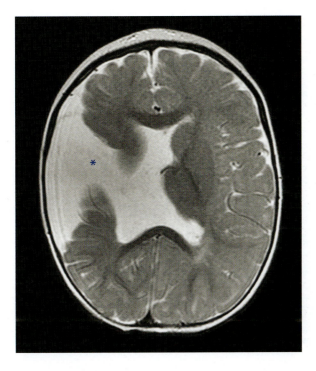

FINDINGS:

Axial T2-weighted MR shows a gaping right frontoparietal transcortical defect lined by gray matter, with intervening CSF (asterisk).

DIAGNOSIS:

Open-lip schizencephaly

DISCUSSION:

Schizencephaly is caused by a full-thickness insult to the cerebral cortex during cortical organization, which produces a gray matter-lined cleft that extends from the ventricular system to the subarachnoid space. Clefts may be small or large, unilateral or bilateral, and classified as type I (closed-lip) or type II (open-lip). In closed-lip schizencephaly, the lips are in contact with each other; in open-lip schizencephaly, the lips are separated by intervening CSF. The gray matter lining the cleft is frequently polymicrogyric (multiple tiny gyri) and can extend into the ventricle, forming subependymal gray matter heterotopia. Schizencephaly should not be confused with porencephaly, in which an acquired insult results in a white matter-lined cavity adjacent to the ventricular system and/or subarachnoid space.

References:

Abdel Razek AA, Kandell AY, Elsorogy LG, et al. Disorders of cortical formation: MR imaging features. *AJNR Am J Neuroradiol.* 2009;30(1):4-11.

Barkovich AJ, Norman D. MR imaging of schizencephaly. *AJR Am J Roentgenol.* 1988;150(6): 1391-1396.

PARALLEL VENTRICLES, RACING CAR

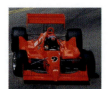

Modalities:
US, CT, MR

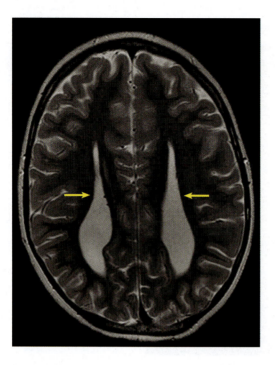

FINDINGS:

Axial T2-weighted MR shows widely spaced and parallel lateral ventricles (arrows), with pointed frontal horns and dilated occipital horns.

DIAGNOSIS:

Callosal agenesis

DISCUSSION:

Dysgenesis of the corpus callosum is caused by abnormalities in neural development between 12 and 18 weeks of gestation. The sequence of formation is largely ventral to dorsal, beginning with the genu and progressing through the anterior body, posterior body, splenium, and rostrum. In callosal agenesis, there is complete absence of the normal crossing white matter tracts. Instead, nondecussating white matter fibers known as Probst bundles course anteroposteriorly along the medial edges of the lateral ventricles. The lateral ventricles assume a parallel orientation, with narrow elongated frontal horns and dilated occipital horns (colpocephaly, "racing car" appearance). Without crossing fibers to displace and invert them, the cingulate gyri remain everted and the cingulate sulcus is unformed. Other imaging signs of callosal agenesis include high-riding third ventricle, radiating gyri, and "keyhole" temporal horns.

References:

Atlas SW. *Magnetic Resonance Imaging of the Brain and Spine.* 4th ed, vol. 1. Philadelphia: Wolters Kluwer; 2008.

Barkovich AJ, Raybaud C. *Pediatric Neuroimaging.* 5th ed. Philadelphia: Wolters Kluwer; 2011.

PEG, SERGEANT STRIPES, TAIL, TONGUE

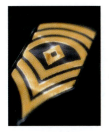

Modalities:
CT, MR

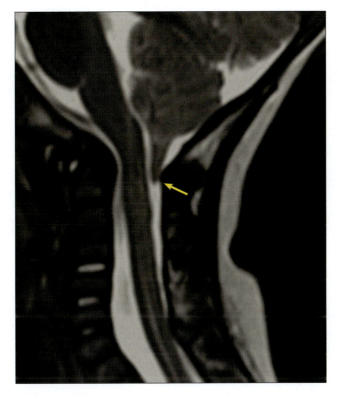

FINDINGS:

Sagittal T2-weighted MR shows inferior descent of the cerebellar tonsils below the foramen magnum, with a pointed appearance (arrow).

DIAGNOSIS:

Chiari malformation

DISCUSSION:

Chiari malformations involve a spectrum of complex congenital anomalies, characterized by posterior fossa hypoplasia and descent of the cerebellar tonsils over 3 to 5 mm below the foramen magnum. In Chiari I, isolated tonsillar displacement may cause syringohydromyelia secondary to obstruction of CSF flow. With Chiari II, a lumbosacral myelomeningocele produces additional traction on the spinal cord, resulting in a hypoplastic posterior fossa. In Chiari III, there is also an occipital or high cervical encephalocele. Characteristic pointing ("peg" or "sergeant stripes" appearance) of the cerebellar tonsils reflects dysplasia of the cerebellar pyramis, uvula, and nodulus. This is a specific sign that can distinguish Chiari malformations from other causes of low-lying tonsils, such as tonsillar ectopia or tonsillar herniation.

Reference:

Naidich TP, McLone DG, Fulling KH. The Chiari II malformation, part IV: the hindbrain deformity. *Neuroradiology.* 1983;25(4):179-197.

PLASTIC, TONGUE, TOOTHPASTE

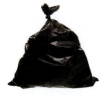

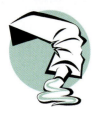

Modalities:
CT, MR

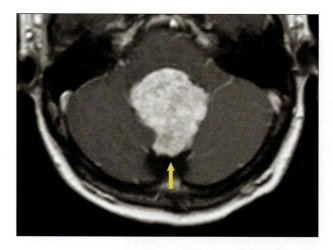

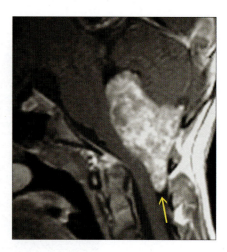

FINDINGS:

Axial and sagittal contrast-enhanced T1-weighted MR show a heterogeneously enhancing, lobulated mass filling the fourth ventricle and extending through the foramen of Magendie (thick arrow) into the cisterna magna and posterior cervical canal (thin arrow).

DIAGNOSIS:

Ependymoma

DISCUSSION:

Ependymomas are benign tumors that arise from ependymal cells lining the ventricles and central canal of the spinal cord. These have a heterogeneous appearance with variable degrees of enhancement, cystic changes, hemorrhage, and calcification. The floor of the fourth ventricle is the most common location, with tumor filling the ventricle and insinuating into foramina—the so-called "plastic" appearance. Classically, extension occurs through the foramen of Magendie into the cisterna magna, and through the foramina of Luschka into the cerebellopontine angles. Ventricular obstruction can result in hydrocephalus and/or syringomyelia. There is an association with neurofibromatosis type II (MISME: multiple inherited schwannomas, meningiomas, and ependymomas). Denser intraventricular neoplasms such as medulloblastoma, choroid plexus tumor, and metastases grow by direct extension, rather than conforming to the shape of the ventricles.

Reference:

Koeller KK, Sandberg GD. From the archives of the AFIP. Cerebral intraventricular neoplasms: radiologic-pathologic correlation. *Radiographics*. 2002;22(6):1473-1505.

POINT, WEDGE

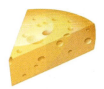

Modality:
MR

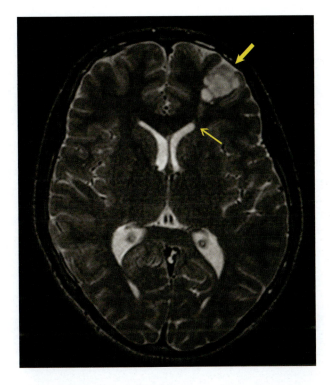

FINDINGS:

Axial T2-weighted MR shows a hyperintense wedge-shaped mass in the left middle frontal gyrus, extending from frontal horn (thin arrow) to cortex (thick arrow).

DIAGNOSIS:

Dysembryoplastic neuroepithelial tumor

DISCUSSION:

Dysembryoplastic neuroepithelial tumors (DNETs) are benign, slow-growing neuroepithelial tumors arising from cortical or deep gray matter. Patients are typically male and under age 20. The temporal lobe is the most common location, followed by the frontal lobe. Simple DNETs are T2-hyperintense multiseptated "bubbly" masses with little vasogenic edema, enhancement, or mass effect. On FLAIR MR, there is nulling of the cystic components of tumor with a characteristic "bright rim," which may be complete or incomplete. Pathologically, this corresponds to peripheral loose neuroglial elements, and suggests residual or recurrent tumor in the postoperative setting. Complex DNETs have varying amounts of solid tissue and low-level enhancement. Lesions typically have a wedge-shaped morphology, in which the apex points toward the ventricle, and the outer surface extends to cortex with remodeling of the inner table. Associated cortical dysplasia is common.

Reference:

Koeller KK, Henry JM. From the archives of the AFIP: superficial gliomas: radiologic-pathologic correlation. Armed Forces Institute of Pathology. *Radiographics*. 2001;21(6):1533-1556.

POINTING, RADIAL, SPOKE, SUNBURST

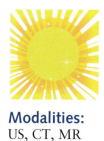

Modalities:
US, CT, MR

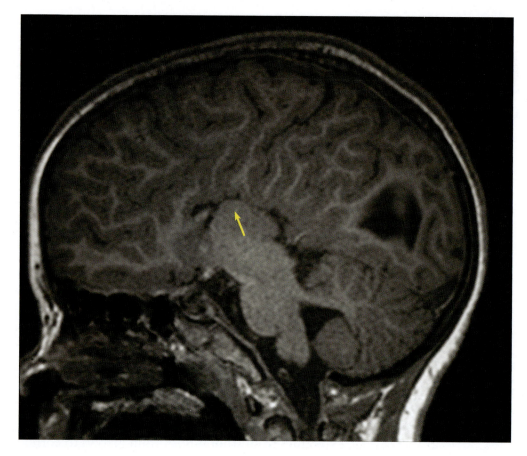

FINDINGS:

Sagittal T1-weighted MR shows a high-riding third ventricle (arrow), with gyri radiating outward to the cortical surface.

DIAGNOSIS:

Callosal agenesis

DISCUSSION:

Dysgenesis of the corpus callosum is caused by abnormalities in neural development between 12 and 18 weeks of gestation. The sequence of formation is largely ventral to dorsal, beginning with the genu and progressing through anterior body, posterior body, splenium, and rostrum. In callosal agenesis, there is nonconvergence of the major fissures. As a result, gyri radiate outward from the third ventricle and extend to the cortical surface in a "sunburst" pattern. Other imaging signs of callosal agenesis include parallel lateral ventricles, colpocephaly, and "keyhole" temporal horns.

References:

Atlas SW. *Magnetic Resonance Imaging of the Brain and Spine*. 4th ed, vol. 1. Philadelphia: Wolters Kluwer; 2008.

Barkovich AJ, Raybaud C. *Pediatric Neuroimaging*. 5th ed. Philadelphia: Wolters Kluwer; 2011.

PSEUDOHYDROCEPHALUS

Modality:
US

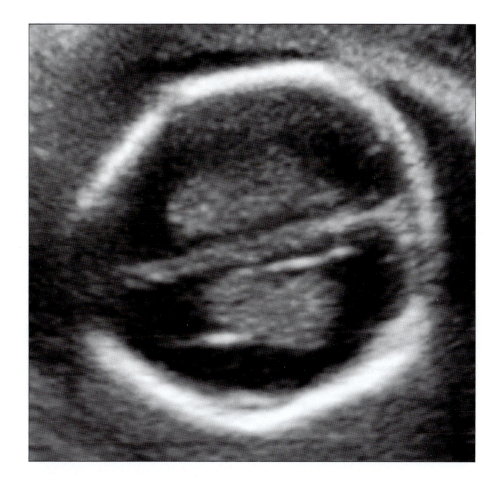

FINDINGS:

Fetal US, axial plane, shows diffusely hypoechoic cerebral tissue. The choroid plexi remain parallel to the interhemispheric fissure.

DIAGNOSIS:

Normal fetal brain

DISCUSSION:

In the second trimester of pregnancy, the cerebral hemispheres appear hypoechoic and can mimic hydrocephalus. In true ventriculomegaly, the choroid angles increase and the free-hanging choroid "dangles" from the foramen of Monro. Absence of these imaging signs, with choroid plexi remaining parallel to the interhemispheric fissure, confirms this normal variant.

References:

Cardoza JD, Filly RA, Podrasky AE. The dangling choroid plexus: a sonographic observation of value in excluding ventriculomegaly. *AJR Am J Roentgenol.* 1988;151(4):767-770.

Nyberg DA, McGahan JP, Pretorius DH, et al. *Diagnostic Imaging of Fetal Anomalies.* 2nd ed. Philadelphia: Lippincott Williams & Wilkins; 2002.

SPOKE WHEEL

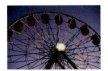

Modalities:
US, CT, MR

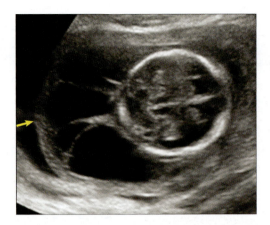

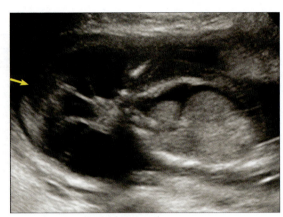

FINDINGS:

Fetal US, axial and coronal planes, show a multiloculated cystic structure arising from the posterior neck (arrows).

DIAGNOSIS:

Cystic hygroma

DISCUSSION:

Cystic hygroma (lymphangioma) is a congenital lymphatic malformation that usually involves the head and neck. The classic imaging appearance is a multiloculated, septated cystic structure that can extend into multiple compartments. Internal contents include serous fluid with varying amounts of protein and hemorrhage, producing fluid-fluid levels. The most common location is the posterior triangle of the neck, with multiple septa radiating out in a "spoke-wheel" pattern. There is an association with hydrops fetalis, Turner and Noonan syndromes, and trisomies.

Reference:

Ibrahim M, Hammoud K, Maheshwari M, et al. Congenital cystic lesions of the head and neck. *Neuroimaging Clin N Am.* 2011;21(3):621-639.

SWISS CHEESE

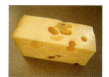

Modalities:
US, CT, MR

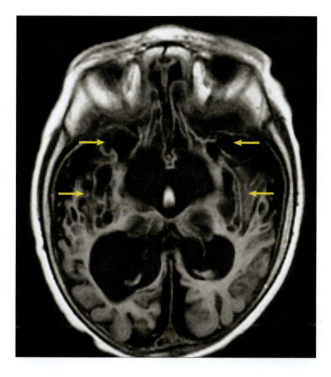

FINDINGS:

Axial FLAIR MR shows advanced encephalomalacia with multiple periventricular cystic spaces (arrows), white matter volume loss, and ventriculomegaly.

DIAGNOSIS:

Periventricular leukomalacia, end-stage

DISCUSSION:

In premature infants, the periventricular white matter is most susceptible to hypoxic injury because it is supplied by ventriculopetal penetrating arteries from the cortical surface. Periventricular leukomalacia (PVL) is the most common preterm brain injury, manifesting with periventricular white matter changes that appear echogenic on US, hypodense on CT, and hyperintense on T2-weighted MR. Localized venous infarctions produce "fan" or "triangle"-shaped abnormalities, reflecting the vascular borderzones in this age group. After 2-6 weeks, the white matter begins to involute, with ex vacuo dilation of the ventricles creating an "angular" or "scalloped" morphology. End-stage PVL is characterized by cystic encephalomalacia ("Swiss cheese" brain) with severe white matter loss and ventriculomegaly.

References:

Chao CP, Zaleski CG, Patton AC. Neonatal hypoxic-ischemic encephalopathy: multimodality imaging findings. *Radiographics*. 2006;26(Suppl 1):S159-S172.

Nakamura Y, Okudera T, Hashimoto T. Vascular architecture in white matter of neonates: its relationship to periventricular leukomalacia. *J Neuropathol Exp Neurol*. 1994;53(6):582-589.

TEARDROP

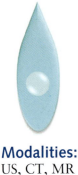

Modalities:
US, CT, MR

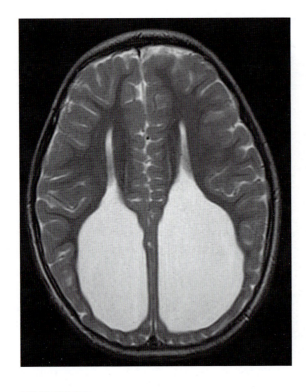

FINDINGS:

Axial T2-weighted MR shows parallel lateral ventricles with pointed frontal horns and massively dilated, rounded atria and occipital horns.

DIAGNOSIS:

Callosal agenesis

DISCUSSION:

Dysgenesis of the corpus callosum is caused by abnormalities in neural development between 12 and 18 weeks of gestation. The sequence of formation is largely ventral to dorsal, beginning with the genu and progressing through the anterior body, posterior body, splenium, and rostrum. In callosal agenesis, there is complete absence of the normal crossing white matter tracts. Instead, nondecussating white matter fibers known as Probst bundles course anteroposteriorly along the medial edges of the lateral ventricles. The lateral ventricles assume a parallel orientation, with narrow elongated frontal horns and dilated occipital horns (colpocephaly, "teardrop" appearance). Without crossing fibers to displace and invert them, the cingulate gyri remain everted and the cingulate sulcus is unformed. Other imaging signs of callosal agenesis include high-riding third ventricle, radiating gyri, and "keyhole" temporal horns.

References:

Atlas SW. *Magnetic Resonance Imaging of the Brain and Spine*. 4th ed, vol. 1. Philadelphia: Wolters Kluwer; 2008.

Barkovich AJ, Raybaud C. *Pediatric Neuroimaging*. 5th ed. Philadelphia: Wolters Kluwer; 2011.

TECTAL BEAK/POINT/SPUR

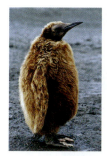

Modalities:
US, CT, MR

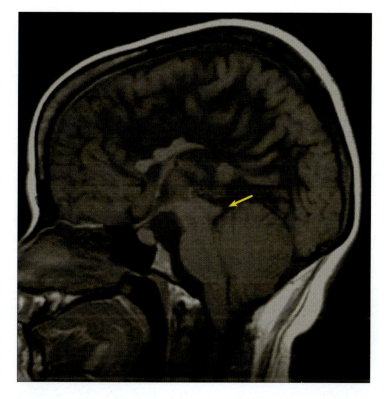

FINDINGS:

Sagittal T1-weighted MR shows posterior beaking of the tectal plate (arrow). There is also a low-lying tentorium cerebelli, hypoplastic posterior fossa with tonsillar descent, cervicomedullary kink, and callosal dysgenesis.

DIAGNOSIS:

Chiari II malformation

DISCUSSION:

The Chiari II malformation is a complex congenital anomaly consisting of small posterior fossa, inferior displacement of the cerebellum and brainstem, and lumbosacral myelomeningocele. The characteristic tectal "beak" reflects fusion of the superior and/or inferior colliculi, with formation of an elongated conical mass that extends up between the cerebellar hemispheres. Other characteristic imaging signs of Chiari II malformation include cervicomedullary kink, wide incisura with towering cerebellum, and fenestrated falx with interdigitating gyri. In the Chiari III malformation, there is also an occipital or high cervical encephalocele.

References:

Geerdink N, van der Vliet T, Rotteveel JJ, et al. Essential features of Chiari II malformation in MR imaging: an interobserver reliability study—part 1. *Childs Nerv Syst.* 2012;28(7):977-985.

Naidich TP, Pudlowski RM, Naidich JB. Computed tomographic signs of Chiari II malformation, II: midbrain and cerebellum. *Radiology.* 1980;134(2):391-398.

TOO-FAR-BACK VENTRICLE

Modalities:
US, MR

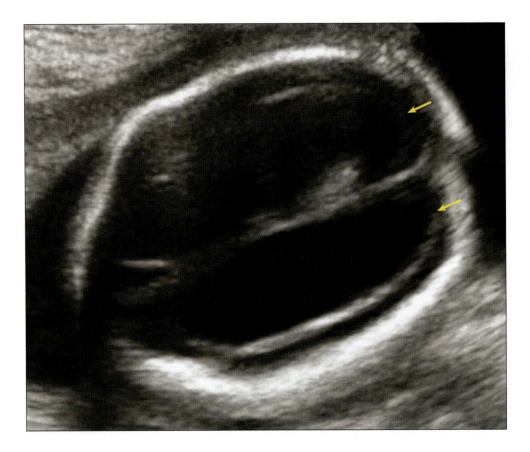

FINDINGS:

Fetal US, axial plane, shows dilated lateral ventricles with decreased ventricle-to-occiput distance (arrows).

DIFFERENTIAL DIAGNOSIS:

- Fetal Chiari II
- Spinal dysraphism

DISCUSSION:

Accurate diagnosis of fetal neural tube defects is crucial for guiding further imaging evaluation, genetic workup, and prenatal counseling. The Chiari II malformation is a complex congenital deformity involving a small posterior fossa and lumbosacral myelomeningocele. Infratentorial abnormalities can be difficult to detect in early pregnancy. Before 24 weeks of gestational age, there is ventriculomegaly with characteristic posterior displacement ("too-far-back" ventricle) and pointing of the occipital horns ("angular" appearance). Fetal MR may help to further characterize the spectrum of anatomic abnormalities.

Reference:

Filly MR, Filly RA, Barkovich AJ, et al. Supratentorial abnormalities in the Chiari II malformation, IV: the too-far-back ventricle. *J Ultrasound Med.* 2010;29(2):243-248.

TRANSMANTLE

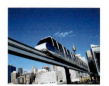

Modality:
MR

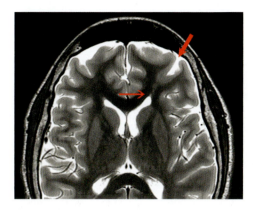

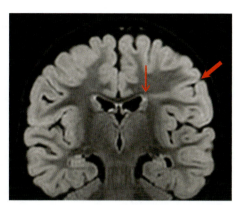

FINDINGS:

Axial T2-weighted and coronal FLAIR MR show left frontal cortical thickening and loss of gray-white distinction (thick arrows). A band of hyperintense signal extends from the cortex to the frontal horn (thin arrows).

DIAGNOSIS:

Focal cortical dysplasia, type II (transmantle dysplasia)

DISCUSSION:

Focal cortical dysplasia (FCD), first described by Taylor et al. in 1971, is a common cause of intractable childhood epilepsy. FCD represents a spectrum of developmental migrational anomalies with varying embryologic, genetic, histopathologic, and imaging features. In 2011, the International League Against Epilepsy (ILAE) reclassified the disease into three tiers: FCD type I refers to isolated cortical dyslamination in the radial (type Ia), tangential (type Ib), or both (type Ic) directions. FCD type II involves dysmorphic neurons, either without (type IIa) or with (type IIb) balloon cells. FCD type III occurs adjacent to a principal lesion such as hippocampal sclerosis (type IIIa), tumor (type IIIb), vascular malformation (type IIIc), or other acquired conditions such as trauma/ischemia/infection (type IIId). On MR, imaging features include cortical thickening and expansion, loss of gray-white distinction, and T2-hyperintense signal. The "transmantle" sign refers to T2 signal abnormality extending across the cerebral mantle, from cortical surface to ventricle. Morphology may be linear, curvilinear, radial, or funnel-shaped. This finding is most often associated with FCD type II, and characteristically seen in the frontal lobes. The imaging differential includes dysembryoplastic neuroepithelial tumor ("wedge" appearance), radial bands of tuberous sclerosis, and other migrational anomalies.

References:

Barkovich AJ, Kuzniecky RI, Bollen AW, et al. Focal transmantle dysplasia: a specific malformation of cortical development. *Neurology*. 1997;49(4):1148-1152.

Blümcke I, Thom M, Aronica E, et al. The clinicopathologic spectrum of focal cortical dysplasias: a consensus classification proposed by an ad hoc Task Force of the ILAE Diagnostic Methods Commission. *Epilepsia*. 2011;52(1):158-174.

ANTRAL, HOLMAN-MILLER, HONDOUSA

Modalities:
XR, CT, MR

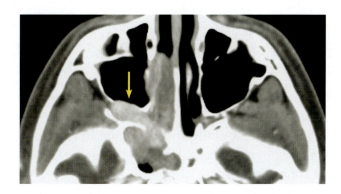

FINDINGS:

Axial contrast-enhanced CT shows an avidly enhancing mass centered in the right sphenopalatine foramen. This extends laterally into the pterygopalatine fossa with anterior bowing of the posterior maxillary sinus wall (arrow), anteriorly into the nasal cavity, and posteriorly into the sphenoid sinus.

DIAGNOSIS:

Juvenile nasopharyngeal angiofibroma

DISCUSSION:

Juvenile nasopharyngeal angiofibroma (JNA) is a benign, locally aggressive tumor seen in adolescent males presenting with unilateral nasal obstruction, rhinorrhea, and epistaxis. It originates in the region of the sphenopalatine foramen and extends anteriorly into the nasal cavity, laterally toward the pterygopalatine fossa, posteriorly into the sphenoid sinus, and inferiorly into the infratemporal fossa. Pterygopalatine fossa involvement produces the antral or Holman-Miller sign, represented by anterior bowing of the posterior wall of the maxillary sinus (antrum of Highmore). Infratemporal fossa involvement produces the Hondousa sign, which refers to widening of the gap between the mandibular ramus and maxillary body. Tumors are highly vascular, with avid enhancement and flow voids on MR. Treatment is total surgical resection, often preceded by angiographic embolization of the feeding vessel (internal maxillary branch of the ECA) to reduce bleeding, followed by adjuvant radiation. Other nasal cavity tumors in this age group include rhabdomyosarcoma, lymphoma, and hemangioma, which are typically less vascular and have different growth patterns.

Reference:

Ludwig BJ, Foster BR, Saito N, et al. Diagnostic imaging in nontraumatic pediatric head and neck emergencies. *Radiographics*. 2010;30(3):781-799.

APPLE TREE, BEADED, MULBERRY, ROSARY, SAUSAGE STRING/LINK, WINTER TREE

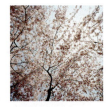
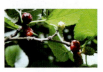

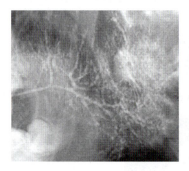
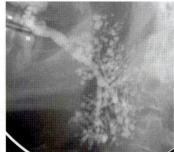
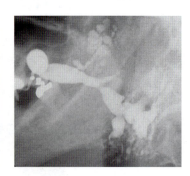

Modalities:
XR, US, MR

FINDINGS:

- Sialogram in mild sialadenitis shows smooth parotid ducts with peripheral pruning and innumerable tiny contrast collections throughout the gland.
- Moderate sialadenitis shows segmental ductal stricturing and dilation, with several globular contrast collections.
- End-stage sialadenitis shows severe distortion of the parotid ductal system, with large bizarre extraductal collections.

DIAGNOSIS:

Chronic sialadenitis

DISCUSSION:

Sialography is a radiographic technique used to visualize salivary gland ducts (parotid: Stensen duct, submandibular: Wharton duct, sublingual: Gartner duct). The procedure involves evoked salivation, direct cannulation with a microcatheter, and injection of contrast under fluoroscopy. Noninvasive imaging techniques include US or MR sialography using high-resolution, heavily T2-weighted sequences. Normal salivary ducts are smooth and branch to the gland periphery. With recurrent sialadenitis, ductal irregularity progresses through four stages. In the punctate stage, tiny (<1 mm) contrast collections are seen throughout the gland, with normal ducts. Significant gland edema can compress peripheral ducts producing a pruned or "winter tree" appearance. Next is the globular stage, in which larger contrast collections (1-2 mm) develop, with duct strictures and dilations creating a "beaded" or "sausage string" pattern. Acinar spill may produce a patchy blurred appearance, resembling an "apple tree in bloom." The "mulberry" or "branchless fruit-laden tree" appearance occurs when connections to the ductal system are not well defined. In the cavitary stage, few large irregular contrast collections (up to 1 cm) are haphazardly distributed in the gland. The destructive phase represents end-stage disease with total gland destruction and duct sclerosis, yielding abrupt cutoffs and bizarre pooling of contrast.

Reference:

Graamans K, Van den Akker HP. *Diagnosis of salivary gland disorders*. Philadelphia: Kluwer; 1991.

BAG/SAC OF MARBLES

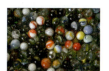

Modalities:
US, CT, MR

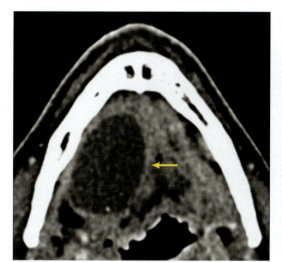
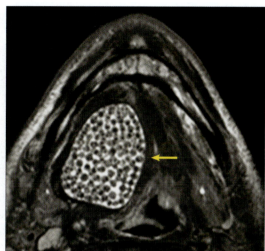

FINDINGS:

Axial CT and T2-weighted MR with fat saturation show an encapsulated fluid-filled sac with multiple fatty nodules in the right floor of mouth (arrows).

DIAGNOSIS:

Dermoid cyst

DISCUSSION:

Congenital inclusion cysts in the head and neck may be composed of pure epithelial (epidermoid) or mixed epithelial and dermal (dermoid) elements. In the floor of mouth, these typically present as thin-walled unilocular masses in the submandibular and sublingual spaces. Dermoids are more often located at midline and contain heterogeneous internal contents including fat, hair, and/or calcification. Fat nodules may coalesce within the fluid-filled cyst, creating a pathognomonic "sac-of-marbles" appearance. Nodules are echogenic on US, hypodense on CT, and hyperintense on T1-weighted MR, with signal dropout on fat-saturated sequences.

Reference:

Koeller KK, Alamo L, Adair CF, et al. Congenital cystic masses of the neck: radiologic-pathologic correlation. *Radiographics*. 1999;19(1):121-146.

BEAK, NOTCH, TAIL

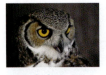

Modalities:
US, CT, MR

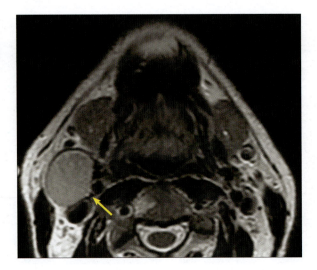

FINDINGS:

Axial T2-weighted MR shows a cystic lesion posterior to the submandibular gland and anterior to the sternocleidomastoid muscle, insinuating between the ICA and ECA (arrow).

DIAGNOSIS:

Second branchial cleft cyst

DISCUSSION:

Branchial cleft anomalies are congenital defects of the head and neck. In utero, there are six branchial arches, which form pouches on the endodermal surface and grooves (clefts) on the ectodermal surface. Branchial fistulae, sinuses, and cysts are congenital anomalies that are thought to arise from vestigial remnants or trapped cell rests. Second branchial cleft anomalies are the most common and occur along the course of the second branchial apparatus, which begins from the lateral neck at the anterior border of the sternocleidomastoid muscle, passes through the carotid bifurcation between the ICA and ECA, and ends at the palatine tonsillar fossa. Second branchial cleft cysts (BCCs) are well-circumscribed mucoid lesions, typically seen below the angle of the mandible and anterior to the sternocleidomastoid muscle. Extension of the cyst wall between the ICA and ECA ("beak" sign) is pathognomonic. In this location, the differential for cystic masses includes necrotic lymph nodes (metastases from squamous cell and thyroid carcinoma are leading considerations in adults), vascular lesions, and neurogenic tumors. These lack a "notch" sign and tend to enhance more avidly than BCCs, except when superinfected.

References:

Ahuja AT, King AD, Metreweli C. Second branchial cleft cysts: variability of sonographic appearances in adult cases. *AJNR Am J Neuroradiol.* 2000;21(2):315-319.

Koeller KK, Alamo L, Adair CF, Smirniotopoulos JG. Congenital cystic masses of the neck: radiologic-pathologic correlation. *Radiographics.* 1999;19:121-146.

BLACK SINUS, BLACK TURBINATE

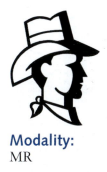

Modality:
MR

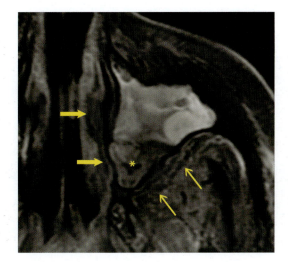 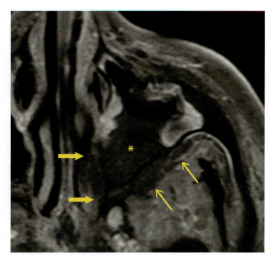

FINDINGS:

Axial T2-weighted and contrast-enhanced T1-weighted MR with fat saturation show T2-hypointense, nonenhancing necrotic tissue in the left posterior maxillary sinus (asterisk), inferior turbinate (thick arrows), and pterygopalatine fossa (thin arrows). There is surrounding bone invasion with involvement of the greater wing and pterygoid processes of the sphenoid.

DIAGNOSIS:

Invasive fungal sinusitis

DISCUSSION:

Invasive fungal sinusitis is a feared condition in immunocompromised patients, particularly those with diabetes, hematologic malignancy, or organ transplantation. Zygomycotic or aspergillotic fungi may spread into submucosa, bone, blood vessels, and nerves. Angioinvasion results in tissue ischemia and necrosis, producing a black "eschar" on clinical examination. On MR, nonviable tissue within the nasal turbinates and/or paranasal sinuses demonstrates decreased T2 signal, hypoenhancement ("black turbinate" sign), and/or reduced diffusion.

Reference:

Safder S, Carpenter JS, Roberts TD, et al. The "black turbinate" sign: an early MR imaging finding of nasal mucormycosis. *AJNR Am J Neuroradiol.* 2010;31(4):771-774.

BOSSELATED

Modalities:
US, CT, MR

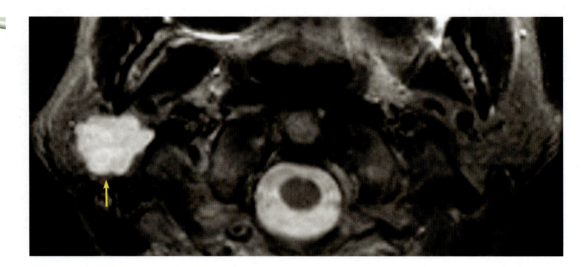

FINDINGS:

Axial T2-weighted MR shows a lobulated hyperintense mass in the right parotid gland, extending through the stylomandibular foramen (arrow).

DIAGNOSIS:

Pleomorphic adenoma

DISCUSSION:

Pleomorphic adenoma (benign mixed tumor) is a benign mass composed of epithelial, myoepithelial, and stromal tissue. When small, lesions are well circumscribed and ovoid. Larger tumors may have a lobulated (bosselated) surface and heterogeneous contents with calcification. MR signal is primarily T2-hyperintense and T1-hypointense, with mild-to-moderate enhancement. The recommended treatment is complete parotidectomy with preservation of the tumor capsule, as intraoperative capsule rupture seeds the surgical bed. If untreated, there is a 10%-25% risk of malignant transformation, known as carcinoma ex pleomorphic adenoma (malignant mixed tumor). Imaging features suggestive of malignant transformation include T2-hypointense or heterogeneous signal, irregular margins, infiltrative growth, rapidly increasing size, and lymphadenopathy.

References:

Kakimoto N, Gamoh S, Tamaki J, et al. CT and MR images of pleomorphic adenoma in major and minor salivary glands. *Eur J Radiol.* 2009;69(3):464-472.

Kashiwagi N, Murakami T, Chikugo T, et al. Carcinoma ex pleomorphic adenoma of the parotid gland. *Acta Radiol.* 2012;53(3):303-306.

BOW TIE, OVAL, RECTANGLE

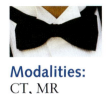

Modalities:
CT, MR

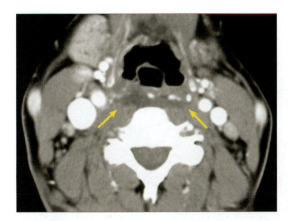 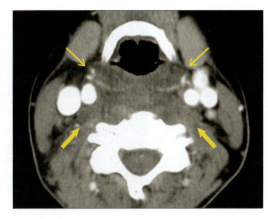

FINDINGS:

- Axial contrast-enhanced CT shows mild symmetric retropharyngeal edema (arrows).
- Axial contrast-enhanced CT in a different patient shows a multiloculated fluid collection distending the retropharyngeal (thick arrows) and pharyngeal mucosal spaces (thin arrows).

DIFFERENTIAL DIAGNOSIS:

- Retropharyngeal edema
- Retropharyngeal abscess

DISCUSSION:

The retropharyngeal space (RPS) extends from the clivus to the upper thoracic spine (T1-T6), posterior to the pharynx/esophagus and anterior to the prevertebral muscles. Its boundaries include the visceral fascia anteriorly, alar/prevertebral fascia posteriorly, and carotid sheaths laterally. Retropharyngeal edema is nonsuppurative inflammation caused by venolymphatic obstruction, longus colli calcific tendinitis, radiation therapy, or adjacent infection. At imaging, there is smooth symmetric expansion of the RPS with a "bow tie," "ovoid," or "rectangular" configuration. No wall thickening or enhancement is present, and the condition resolves with correction of the underlying cause. Retropharyngeal abscess is a purulent fluid collection originating from direct or hematogenous spread of infection. At imaging, a large rim-enhancing fluid collection distends the RPS, causing mass effect on adjacent structures. Prompt surgical drainage is indicated to prevent airway compromise and spread of infection into the perivertebral, carotid, and mediastinal spaces.

Reference:

Hoang JK, Branstetter BF 4th, Eastwood JD, et al. Multiplanar CT and MRI of collections in the retropharyngeal space: is it an abscess? *AJR Am J Roentgenol.* 2011;196(4):W426-W432.

BUCKLED, KINKED, TWISTED

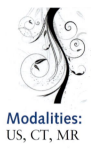

Modalities:
US, CT, MR

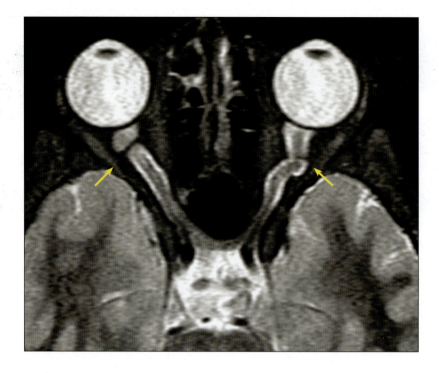

FINDINGS:

Axial T2-weighted MR shows bilateral elongation and kinking of the optic nerves (arrows).

DIAGNOSIS:

Optic nerve gliomas

DISCUSSION:

Optic glioma is the most common optic nerve tumor. There are three subtypes: childhood syndromic (neurofibromatosis type I), childhood sporadic, and adult. Gliomas in children are low grade (WHO I-II), whereas in adults they are higher grade (WHO grade III-IV). These manifest with enlargement and elongation of the optic nerves ("buckled" appearance), chiasm, and/or radiations. MR signal is generally T2-hyperintense ("pseudo-CSF" appearance). Syndromic gliomas are smooth, focally tortuous, and minimally enhancing. Sporadic gliomas are larger, nodular/cystic, and moderately enhancing. Adult gliomas are diffuse, invasive, and heterogeneously enhancing. Other conditions affecting the optic nerve include optic neuritis (nerve edema and enhancement), optic nerve meningioma (tumor of the nerve sheath), orbital pseudotumor (localized inflammation of periorbital structures), and sarcoidosis (multifocal orbital and intracranial manifestations).

References:

Millar WS, Tartaglino LM, Sergott RC, et al. MR of malignant optic glioma of adulthood. *AJNR Am J Neuroradiol.* 1995;16(8):1673-1676.

Taylor T, Jaspan T, Milano G, et al. Radiological classification of optic pathway gliomas: experience of a modified functional classification system. *Br J Radiol.* 2008;81(970):761-766.

BULL NECK

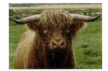

Modalities:
CT, MR

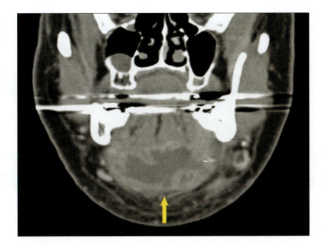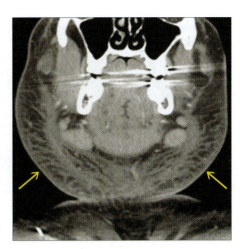

FINDINGS:

Coronal contrast-enhanced CT shows a lobulated, rim-enhancing fluid collection (thick arrow) in the floor of mouth. Surrounding fat stranding extends into the subcutaneous tissues of the face and neck (thin arrows).

DIAGNOSIS:

Ludwig angina

DISCUSSION:

Ludwig angina is an aggressive cellulitis of the floor of mouth, usually secondary to untreated dental infection. Progression of disease leads to extensive facial/cervical cellulitis, fasciitis, and/or abscess formation ("bull neck" appearance). Elevation and posterior displacement of the tongue can cause critical airway compromise. Other potential complications include jugular thrombophlebitis (Lemierre syndrome), mandibular osteomyelitis, mediastinitis, and pleuritis.

References:

Bosemani T, Izbudak I. Head and neck emergencies. *Semin Roentgenol.* 2013;48(1):4-13.

Branstetter BF 4th, Weissman JL. Infection of the facial area, oral cavity, oropharynx, and retropharynx. *Neuroimaging Clin N Am.* 2003;13(3):393-410, ix.

BULLSEYE, CLAW, INTRACYSTIC NODULE, POSTERIOR LEDGE

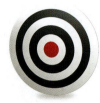

Modality:
MR

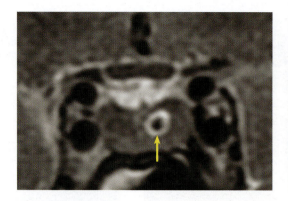
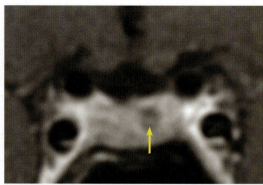

FINDINGS:

Coronal T2-weighted and contrast-enhanced T1-weighted MR with fat saturation show a left pituitary cystic lesion with T2-hypointense, T1-hyperintense central nodule (arrows).

DIAGNOSIS:

Rathke cleft cyst

DISCUSSION:

The Rathke pouch is an ectodermal outpouching of the primitive oral cavity that separates to form the anterior pituitary gland. The anterior wall of the pouch proliferates to form the pars distalis, which comprises the majority of the anterior gland; and the pars tuberalis, which wraps around the pituitary stalk. The posterior wall of the pouch does not proliferate and forms the pars intermedia. The lumen of the pouch normally involutes, but may persist as the Rathke cleft. Rathke cleft cyst (RCC) is a benign expansion of this residual cavity, and is usually asymptomatic. At imaging, it appears as a nonenhancing, noncalcified cystic lesion with a surrounding rim of enhancing pituitary gland ("claw" sign). MR signal varies depending on whether cyst contents are serous (T1-hypointense, T2-hyperintense) or mucoid (T1-hyperintense, T2-hypointense). Rathke cleft cyst usually measures less than 1.5 cm in size and may be difficult to distinguish from a small craniopharyngioma with cystic components. Characteristic imaging features include the "intracystic nodule" and "posterior ledge" signs. Within the cyst, there may be a mucin-containing nodule with variably T1-hyperintense and T2-hypointense signal. Occasionally, the cyst can extend superiorly through the diaphragma sellae and drape over the posterior pituitary, forming the "posterior ledge" sign.

Reference:

Byun WM, Kim OL, Kim D. MR imaging findings of Rathke's cleft cysts: significance of intracystic nodules. *AJNR Am J Neuroradiol.* 2000;21(3):485-488.

CANDLE DRIPPING, FUZZY, SHAGGY

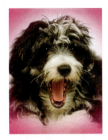

Modalities:
XR, CT

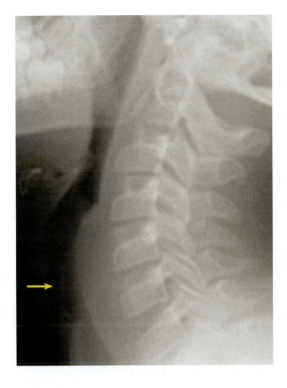

FINDINGS:

Lateral neck radiograph shows tracheal wall thickening and irregularity, with sloughing of membranes (arrow).

DIAGNOSIS:

Bacterial tracheitis

DISCUSSION:

Bacterial tracheitis (exudative tracheitis, membranous croup, membranous laryngotracheobronchitis) is a purulent infection that can be caused by *Staphylococcus aureus*, *Streptococcus pneumoniae*, *Haemophilus influenzae*, and *Moraxella catarrhalis*. It usually affects children between 6 and 10 years of age. Severe inflammation results in exudative plaques and sloughing of membranes in the larynx, trachea, and/or bronchi with a "shaggy" appearance. On frontal radiographs, there is subglottic airway narrowing, which is typically more asymmetric and irregular than in croup. On lateral radiographs, tracheal wall irregularity and intraluminal filling defects are diagnostic. Because of the risk of airway obstruction and respiratory failure, there is need for prompt airway management, antibiotics, and endoscopic membrane stripping. In comparison, croup affects younger patients (6 months to 3 years), is a self-limited infection, and shows smooth symmetric subglottic narrowing.

Reference:

Sammer M, Pruthi S. Membranous croup (exudative tracheitis or membranous laryngotracheobronchitis). *Pediatr Radiol.* 2010;40(5):781.

CEREBRIFORM, CONVOLUTED, STRIATED

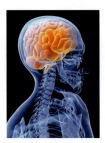

Modalities:
CT, MR

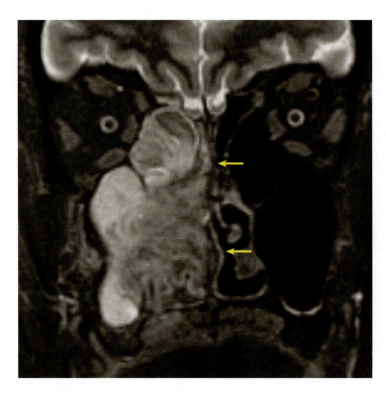

FINDINGS:

Coronal T2-weighted MR shows a right nasal cavity mass (arrows) extending into the right maxillary sinus with a convoluted and double-layered appearance.

DIFFERENTIAL DIAGNOSIS:

- Inverted papilloma
- Oncocytic papilloma
- Sinonasal carcinoma

DISCUSSION:

The Schneiderian membrane is ciliated mucosa of ectodermal origin that lines the sinonasal tract, and is distinct from the endodermally derived mucosa of the upper respiratory tract. Benign neoplasms of the Schneiderian membrane are known as Schneiderian papillomas and classified into three types: fungiform, inverted, and oncocytic. Fungiform (exophytic, septal) papillomas grow out from the nasal septum and do not involve the paranasal sinuses. Inverted (endophytic) papillomas arise from the lateral nasal wall (classically at the hiatus semilunaris) and extend into the sinuses (typically maxillary or ethmoid). Focal hyperostosis and entrapped bone can be seen at the point of tumor attachment. On T2-weighted MR, contrast-enhanced T1-weighted MR, and contrast-enhanced CT, tumors may demonstrate a convoluted and layered "cerebriform" appearance. Oncocytic (cylindrical cell) papillomas are the rarest subtype, occurring in the lateral nasal wall or sinuses. They appear similar to inverted papillomas on imaging, but show both exo- and endophytic growth patterns at histology. Treatment of papillomas involves complete resection because associated synchronous and/or metachronous carcinomas (particularly squamous cell carcinoma) are seen in 10% of cases. At imaging, the presence of carcinoma is suggested by loss of the "cerebriform" pattern, central necrosis, irregular margins, and bone destruction.

References:

Barnes L. Schneiderian papillomas and nonsalivary glandular neoplasms of the head and neck. *Mod Pathol.* 2002;15(3):279-297.

Jeona TY, Kima HJ, Chungb SK, et al. Sinonasal inverted papilloma: value of convoluted cerebriform pattern on MR imaging. *Am J Neuroradiol.* 2008;29:1556-1560.

CLAW

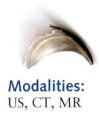

Modalities:
US, CT, MR

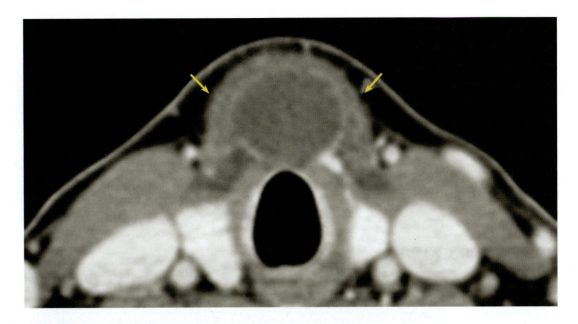

FINDINGS:

Axial contrast-enhanced CT shows a midline cystic lesion deep to and partially embedded in the strap muscles (arrows).

DIAGNOSIS:

Thyroglossal duct cyst

DISCUSSION:

Thyroglossal duct cyst (TGDC) is the most common congenital neck lesion. It represents remnant thyroglossal duct tissue along the path of migration between the foramen cecum at the base of tongue and the thyroid bed in the infrahyoid neck. TGDCs are typically located close to midline (within 2 cm) and may occur in the infrahyoid, hyoid, or suprahyoid regions. Infrahyoid TGDCs that extend anteriorly become embedded in the strap muscles (sternohyoid, sternothyroid, thyrohyoid, and omohyoid), creating the pathognomonic "claw" sign. At imaging, TGDCs appear as thin-walled cystic lesions, though thicker enhancing walls may develop with superinfection. Nodularity and coarse calcifications are concerning for malignant transformation into thyroid carcinoma. The treatment of choice is resection of the entire cyst, remnant tract, and central hyoid bone (Sistrunk procedure).

References:

Glastonbury CM, Davidson HC, Haller JR, et al. The CT and MR imaging features of carcinoma arising in thyroglossal duct remnants. *AJNR Am J Neuroradiol.* 2000;21(4):770-774.

Koeller KK, Alamo L, Adair CF, et al. Congenital cystic masses of the neck: radiologic-pathologic correlation. *Radiographics.* 1999;19(1):121-146; quiz 152-153.

COCA-COLA BOTTLE

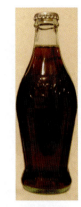

Modalities:
US, CT, MR

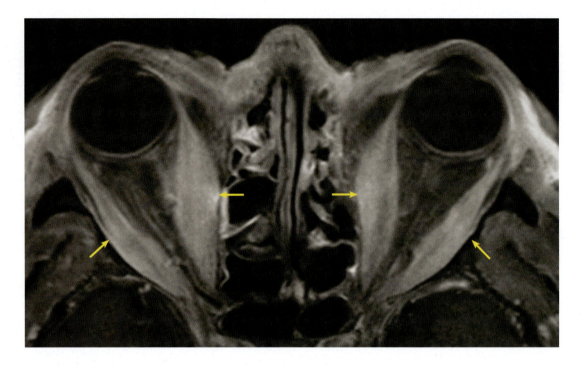

FINDINGS:

Axial contrast-enhanced T1-weighted MR with fat saturation shows fusiform enlargement and hyperenhancement of the extraocular muscles (arrows), with sparing of the tendinous insertions. There is bilateral proptosis and increased periorbital fat.

DIAGNOSIS:

Thyroid ophthalmopathy

DISCUSSION:

Thyroid ophthalmopathy is the most common cause of proptosis in adults and is usually seen in patients with thyroid disease, particularly Graves disease. It is postulated that antibodies to thyroid-stimulating hormone cross-react with orbital antigens, resulting in inflammation and fibrosis with mucopolysaccharide/collagen deposition in the extraocular muscles and orbital fat. There is fusiform enlargement of the extraocular muscle bellies with sparing of the tendinous insertions, resembling the contour of a Coca-Cola bottle. The mnemonic "I'M SLO" describes the typical order of involvement: inferior rectus, medial rectus, superior rectus, lateral rectus, and superior/inferior obliques. Severe muscle enlargement can compress the optic nerve and superior ophthalmic vein at the orbital apex, leading to optic nerve dysfunction and venous congestion of the periorbital fat. Treatment options include radioactive iodine ablation, antithyroid medications, and orbital decompression.

Reference:

Parmar H, Ibrahim M. Extrathyroidal manifestations of thyroid disease: thyroid ophthalmopathy. *Neuroimaging Clin N Am.* 2008;18(3):527-536, viii-ix.

COCHLEAR CLEFT

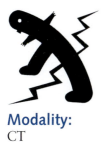

Modality:
CT

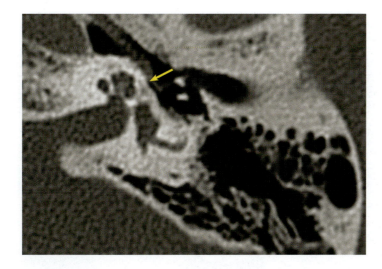

FINDINGS:

Axial temporal bone CT shows an ill-defined lucency posterior to the tensor tympani and anterior to the vestibule, in the region of the fissula ante fenestram (arrow).

DIFFERENTIAL DIAGNOSIS:

- Bone dyscrasia
- Fracture
- Normal variant

DISCUSSION:

Lucencies of the otic capsule are commonly seen in children, and reflect incomplete endochondral ossification with cartilaginous remnants. A normal variant is the cochlear cleft, which is C-shaped and courses parallel to the basal turn of the cochlea. This occurs in close association with the fissula ante fenestram, a fibrocartilaginous region just anterior to the oval window. Otic capsule-violating temporal bone fractures can also occur here. In the adult, the mature bony labyrinth is avascular and undergoes virtually no remodeling. Ill-defined lucencies suggest a bone dyscrasia such as otospongiosis, osteogenesis imperfecta, or Paget disease. Otospongiosis, which exclusively affects the otic capsule and auditory ossicles, is a leading cause of adult-onset hearing loss. The normally dense avascular endochondral bone is replaced by spongy vascular haversian bone. This manifests as hypodensity on CT, most commonly at the fissula ante fenestram (fenestral otospongiosis), and in advanced cases surrounding the cochlea (retrofenestral otospongiosis). Sclerosis occurring in the chronic (healing) phase is known as otosclerosis. Osteogenesis imperfecta and Paget disease show more diffuse involvement of the temporal bone, as well as evidence of systemic disease.

References:

Chadwell JB, Halsted MJ, Choo DI, et al. The cochlear cleft. *AJNR Am J Neuroradiol*. 2004;25(1): 21-24.

Mafee MF, Valvassori GE, Dcitch RL, et al. Use of CT in the evaluation of cochlear otosclerosis. *Radiology*. 1985;156(3):703-708.

COMET, PEAR, TAIL

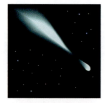

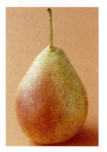

Modalities:
US, CT, MR

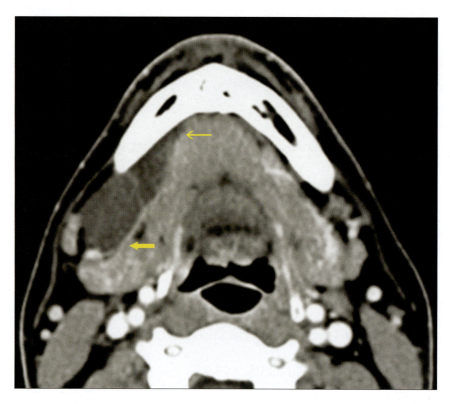

FINDINGS:

Axial contrast-enhanced CT shows an elongated cystic structure originating from the right sublingual space (thin arrow) and tracking posteriorly into the right submandibular space (thick arrow).

DIAGNOSIS:

Diving ranula

DISCUSSION:

Ranulas are mucus retention cysts of the minor salivary glands, most commonly the sublingual gland. They may be congenital, inflammatory, or traumatic. Simple ranulas are lined by epithelium and confined to the sublingual space, above the mylohyoid muscle. Diving (plunging, deep) ranulas are pseudocysts with contained rupture into the submandibular space. The "tail" sign represents the collapsed portion of the cyst within the sublingual space. Ruptures usually track posteriorly over the back of the mylohyoid muscle to terminate in the posteromedial submandibular space. Less commonly, they can extend laterally through a mylohyoid defect (boutonnière) into the anterior submandibular space. Rarely, large ranulas may ascend into the parapharyngeal space.

Reference:

La'porte SJ, Juttla JK, Lingam RK. Imaging the floor of the mouth and the sublingual space. *Radiographics*. 2011;31(5):1215-1230.

CONE, FUNNEL, MARTINI/WINE GLASS, TRIANGLE, TUBULAR

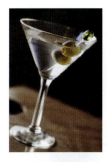

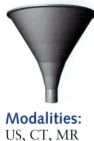

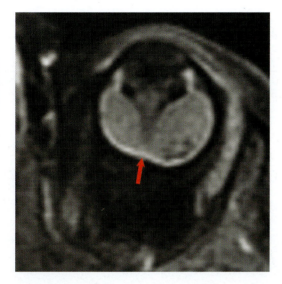

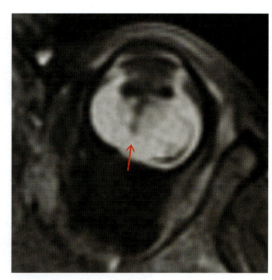

Modalities:
US, CT, MR

FINDINGS:

Axial fat-saturated T2-weighted MR shows a conical soft-tissue mass extending from the lens to the optic nerve head (thick arrow). There is a linear area of low signal intensity within the mass (thin arrow), representing remnant hyaloid vasculature.

DIAGNOSIS:

Persistent hyperplastic primary vitreous

DISCUSSION:

The fetal intraocular vascular system consists of anterior and posterior divisions. The anterior system supplies the iris anterior to the lens, whereas the posterior system has three components: hyaloid artery supplying the central primary vitreous, vasa hyaloidea propria supplying the peripheral primary vitreous, and tunica vasculosa lentis supplying the iris and lens. The primary vitreous forms between the lens and the retina around 7 weeks of gestation, and begins involuting by 20 weeks as it is replaced by the secondary vitreous. Persistent hyperplastic primary vitreous (PHPV) refers to persistence of this system, which can affect the anterior and/or posterior compartments. In anterior PHPV, there is a shallow anterior chamber and retrolental fibrovascular membrane. In posterior PHPV, there is a retrolental mass, funnel-shaped retinal detachment, and a stalk extending from the optic nerve to the posterior lens (remnant of hyaloid canal carrying the hyaloid artery) creating the "martini glass" appearance. Bilateral PHPV is associated with trisomy 13 (Patau syndrome), Norrie disease, and Walker-Warburg syndrome.

References:

Castillo M, Wallace DK, Mukherji SK. Persistent hyperplastic primary vitreous involving the anterior eye. *AJNR Am J Neuroradiol*. 1997;18(8):1526-1528.

Kaste SC, Jenkins JJ 3rd, Meyer D, et al. Persistent hyperplastic primary vitreous of the eye: imaging findings with pathologic correlation. *AJR Am J Roentgenol*. 1994;162(2):437-440.

COW/OX EYE

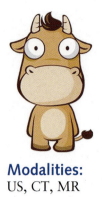

Modalities:
US, CT, MR

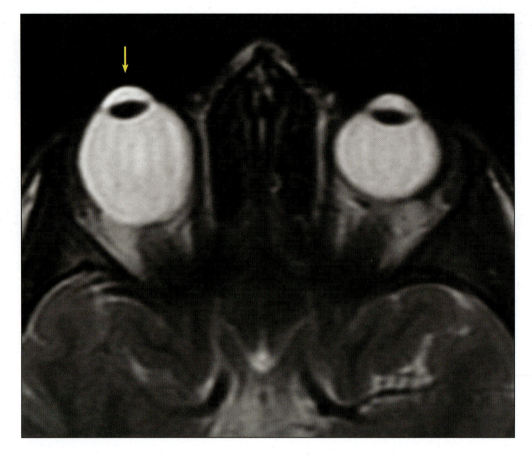

FINDINGS:

Axial T2-weighted MR shows an asymmetrically enlarged right globe (arrow).

DIAGNOSIS:

Macrophthalmos

DISCUSSION:

Macrophthalmos refers to enlargement of the globe, which usually presents in the first 3 months of life. Buphthalmos (Greek for "ox or cow eye") is enlargement due to increased intraocular pressure in the first 3-4 years of life, when the sclera is still malleable. This occurs in congenital glaucoma and acquired glaucoma secondary to aniridia, neurofibromatosis type I, Sturge-Weber syndrome, Proteus syndrome, Peter anomaly, retinoblastoma, and melanoma. Patients with connective tissue disorders have floppy sclerae and can present with ocular enlargement at any age. Megalophthalmos has been used to denote globe enlargement with normal intraocular pressures. Nonglaucomatous causes of globe enlargement include axial myopia, staphyloma, coloboma, and anophthalmos with cyst (congenital cystic eye).

Reference:

Som PM, Curtin HD. *Head and Neck Imaging*. 5th ed. St Louis, MO: Mosby; 2011.

CRESCENT, DODD

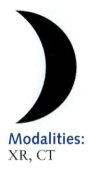

Modalities:
XR, CT

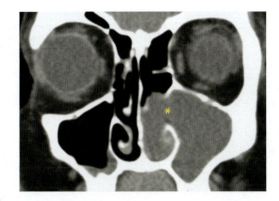
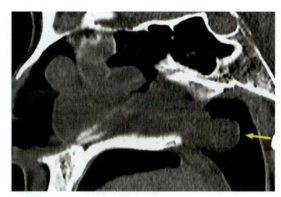

FINDINGS:

Axial and sagittal CT show a soft-tissue mass arising in the left maxillary sinus and expanding the antrum (asterisk). This extends posteriorly through the nasal cavity and choana into the nasopharynx, where it is outlined by a crescent of air (arrow).

DIAGNOSIS:

Choanal polyp

DISCUSSION:

Choanal (Killian) polyps are inflammatory polyps that produce unilateral nasal obstruction in teenagers and young adults. They arise from the sinonasal mucosa and herniate through the sinus ostium into the nasal cavity, causing smooth bone remodeling. Polyps that are sufficiently large can prolapse through the choana into the nasopharynx. Antrochoanal polyps are the most common, appearing as dumbbell-shaped mucoid masses at the maxillary sinus antrum that extend through an accessory or major ostium into the ipsilateral nasal cavity. Continued growth through the choana yields a bulbous nasopharyngeal component, which rests on the soft palate and is surrounded by a crescent of air (Dodd sign). In contrast, sinonasal inverted papillomas arise from the lateral nasal wall near the hiatus semilunaris and demonstrate peripheral growth into the sinuses, with a "cerebriform" pattern at imaging. Less common types of choanal polyps are nasochoanal, sphenochoanal, frontochoanal, and ethmochoanal.

References:

Aydin O, Keskin G, Ustündağ E, et al. Choanal polyps: an evaluation of 53 cases. *Am J Rhinol.* 2007;21(2):164-168.

Chung SK, Chang BC, Dhong HJ. Surgical, radiologic, and histologic findings of the antrochoanal polyp. *Am J Rhinol.* 2002;16(2):71-76.

CRESCENT, FUNNEL, V

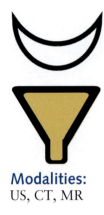

Modalities:
US, CT, MR

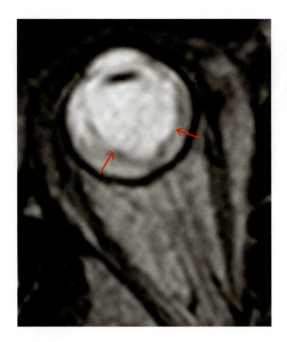
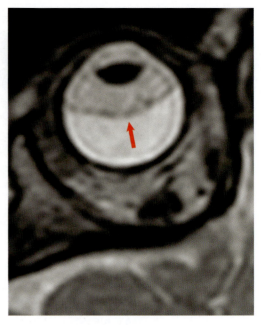

FINDINGS:

- Axial T2-weighted MR shows partial retinal detachment, with the detached leaves of the retina (thin arrows) converging toward the optic disc.
- Axial T2-weighted MR in a different patient shows complete retinal detachment, in which the outer retinal membrane (thick arrow) has completely separated from the inner sensory layer.

DIAGNOSIS:

Retinal detachment

DISCUSSION:

The globes are lined by three concentric coverings: the internal nervous, middle vascular, and external fibrous tunics. The retina contains photoreceptors (rods, cones, and photosensitive ganglion cells) that process light stimuli and send impulses through the optic nerve to the brain. The choroid consists of vascular pigmented connective tissue, which is responsible for nutrition and gas exchange, and forms the uveal tract along with the ciliary body and iris. The sclera, which is composed of protective fibrous tissue, is continuous anteriorly with the cornea. Retinal detachment (RD) refers to separation of the retina from the choroid, which can occur following inflammation (tractional), fluid accumulation (exudative), or trauma (rhegmatogenous). In partial RD, the leaves of the retina converge toward the optic disc ("V" appearance). In complete RD, the optic attachment is also disrupted ("crescent" appearance). Therapeutic options include pneumatic, silicone, laser, or cryoretinopexy and scleral buckle.

Reference:

Mafee MF, Peyman GA. Retinal and choroidal detachments: role of magnetic resonance imaging and computed tomography. *Radiol Clin North Am.* 1987;25(3):487-507.

DANGER SPACE

Modalities:
CT, MR

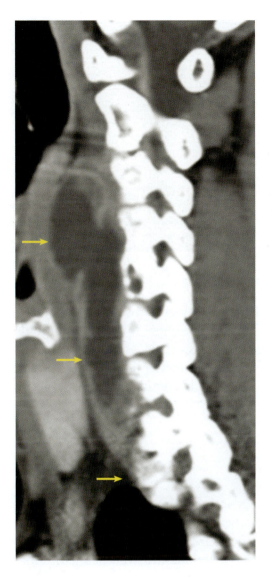

FINDINGS:

Sagittal contrast-enhanced CT shows a rim-enhancing prevertebral fluid collection that extends inferiorly into the upper thorax (arrows).

DIFFERENTIAL DIAGNOSIS:

- Danger space abscess
- Retropharyngeal abscess

DISCUSSION:

The danger space is a potential space between the alar and prevertebral fasciae, extending from the level of the skull base to the posterior diaphragm. This is a conduit for spread of infection and tumor between the neck and the mediastinum. Danger space infections can be difficult to distinguish from infections of the retropharyngeal space, which are located more anteriorly between the visceral (buccopharyngeal) and alar fasciae. Collections are often unilateral because of the presence of a midline raphe, and do not extend beyond the upper mediastinum.

Reference:

Bosemani T, Izbudak I. Head and neck emergencies. *Semin Roentgenol.* 2013;48(1):4-13.

DEFORMABLE, VANISHING

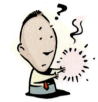

Modality:
MR

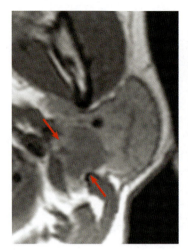 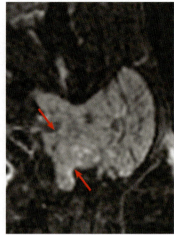 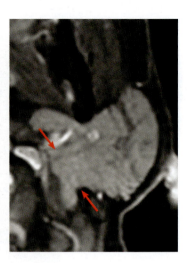

FINDINGS:

- Axial T1-weighted MR shows a well-circumscribed hypointense mass in the left parotid (arrows), which extends through the stylomandibular foramen and is deformed by surrounding structures.
- Axial T2-weighted MR and contrast-enhanced T1-weighted MR with fat saturation show the mass (arrows) becoming isointense to parotid parenchyma.

DIAGNOSIS:

Parotid oncocytoma

DISCUSSION:

Parotid oncocytoma (oncocytic adenoma, oxyphilic granular cell adenoma, oxyphilic adenoma) is a rare benign epithelial tumor consisting of mitochondria-rich oncocytes. Imaging features are nonspecific and overlap with other benign parotid tumors. The majority of lesions are well-defined, enhancing, and can be bilateral. There may be internal nonenhancing curvilinear clefts and cystic areas, corresponding histologically to a central scar. On MR, oncocytomas are classically T1-hypointense, becoming isointense on T2-weighted images with fat saturation and contrast-enhanced T1-weighted images ("vanishing" lesions). Nuclear medicine features include high uptake on Tc-99m pertechnetate scans and 18F-FDG PET. Large tumors can be distorted by surrounding structures, creating a "deformable" appearance. Because oncocytes are radioresistant, complete surgical resection is the treatment of choice. There is a low risk of transformation to oncocytic carcinoma.

References:

Patel ND, van Zante A, Eisele DW, et al. Oncocytoma: the vanishing parotid mass. *AJNR Am J Neuroradiol*. 2011;32(9):1703-1706.

Tan TJ, Tan TY. CT features of parotid gland oncocytomas: a study of 10 cases and literature review. *AJNR Am J Neuroradiol*. 2010;31(8):1413-1417.

DOME, MOUND, MUSHROOM

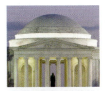

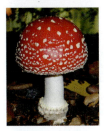

Modalities:
US, CT, MR

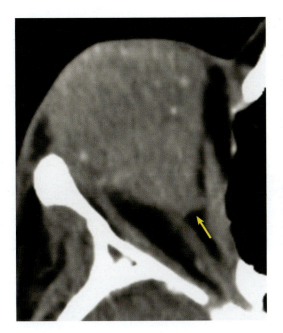

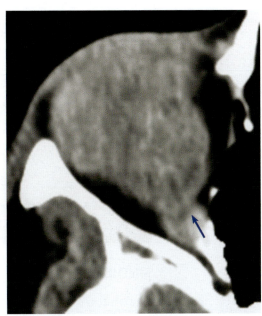

FINDINGS:

Axial noncontrast and contrast-enhanced CT show a partially calcified, heterogeneously enhancing mass that replaces the right globe and invades the optic nerve (arrows).

DIFFERENTIAL DIAGNOSIS:

- Ocular melanoma
- Metastasis

DISCUSSION:

Melanoma is the most common primary intraocular malignancy in adults. It arises from melanocytes within the pigmented uveal tract (choroid, ciliary body, and iris). The typical imaging appearance is a solid, diffusely enhancing mass with intrinsic T1 hyperintensity and T2 hypointensity on MR. The choroid is the most common location, with a "dome" or "mushroom" morphology. The latter appearance implies penetration through the Bruch membrane, a structure that normally separates the choroid and retina. Associated retinal detachment and subretinal effusions may be seen. Further tumor spread can occur posteriorly along the optic nerve and anteriorly into the globe, ciliary body, and iris. Other invasive ocular masses include metastases from breast, lung, thyroid, renal, and gastrointestinal primaries. Retinoblastoma, the most common ocular tumor in children, tends to be more densely calcified.

References:

Peyster RG, Augsburger JJ, Shields JA, et al. Intraocular tumors: evaluation with MR imaging. *Radiology.* 1988;168(3):773-779.

Tong KA, Osborn AG, Mamalis N, et al. Ocular melanoma. *AJNR Am J Neuroradiol.* 1993;14(6): 1359-1366.

DONUT/DOUGHNUT

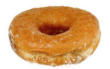

Modalities:
US, CT, MR

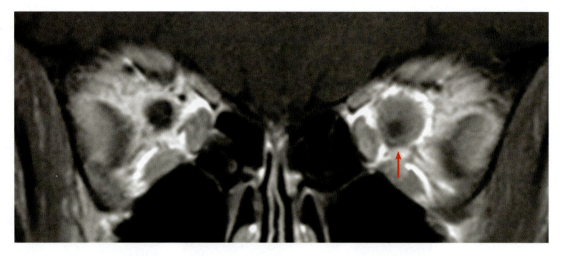

FINDINGS:

Coronal contrast-enhanced T1-weighted MR shows an enhancing mass (arrow) that circumferentially encases and compresses the left optic nerve.

DIAGNOSIS:

Perioptic meningioma

DISCUSSION:

Perioptic meningiomas are benign tumors arising from the arachnoid cap cells in the optic nerve sheath. They may arise within the orbit (optic nerve sheath meningioma), optic nerve canal (intracanalicular meningioma), or optic foramen (foraminal meningioma). Three distinct morphologies have been described: tubular, exophytic, and fusiform. The tubular form symmetrically surrounds and compresses the optic nerve, with associated enhancement and/or calcification. This gives rise to the "doughnut" sign en face and the "tram-track" sign in long axis. In contrast, optic gliomas are infiltrative tumors that are intimately associated with the optic nerve. Other causes of perioptic enhancement include orbital pseudotumor, infection, sarcoidosis, leukemia/lymphoma, and metastases.

Reference:

Kanamalla US. The optic nerve tram-track sign. *Radiology*. 2003;227(3):718-719.

DOTTED I, SAUSAGE

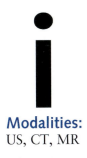

Modalities:
US, CT, MR

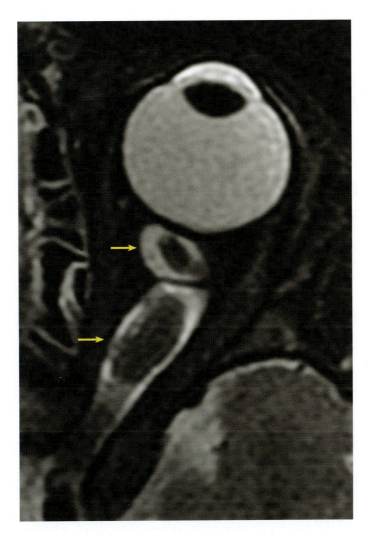

FINDINGS:

Axial T2-weighted MR shows enlargement and kinking of the left optic nerve (arrows).

DIAGNOSIS:

Optic nerve glioma

DISCUSSION:

Optic glioma is the most common optic nerve tumor. There are three subtypes: childhood syndromic (neurofibromatosis type I), childhood sporadic, and adult. Gliomas in children are low-grade (WHO I-II), whereas in adults they are higher grade (WHO grade III-IV). These manifest with fusiform enlargement and elongation of the optic nerve ("dotted i" appearance), chiasm, and/or radiations. MR signal is generally T2-hyperintense ("pseudo-CSF" appearance). Syndromic gliomas are smooth, focally tortuous, and minimally enhancing. Sporadic gliomas are larger, nodular/cystic, and moderately enhancing. Adult gliomas are diffuse, invasive, and heterogeneously enhancing. Other conditions affecting the optic nerve include optic neuritis (nerve edema and enhancement), optic nerve meningioma (tumor of the nerve sheath), orbital pseudotumor (localized inflammation of various periorbital structures), and sarcoidosis (multifocal orbital and intracranial manifestations).

References:

Millar WS, Tartaglino LM, Sergott RC, et al. MR of malignant optic glioma of adulthood. *AJNR Am J Neuroradiol.* 1995;16(8):1673-1676.

Taylor T, Jaspan T, Milano G, et al. Radiological classification of optic pathway gliomas: experience of a modified functional classification system. *Br J Radiol.* 2008;81(970):761-766.

DOUBLE RING/HALO/LUCENT, FOURTH TURN

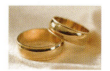

Modality:
CT

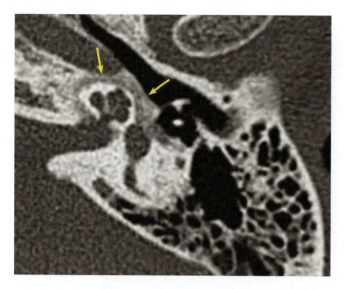

FINDINGS:

Axial temporal bone CT shows a ringlike lucency (arrows) encircling the cochlea. There is also involvement of the fissula ante fenestram.

DIFFERENTIAL DIAGNOSIS:

- Retrofenestral otospongiosis
- Osteogenesis imperfecta

DISCUSSION:

The otic capsule is composed of dense avascular endochondral bone, which ossifies and undergoes virtually no remodeling after development. However, disorganization of bone can be induced by such conditions as otospongiosis, inflammation/infection, radiation, trauma, Paget disease, osteopetrosis, and fibrous dysplasia. Otospongiosis, which exclusively affects the otic capsule and auditory ossicles, is a leading cause of adult-onset hearing loss. The normally dense avascular endochondral bone is replaced by spongy vascular haversian bone. This typically begins at the fissula ante fenestram (fenestral otospongiosis), a fibrocartilaginous region just anterior to the oval window. In the late stages, the disease spreads peripherally to surround the cochlea (retrofenestral or cochlear otospongiosis). This appearance has been termed the "fourth turn" of the cochlea. Sclerosis in the chronic (healing) phase is known as otosclerosis. Osteogenesis imperfecta mimics severe cochlear otospongiosis, but with systemic manifestations. Paget disease diffusely involves the temporal bone and skull base, progressing from peripheral to central. Fibrous dysplasia has an expansile, ground-glass appearance with relative sparing of the otic capsule. Chronic otitis media and cholesteatoma demonstrate middle ear opacification with bone erosion and remodeling. Osteoradionecrosis results in diffuse "moth-eaten" demineralization of the temporal bone.

Reference:

Mafee MF, Valvassori GE, Deitch RL, et al. Use of CT in the evaluation of cochlear otosclerosis. *Radiology.* 1985;156(3):703-708.

DUMBBELL

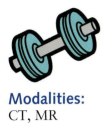

Modalities:
CT, MR

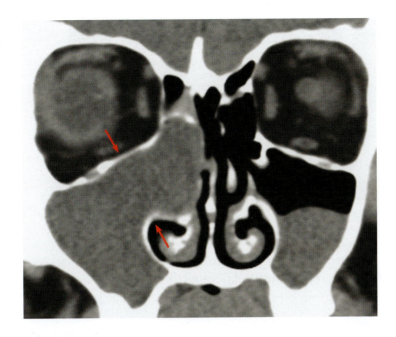

FINDINGS:

Coronal CT shows a soft-tissue mass involving the right maxillary sinus and nasal cavity, with enlargement of the intervening maxillary antrum (arrows).

DIAGNOSIS:

Choanal polyp

DISCUSSION:

Choanal (Killian) polyps are inflammatory polyps that produce unilateral nasal obstruction in teenagers and young adults. They arise from the sinonasal mucosa and herniate through the sinus ostium into the nasal cavity, causing smooth bone remodeling. Polyps that are sufficiently large can prolapse through the choana into the nasopharynx. Antrochoanal polyps are the most common, appearing as "dumbbell"-shaped mucoid masses that extend from the maxillary sinus through an accessory or major ostium into the ipsilateral nasal cavity. In contrast, sinonasal inverted papillomas arise from the lateral nasal wall near the hiatus semilunaris and demonstrate peripheral growth into the sinuses, with a "cerebriform" pattern at imaging. Less common types of choanal polyps are nasochoanal, sphenochoanal, frontochoanal, and ethmochoanal.

References:

Aydin O, Keskin G, Ustündağ E, et al. Choanal polyps: an evaluation of 53 cases. *Am J Rhinol.* 2007;21(2):164-168.

Chung SK, Chang BC, Dhong HJ. Surgical, radiologic, and histologic findings of the antrochoanal polyp. *Am J Rhinol.* 2002;16(2):71-76.

DUMBBELL

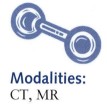

Modalities:
CT, MR

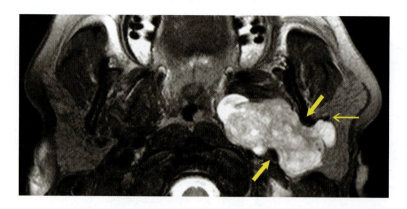

FINDINGS:

Axial T2-weighted MR shows a lobulated hyperintense mass in the left parotid gland, deep to the retromandibular vein (thin arrow). There is extension through the stylomandibular foramen (thick arrows) into the parapharyngeal space.

DIAGNOSIS:

Parotid tumor, deep lobe

DISCUSSION:

The parotid gland is anatomically divided into superficial and deep lobes by the extracranial facial nerve. The superficial lobe represents the palpable, dominant portion of the gland. It constitutes approximately two-thirds of total gland volume and extends from the external auditory canal and mastoid tip to below the angle of the mandible (parotid tail). The deep lobe, which projects into the lateral parapharyngeal space, comprises the remaining one-third of gland volume. Because the intraparotid facial nerve is too small to visualize on conventional imaging, the retromandibular vein (which lies directly medial to CN VII) is used as a marker for its course. Deep lobe tumors can occasionally grow through the stylomandibular tunnel into the parapharyngeal space, creating a "dumbbell" appearance. This behavior is concerning for malignancy, though benign lesions (including pleomorphic adenomas and schwannomas) can have a similar appearance. Symptoms are nonspecific due to containment within an anatomically limited space. This means that metastasis may occur before the primary tumor is diagnosed. If the tumor has not metastasized, definitive therapy involves total parotidectomy with facial nerve preservation. This may require external, transoral, or combined surgical approaches. Resection of the styloid process of the temporal bone is necessary to enlarge the stylomandibular foramen and ensure complete tumor removal.

References:

Christe A, Waldherr C, Hallett R, et al. MR imaging of parotid tumors: typical lesion characteristics in MR imaging improve discrimination between benign and malignant disease. *AJNR Am J Neuroradiol.* 2011;32(7):1202-1207.

Patey DH, Thackray AC. The pathological anatomy and treatment of parotid tumours with retropharyngeal extension (dumb-bell tumours); with a report of 4 personal cases. *Br J Surg.* 1957; 44(186):352-358.

DUMBBELL

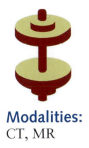

Modalities:
CT, MR

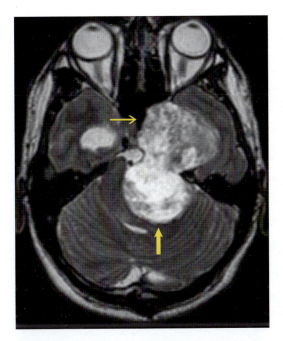
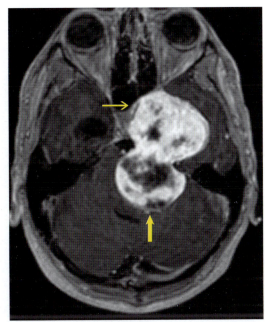

FINDINGS:

Axial T2-weighted and contrast-enhanced T1-weighted MR show a bilobed solid and cystic mass extending from the left cerebellopontine angle (thick arrows) into the Meckel cave and cavernous sinus. There is significant left pontine and cerebellar compression, effacement of the fourth ventricle, and medial deviation of the left cavernous ICA (thin arrows).

DIAGNOSIS:

Trigeminal nerve schwannoma

DISCUSSION:

Schwannomas (neurilemmomas) are benign nerve sheath tumors composed of myelinating Schwann cells. These frequently involve the cranial nerves, with a characteristic fusiform appearance and smooth bony expansion. Large tumors can extend through osseous foramina to create a bilobed or "dumbbell" morphology. Common locations include CN V (trigeminal), VII (facial), VIII (vestibulocochlear), and X (vagal). Multiple schwannomas are seen in schwannomatosis and neurofibromatosis type II (MISME: multiple inherited schwannomas, meningiomas, and ependymomas).

References:

Al-Mefty O, Ayoubi S, Gaber E. Trigeminal schwannomas: removal of dumbbell-shaped tumors through the expanded Meckel cave and outcomes of cranial nerve function. *J Neurosurg.* 2002;96(3):453-463.

Kadri PA, Al-Mefty O. Surgical treatment of dumbbell-shaped jugular foramen schwannomas. *Neurosurg Focus.* 2004;17(2):E9.

Salzman KL, Davidson HC, Harnsberger HR, et al. Dumbbell schwannomas of the internal auditory canal. *AJNR Am J Neuroradiol.* 2001;22(7):1368-1376.

DUMBBELL, FIGURE EIGHT, SNOWMAN

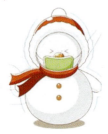

Modalities:
CT, MR

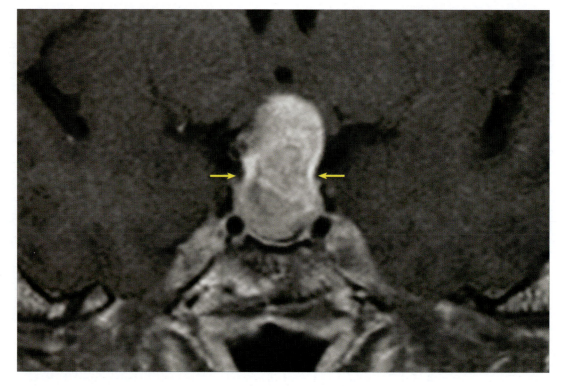

FINDINGS:

Coronal contrast-enhanced T1-weighted MR shows an enhancing sellar/suprasellar mass with focal constriction at the diaphragma sellae (arrows).

DIAGNOSIS:

Pituitary macroadenoma

DISCUSSION:

Pituitary macroadenomas are benign, usually nonfunctioning tumors greater than 1 cm in size. Over time, these gradually replace the pituitary gland, grow up through the diaphragma sellae into the suprasellar region with a "snowman" appearance, and elevate the optic chiasm. Often, there is heterogeneous enhancement with areas of cystic change, necrosis, and hemorrhage. Aggressive adenomas can invade and remodel the sella, sphenoid, clivus, and cavernous sinuses. Other sellar/suprasellar masses include craniopharyngioma, Rathke cleft cyst, and meningioma, which do not typically show focal constriction at the diaphragma sellae. The general mnemonic for suprasellar masses is "SATCHMOE": sellar/parasellar neoplasm, aneurysm, teratoma/germ cell tumor, craniopharyngioma, hypothalamic hamartoma or Langerhans cell histiocytosis, meningioma or metastasis, optic or hypothalamic glioma, and epidermoid or dermoid cyst.

Reference:

Hess CP, Dillon WP. Imaging the pituitary and parasellar region. *Neurosurg Clin N Am.* 2012;23(4): 529-542.

DUMBBELL, WAIST

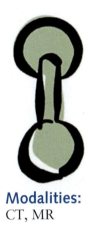

Modalities:
CT, MR

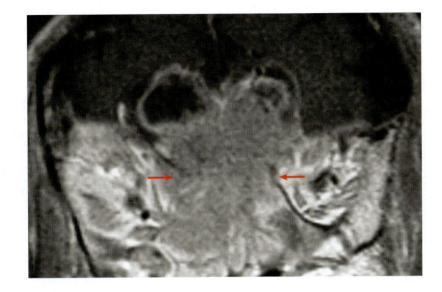

FINDINGS:

Coronal contrast-enhanced T1-weighted MR shows an enhancing mass centered at the cribriform plate (arrows), with intracranial and intranasal extension. Peritumoral cysts are present along the superior margin of the mass.

DIFFERENTIAL DIAGNOSIS:

- Esthesioneuroblastoma
- Sinonasal carcinoma

DISCUSSION:

Esthesioneuroblastoma (olfactory neuroblastoma) is a rare malignant primitive neuroectodermal tumor (PNET) that arises from the olfactory epithelium in the superior nasal cavity. Typically, signal is T2 iso- to hyperintense and T1-hypointense on MR, with avid enhancement. Progressive tumor expansion can cause destruction of surrounding bone with extension into the paranasal sinuses, contralateral nasal cavity, orbits, and/or cranial cavity. Invasion through the cribriform plate produces a "dumbbell" shape, and cystic degeneration may be identified at the tumor-brain junction. The differential includes other sinonasal malignancies (squamous cell carcinoma, adenocarcinoma, non-Hodgkin lymphoma, undifferentiated carcinoma), which usually occur in older patients. On imaging, these tend to demonstrate more irregular morphology, lower-level heterogeneous enhancement, and absence of peritumoral cysts.

References:

Pickuth D, Heywang-Köbrunner SH, Spielmann RP. Computed tomography and magnetic resonance imaging features of olfactory neuroblastoma: an analysis of 22 cases. *Clin Otolaryngol Allied Sci.* 1999;24(5):457-461.

Yu T, Xu YK, Li L, et al. Esthesioneuroblastoma methods of intracranial extension: CT and MR imaging findings. *Neuroradiology.* 2009;51(12):841-850.

EAGLE BEAK/HEAD

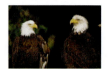

Modalities:
CT, MR

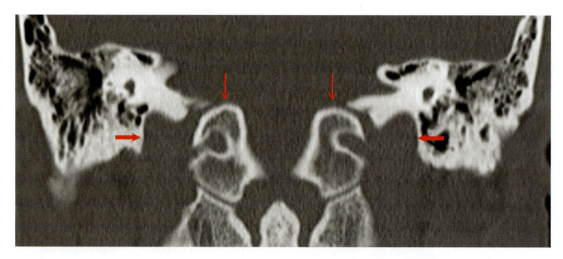

FINDINGS:

Coronal CT shows normal bilateral jugular foramina (thick arrows) and jugular tubercles (thin arrows) curving superiorly over the hypoglossal canals.

DIAGNOSIS:

Normal jugular tubercles

DISCUSSION:

The jugular tubercles are lateral protuberances of the occipital bone that curve posterosuperiorly over the hypoglossal canals. The pointed "eagle beak" appearance was first described on anteroposterior tomographic images, but can now be seen on coronal CT or MR. This appearance may be disrupted by tumors or bone dyscrasias.

Reference:

Osborn AG, Brinton WR, Smith WH. Radiology of the jugular tubercles. *AJR Am J Roentgenol.* 1978;131(6):1037-1040.

EARRING

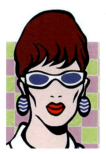

Modalities:
US, CT, MR

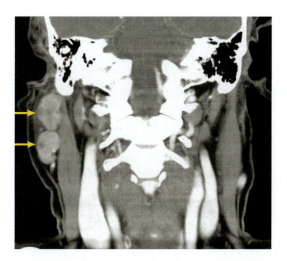 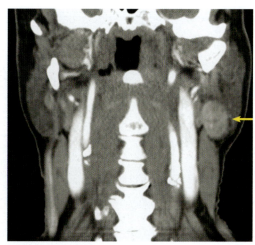

FINDINGS:

Coronal contrast-enhanced CT shows heterogeneously enhancing rounded masses in the bilateral parotid tails (arrows).

DIFFERENTIAL DIAGNOSIS:

- Warthin tumor
- Pleomorphic adenoma
- Lymphoma

DISCUSSION:

The parotid gland is anatomically divided into superficial and deep lobes by the extracranial facial nerve. The superficial lobe represents the palpable, dominant portion of the gland. It constitutes approximately two-thirds of total gland volume and extends from the external auditory canal and mastoid tip to below the angle of the mandible. The parotid tail is the most inferior aspect of the superficial lobe, and lies close to the posterior submandibular space. On axial images, a parotid tail mass can easily be mistaken for a submandibular or jugulodigastric lymph node, particularly if the lesion is pedunculated and/or the parotid gland is atrophic. Review of coronal images is essential to demonstrate a connection to the parotid gland ("earring" appearance). The most common parotid tail lesion is Warthin tumor (papillary cystadenoma lymphomatosum, adenolymphoma, lymphomatous adenoma), which arises from salivary lymphoid tissue in intraparotid and periparotid nodes. This is the second most common benign tumor of the parotid gland, and is typically seen in older male smokers. Lesions have a heterogeneous solid/cystic appearance and can be bilateral. Various other lesions can occur in the parotid tail, including pleomorphic adenoma, lymphoma, metastases, mucoepidermoid carcinoma, lipoma, oncocytoma, infection, venolymphatic malformation, lymphoepithelial cyst, and first branchial cleft cyst. Surgical resection is typically required for tissue diagnosis.

Reference:

Hamilton BE, Salzman KL, Wiggins RH 3rd, et al. Earring lesions of the parotid tail. *AJNR Am J Neuroradiol.* 2003;24(9):1757-1764.

EMPTY NOSE

Modalities:
CT, MR

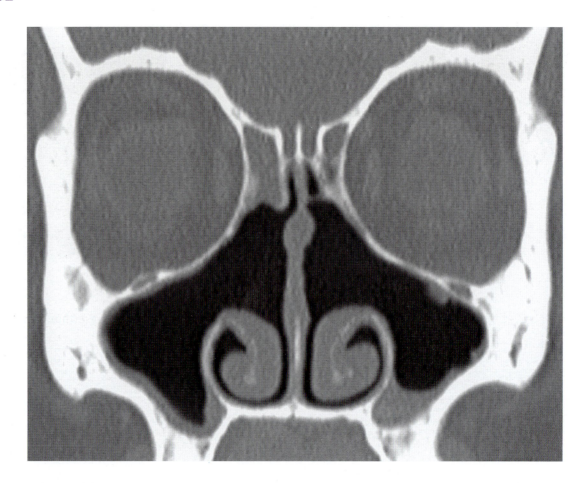

FINDINGS:

Coronal CT shows bilateral maxillary antrostomy, middle turbinectomy, and internal ethmoidectomy.

DIAGNOSIS:

Sinus surgery

DISCUSSION:

The paired nasal turbinates are responsible for controlling, heating, humidifying, and filtering airflow through the nose. Normal nasal cycling occurs every 3-6 hours, in which one side of the nose congests with blood and regenerates, while the other side remains decongested and performs the workload of breathing. In patients with chronic sinusitis, turbinectomy may be performed to alleviate obstruction. In cases of excessive turbinectomy, the remaining mucosa loses the ability to regenerate, becomes inflamed, and eventually atrophies ("empty nose" appearance). Symptoms include chronic dryness and a paradoxical sense of obstruction.

Reference:

Coste A, Dessi P, Serrano E. Empty nose syndrome. *Eur Ann Otorhinolaryngol Head Neck Dis.* 2012;129(2):93-97.

EMPTY PITUITARY FOSSA, EMPTY SELLA

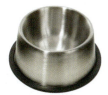

Modalities:
XR, CT, MR

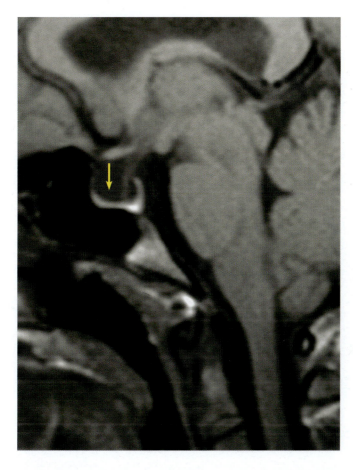

FINDINGS:

Sagittal T1-weighted MR shows increased CSF within the sella, with flattening of the pituitary gland (arrow) against the sellar floor.

DIFFERENTIAL DIAGNOSIS:

- Normal variant
- Idiopathic intracranial hypertension
- Secondary empty sella

DISCUSSION:

The sella turcica is a depression in the sphenoid bone that encloses the pituitary gland. Empty sella refers to a pituitary fossa that is largely devoid of tissue and filled with cerebrospinal fluid. This is thought to represent extension of the subarachnoid space through a defect in the diaphragma sellae. Primary empty sella is a common incidental finding, though there is an association with pseudotumor cerebri (idiopathic intracranial hypertension). Secondary empty sella can occur due to surgery, trauma, radiation, medications, infection, infarction, or hemorrhage. In the days of radiography, "empty sella" denoted the finding of a symmetrically enlarged pituitary fossa with thinned bony margins, for which no mass was identified at pneumoencephalography or surgery. With cross-sectional imaging, enlargement of the CSF space can be seen, with a traversing midline infundibulum and compression of the pituitary gland against the sellar floor.

References:

Haughton VM, Rosenbaum AE, Williams AL, et al. Recognizing the empty sella by CT: the infundibulum sign. *AJR Am J Roentgenol.* 1981;136(2):293-295.

Yuh WT, Zhu M, Taoka T, et al. MR imaging of pituitary morphology in idiopathic intracranial hypertension. *J Magn Reson Imaging.* 2000;12(6):808-813.

ENLARGED/SWOLLEN PITUITARY

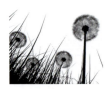

Modalities:
CT, MR

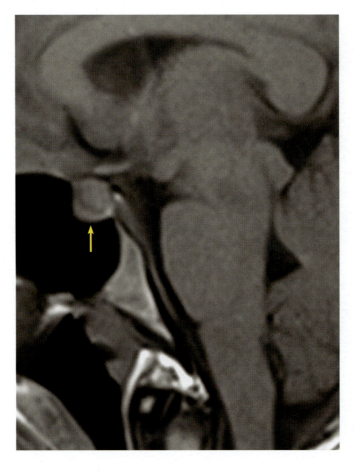

FINDINGS:

Sagittal T1-weighted MR shows an enlarged pituitary gland (arrow) that fills the sella turcica and bulges into the suprasellar region.

DIFFERENTIAL DIAGNOSIS:

- Venous congestion
- Pituitary hyperplasia
- Pituitary tumor
- Pituitary inflammation
- Normal variant

DISCUSSION:

Pituitary size and height vary widely with age, gender, and hormonal status. Pseudoenlargement of the gland can occur with a shallow sella or medialization of the cavernous ICAs. Pituitary hyperplasia is common in patients with elevated hormonal activity. At imaging, there is convex bulging of the gland with homogeneous enhancement. Pituitary cysts and nonfunctioning adenomas ("incidentalomas") can enlarge the gland without symptoms. On dynamic contrast-enhanced MR, these appear as focal nonenhancing or hypoenhancing masses. Pituitary apoplexy, or Sheehan syndrome, refers to acute infarction and/or hemorrhage, usually in association with an underlying adenoma. Other inflammatory and infiltrative processes that enlarge the pituitary gland and/or infundibulum include sarcoidosis, Langerhans cell histiocytosis, lymphocytic hypophysitis, leukemia, lymphoma, and metastases. Rarely, venous congestion from intracranial hypotension (CSF hypovolemia) or a dural arteriovenous fistula can cause pituitary edema.

References:

Argyropoulou MI, Kiortsis DN. MRI of the hypothalamic-pituitary axis in children. *Pediatr Radiol.* 2005;35(11):1045-1055.

Tsunoda A, Okuda O, Sato K. MR height of the pituitary gland as a function of age and sex: especially physiological hypertrophy in adolescence and in climacterium. *AJNR Am J Neuroradiol.* 1997;18(3):551-554.

FIGURE EIGHT, SNOWMAN

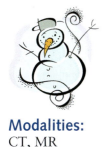

Modalities:
CT, MR

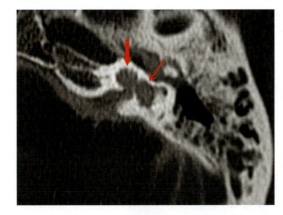
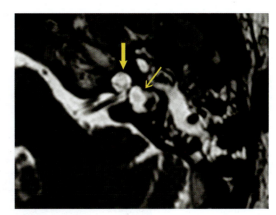

FINDINGS:

Axial CT cisternogram and high-resolution T2-weighted MR of the temporal bone show a bulbous appearance of the cochlea (thick arrows), which consists of a single turn with connection to a dilated vestibule (thin arrows). There is enlargement of the semicircular canals and internal auditory canal. Contrast is seen leaking from the inner ear into the middle ear cavity.

DIAGNOSIS:

Incomplete partition type I (cystic cochleovestibular anomaly)

DISCUSSION:

Cochleovestibular malformations are thought to result from interruptions in inner ear development between the third and seventh weeks of embryogenesis, with earlier insults producing more severe anomalies. Associated findings include enlarged vestibular aqueduct, semicircular canal dysplasia, and cranial nerve deficiency. The spectrum of cochleovestibular abnormalities has been classified by Sennaroglu into six categories. From most to least severe, these are labyrinthine aplasia (Michel deformity), cochlear aplasia, common cavity, incomplete partition type I (cystic cochleovestibular anomaly), cochleovestibular hypoplasia, and incomplete partition type II (Mondini deformity, large endolymphatic sac anomaly). In labyrinthine aplasia, there is complete absence of cochlea and vestibule. In cochlear aplasia, the cochlea is absent and a rudimentary vestibule is present. In common cavity, the cochlea and vestibule are fused into a single large cystic cavity. In IP-I, the cochlea and vestibule are cystic and partially separated, forming a "figure 8" pattern. In cochleovestibular hypoplasia, the cochlea and vestibule are separate and smaller than normal. In IP-II, the cochlea is hypoplastic with a decreased number of turns (classically 1.5), cystic apex (fused middle and apical turns), and deficient modiolus.

References:

Harnsberger HR, Glastonbury CM, Michel MA, et al. *Diagnostic Imaging: Head and Neck*. 2nd ed. Lippincott Williams & Wilkins; 2010.

Sennaroglu L, Saatci I. A new classification for cochleovestibular malformations. *Laryngoscope*. 2002;112(12):2230-2241.

FLAT TIRE, UMBRELLA

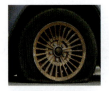

Modalities:
US, CT, MR

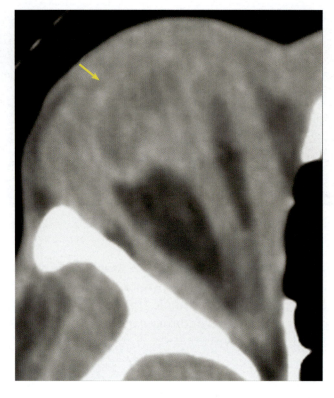

FINDINGS:

Axial CT shows a collapsed and posteriorly flattened right globe (arrow), with intraocular hemorrhage and severe preseptal edema.

DIAGNOSIS:

Scleral rupture

DISCUSSION:

The globes are lined by three concentric coverings: the internal nervous, middle vascular, and external fibrous tunics. The retina contains photoreceptors (rods, cones, and photosensitive ganglion cells) that process light stimuli and send impulses through the optic nerve to the brain. The choroid consists of vascular pigmented connective tissue responsible for nutrition and gas exchange, and forms the uveal tract along with the ciliary body and iris. The sclera is composed of protective fibrous tissue, and is continuous anteriorly with the cornea. Scleral rupture is the most severe form of ocular trauma, and is usually clinically obvious. However, posterior ruptures may be occult and identified on CT as flattening and posterior thickening of the globe ("flat tire" or "umbrella"). Vitreous hemorrhage, intraocular gas, and foreign bodies may also be present. Therapy involves prompt wound closure and ocular reconstruction.

Reference:

Sevel D, Krausz H, Ponder T, et al. Value of computed tomography for the diagnosis of a ruptured eye. *J Comput Assist Tomogr.* 1983;7(5):870-875.

HIGH HEEL FOOTPRINT

Modality:
CT

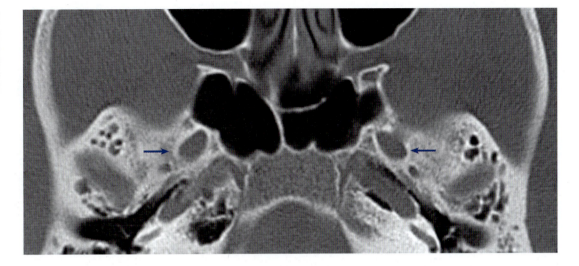

FINDINGS:

Axial CT of the skull base shows the elongated foramina ovale anteromedially (arrows) and the punctate foramina spinosum posterolaterally.

DIAGNOSIS:

Normal foramen ovale and foramen spinosum

DISCUSSION:

The skull base transmits several important neurovascular foramina. Within the greater wing of the sphenoid, the foramen rotundum, ovale, and spinosum are seen from anteromedial to posterolateral. The foramen rotundum has a small rounded shape, courses anteroposteriorly, and contains the maxillary nerve (CN V2). The foramen ovale is large and ovoid, transmitting several structures per the mnemonic "OVALE": otic ganglion, CN V3 (mandibular nerve), accessory meningeal artery, lesser petrosal nerve (of CN IX), and emissary veins. The punctate foramen spinosum, which is adjacent to the foramen ovale, contains the recurrent meningeal nerve, middle meningeal artery, and middle meningeal vein. On axial images, the foramina ovale and spinosum resemble a "high heel footprint."

References:

Barra FR, Gonçalves FG, Matos VL, et al. Signs in neuroradiology—part 2. *Radiol Bras.* 2011;44(2): 129-133.

Ginsberg LE, Pruett SW, Chen MY, et al. Skull-base foramina of the middle cranial fossa: reassessment of normal variation with high-resolution CT. *AJNR Am J Neuroradiol.* 1994;15(2):283-291.

HONEYCOMB, SALT AND PEPPER, STIPPLED

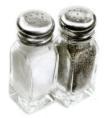

Modalities:
CT, MR

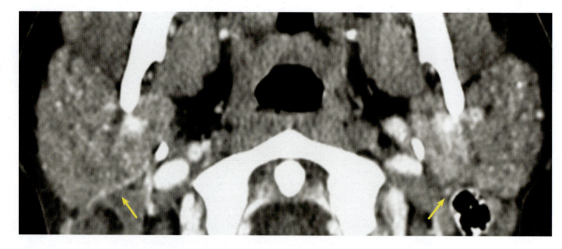

FINDINGS:

Axial contrast-enhanced CT shows heterogeneous enhancement of both parotid glands (arrows), with multiple specks of fat and calcification.

DIAGNOSIS:

Sjögren syndrome

DISCUSSION:

Sjögren (sicca) syndrome is a systemic autoimmune disorder affecting the salivary and lacrimal glands. The primary form occurs in isolation, while the secondary form is seen in conjunction with other autoimmune disorders such as lupus, rheumatoid arthritis, or scleroderma. In the acute phase, the parotid glands appear swollen and edematous. In early subacute disease, numerous lymphoepithelial cysts can be seen in a miliary distribution. In late subacute disease, there is a mixed cystic and solid appearance with calcifications. Discrete nodules in the gland may represent inflammatory pseudomasses (Kuttner tumor, or chronic sclerosing sialadenitis), lymphoid hyperplasia, or lymphoma. In the chronic phase, there is diffuse gland atrophy with fatty replacement and fibrosis. The combination of parotid parenchyma, cysts, calcification, and fat produces a "salt and pepper" appearance on both CT and MR.

References:

Takashima S, Takeuchi N, Morimoto S, et al. MR imaging of Sjögren syndrome: correlation with sialography and pathology. *J Comput Assist Tomogr*. 1991;15(3):393-400.

Yousem DM, Kraut MA, Chalian AA. Major salivary gland imaging. *Radiology*. 2000;216(1):19-29.

HONEYCOMB, SPECKLED, STIPPLED

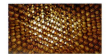

Modality:
CT

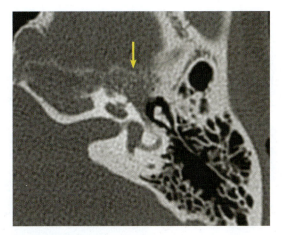

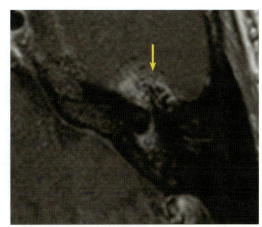

FINDINGS:

- Axial temporal bone CT shows an expansile lytic lesion with punctate sclerotic foci in the perigeniculate region (arrow).
- Axial contrast-enhanced T1-weighted MR shows speckled enhancement with central low-signal foci in the geniculate ganglion (arrow).

DIFFERENTIAL DIAGNOSIS:

- Facial nerve venous malformation
- Geniculate ganglion meningioma

DISCUSSION:

Facial nerve venous malformation (previously known as ossifying hemangioma) is a benign developmental vascular lesion of CN VII that frequently occurs in the region of the geniculate ganglion, and rarely in the internal auditory canal. These are avidly enhancing, irregular masses that induce reactive changes in the surrounding bone, with amorphous "honeycomb" matrix and high-density flecks or spicules. Geniculate ganglion meningiomas are rare tumors that arise from ectopic arachnoid cell rests. As they grow, they tend to infiltrate the temporal bone with a permeative and sclerotic appearance. Facial nerve schwannomas are tubular masses that smoothly enlarge the facial nerve canal. Perineural spread of malignancy shows contiguous enlargement and enhancement of CN VII, extending proximally through the stylomastoid foramen.

References:

Curtin HD, Jensen JE, Barnes L Jr, et al. "Ossifying" hemangiomas of the temporal bone: evaluation with CT. *Radiology.* 1987;164(3):831-835.

Mijangos SV, Meltzer DE. Case 171: facial nerve hemangioma. *Radiology.* 2011;260(1):296-301.

ICE CREAM CONE

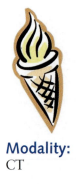

Modality:
CT

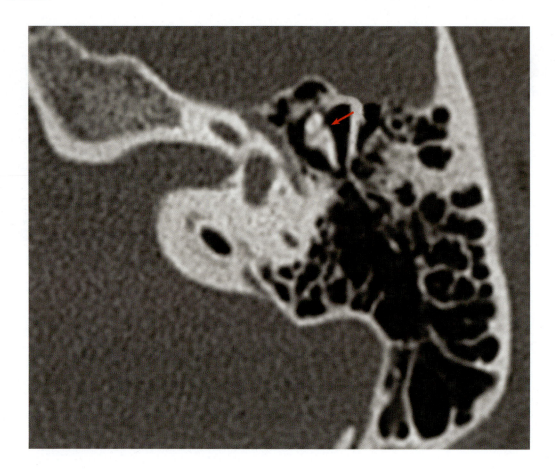

FINDINGS:

Axial temporal bone CT shows a normal incudomalleal joint (arrow), with the head of the malleus articulating with the body of the incus.

DIAGNOSIS:

Normal incus-malleus configuration

DISCUSSION:

The auditory ossicles are a chain of movable bones in the middle ear, which transmit vibrations from the external auditory canal to the inner ear. The malleus (Latin for "hammer") consists of a head, neck, lateral process, anterior process, and manubrium. The manubrium (Latin for "handle") contacts the tympanic membrane at its lateral margin. The oval head of the malleus ("ice cream") articulates posteriorly with the body of the incus ("cone"). The incus (Latin for "anvil") consists of a body, short process, long process, and lenticular process. The stapes (Latin for "stirrup") consists of a head, neck, anterior and posterior crura, and a base (footplate) that articulates directly with the oval window.

Reference:

Gray H. *Anatomy of the Human Body*. Bartleby; 1918.

ICE CREAM CONE, MUSHROOM, TRUMPET, TAIL

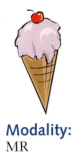

Modality:
MR

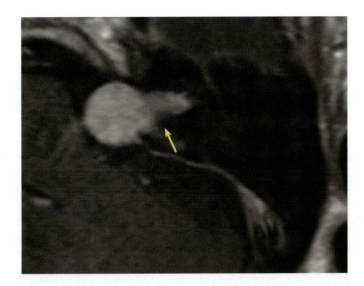

FINDINGS:

Axial contrast-enhanced T1-weighted MR shows an enhancing mass extending from the left cerebellopontine angle through the porus acousticus (arrow) into the internal auditory canal.

DIAGNOSIS:

Vestibular schwannoma

DISCUSSION:

Vestibular schwannomas (acoustic neuromas) are benign Schwann cell tumors arising from the vestibular portion of CN VIII at the glial-Schwann cell junction. Small intracanalicular schwannomas may appear as ovoid or cylindrical masses with punctate enhancement in the internal auditory canal. Larger lesions can fill the cerebellopontine angle and IAC, bulging through the porus acousticus ("ice cream cone" sign). Cystic change is common, while hemorrhage and calcification are rare in untreated tumors. Patients present with unilateral sensorineural hearing loss, for which stereotactic radiosurgery is the recommended therapy. If surgery is planned, a middle cranial fossa approach can be used for small intracanalicular masses to preserve CN VII and VIII. A suboccipital (retrosigmoid) or translabyrinthine approach is required to access CPA and deep IAC locations. Bilateral vestibular schwannomas should suggest the diagnosis of neurofibromatosis type II (MISME: multiple inherited schwannomas, meningiomas, and ependymomas). The differential for cerebellopontine angle masses is wide and includes schwannoma, meningioma, epidermoid cyst, arachnoid cyst, metastasis, aneurysm, and lipoma. Facial nerve schwannomas have a similar appearance within the IAC, but can extend peripherally into the labyrinthine segment and geniculate ganglion of CN VII ("dumbbell" lesion). Meningiomas are usually dural-based, eccentric to the porus acousticus, and may be calcified. Epidermoid cysts have an insinuating "cauliflower" morphology with reduced diffusion. Arachnoid cysts are well marginated and follow the intensity of CSF. Metastases are enhancing and multifocal. Aneurysms occur along the course of the vertebrobasilar circulation and follow blood pool signal. Lipomas follow fat signal on all sequences.

References:

Silk PS, Lane JI, Driscoll CL. Surgical approaches to vestibular schwannomas: what the radiologist needs to know. *Radiographics.* 2009;29(7):1955-1970.

Smirniotopoulos JG, Yue NC, Rushing EJ. Cerebellopontine angle masses: radiologic-pathologic correlation. *Radiographics.* 1993;13(5):1131-1147.

INFUNDIBULUM, PITUITARY STALK DEVIATION/TILT

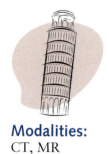

Modalities:
CT, MR

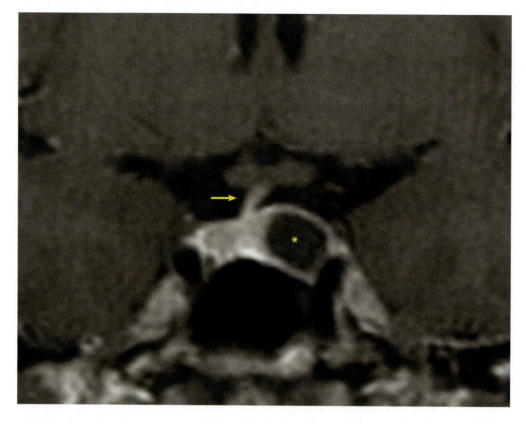

FINDINGS:

Coronal contrast-enhanced T1-weighted MR shows a hypoenhancing mass in the left pituitary gland (asterisk), with contralateral infundibular deviation (arrow).

DIFFERENTIAL DIAGNOSIS:

- Sellar mass
- Normal variant

DISCUSSION:

The pituitary stalk (infundibulum) connects the hypothalamus to the posterior pituitary gland (neurohypophysis). It carries neurosecretory axons down to the posterior pituitary, where the hormones oxytocin and vasopressin (antidiuretic hormone) are released into the blood. In the presence of sellar enlargement, visualization of a midline infundibulum extending to the sellar floor is compatible with the diagnosis of an empty sella. Deviation of the infundibulum to one side suggests displacement by a pituitary cyst or mass, though normal patients can have a small degree of tilt.

References:

Ahmadi H, Larsson EM, Jinkins JR. Normal pituitary gland: coronal MR imaging of infundibular tilt. *Radiology.* 1990;177(2):389-392.

Haughton VM, Rosenbaum AE, Williams AL et al. Recognizing the empty sella by CT: the infundibulum sign. *AJR Am J Roentgenol.* 1981;136(2):293-295.

INVERTED V, PENCIL TIP, STEEPLE

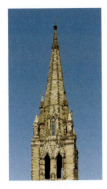

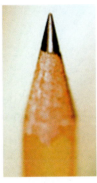

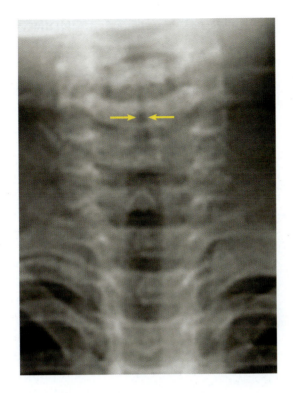

Modalities:
XR, CT

FINDINGS:

Frontal radiograph shows tracheal wall edema with loss of the lateral convexities and smooth symmetric subglottic narrowing (arrows).

DIFFERENTIAL DIAGNOSIS:

- Croup
- Bacterial tracheitis

DISCUSSION:

Croup (acute laryngotracheobronchitis) refers to viral airway inflammation, usually caused by parainfluenza or respiratory syncytial virus, and seen in children between 6 months and 3 years of age. There is diffuse tracheal wall edema, with loss of the normal lateral convexities ("shoulders") of the true vocal cords. Below the vocal cords, smooth symmetric luminal narrowing produces the characteristic "steeple" shape. This can cause proximal obstruction with dilation of the hypopharynx and laryngeal ventricles. Treatment is supportive and the condition is self-limiting. In contrast, bacterial tracheitis is an aggressive infection that occurs in older children (6-10 years) who present with toxic symptoms. Subglottic airway narrowing is also present, but tends to be more irregular and asymmetric. Additional causes of the steeple sign are epiglottitis, thermal injury, and angioedema. Therefore, clinical evaluation is key for diagnosis.

Reference:

Salour M. The steeple sign. *Radiology.* 2000;216(2):428-429.

KISSING CHOROID, LENTIFORM

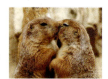

Modalities:
US, CT, MR

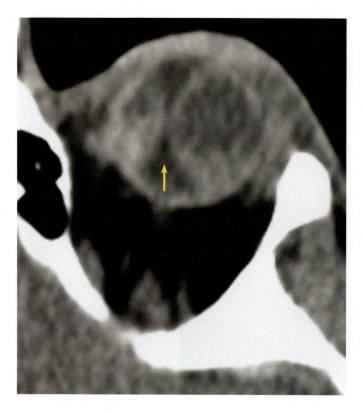

FINDINGS:

Axial CT shows hemorrhagic choroidal detachment along the medial and lateral walls of the globe, with contact in the midline (arrow).

DIAGNOSIS:

Choroidal detachment

DISCUSSION:

The globes are lined by three concentric coverings: the internal nervous, middle vascular, and external fibrous tunics. The retina contains photoreceptors (rods, cones, and photosensitive ganglion cells) that process light stimuli and send impulses through the optic nerve to the brain. The choroid consists of vascular pigmented connective tissue, which is responsible for nutrition and gas exchange and forms the uveal tract along with the ciliary body and iris. The sclera is composed of protective fibrous tissue and is continuous anteriorly with the cornea. Choroidal detachment refers to separation of the choroid from the sclera, due to either fluid transudation (serous) or trauma with rupture of choroidal vessels (hemorrhagic). The uveal tract is anchored anteriorly at the scleral spur and posteriorly by the posterior ciliary vessels. Therefore, fluid fills zones of loose attachment along the medial and lateral walls of the globe, known as the suprachoroidal space. In severe cases, the detached leaves can contact each other in the midline ("kissing" appearance). Therapy includes topical corticosteroids, cycloplegics, mydriatics, and intraocular pressure-lowering drugs. Suprachoroidal paracentesis is performed in medically refractory cases.

References:

Berrocal T, de Orbe A, Prieto C, et al. US and color Doppler imaging of ocular and orbital disease in the pediatric age group. *Radiographics.* 1996;16(2):251-272.

Mafee MF, Peyman GA. Retinal and choroidal detachments: role of magnetic resonance imaging and computed tomography. *Radiol Clin North Am.* 1987;25(3):487-507.

KISSING TONSILS, STRIATED, TIGROID

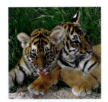

Modalities:
CT, MR

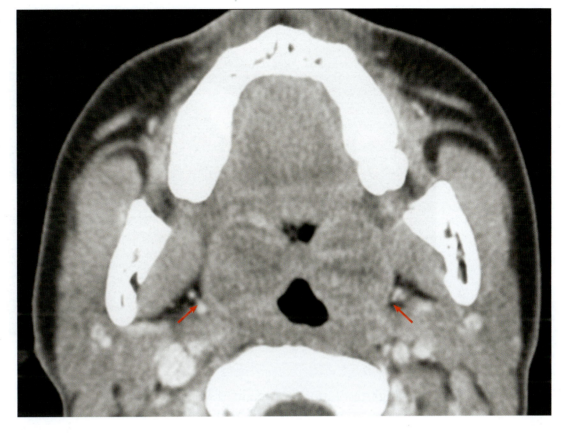

FINDINGS:

Axial contrast-enhanced CT shows enlarged kissing palatine tonsils (arrows) with striated enhancement.

DIAGNOSIS:

Tonsillitis

DISCUSSION:

Tonsillitis and peritonsillar abscesses are the most common deep neck infections in adolescents and young adults. Causative organisms include β-hemolytic *Streptococcus*, *Staphylococcus aureus*, *Pneumococcus*, *Haemophilus influenzae*, and Epstein-Barr virus. On CT, the tonsils appear enlarged with linear striated enhancement ("tigroid" appearance). Intervening areas of hypodensity suggest edema and suppurative changes; true intratonsillar abscesses are rare. However, infection that penetrates the tonsillar capsule can produce a peritonsillar abscess and require drainage.

Reference:

Capps EF, Kinsella JJ, Gupta M, et al. Emergency imaging assessment of acute, nontraumatic conditions of the head and neck. *Radiographics.* 2010;30(5):1335-1352.

LOOP

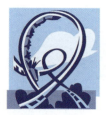

Modality:
MR

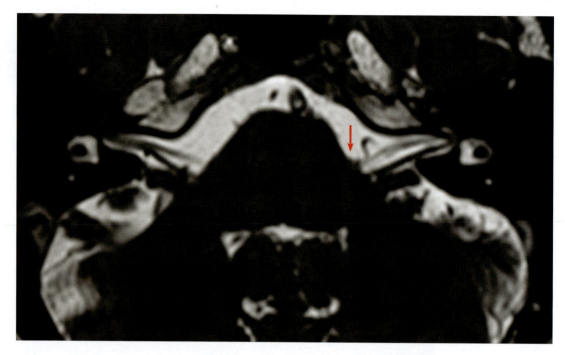

FINDINGS:

Axial high-resolution T2-weighted MR in a patient with left hemifacial spasm shows bilateral tortuous AICAs, contacting the CN VII root entry zone on the left (arrow).

DIAGNOSIS:

Neurovascular compression syndrome

DISCUSSION:

Neurovascular compression syndrome refers to abnormal contact between an intracranial vessel and cranial nerve at the root entry/exit zone or CNS segment. At imaging, a tortuous vascular "loop" or aneurysm may be identified. Involvement of cranial nerves V, VII, VIII, and IX has been associated with trigeminal neuralgia, hemifacial spasm, vestibular paroxysmia, and glossopharyngeal neuralgia, respectively. Treatment options include neuropathic medications, microvascular decompression with placement of a spacer between the nerve and blood vessel, and direct neurectomy or rhizotomy. For hemifacial spasm, superficial injections of botulinum toxin can provide temporary relief.

References:

De Ridder D, Møller A, Verlooy J, et al. Is the root entry/exit zone important in microvascular compression syndromes? *Neurosurgery.* 2002;51(2):427-433.

Langner S, Schroeder HW, Hosten N, et al. Diagnosing neurovascular compression syndromes. *Rofo.* 2012;184(3):220-228.

LYRE, OMEGA, SPLAYED

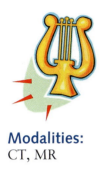

Modalities:
CT, MR

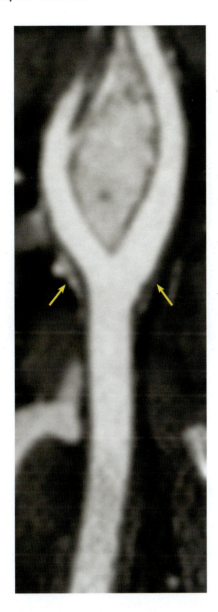

FINDINGS:

Sagittal contrast-enhanced CT shows an avidly enhancing carotid bifurcation mass, splaying the ICA and ECA (arrows).

DIAGNOSIS:

Carotid body tumor

DISCUSSION:

Glomus tumors (paragangliomas, chemodectomas, glomangiomas) are neuroendocrine neoplasms in the head and neck region originating from paraganglia. Lesions are frequently multiple and occur in characteristic locations: carotid body (glomus caroticum or carotid body tumor), middle ear (glomus tympanicum), jugular foramen (glomus jugulare), vagus nerve (glomus vagale), and facial nerve canal (glomus faciale). The carotid body is located at the carotid bifurcation and detects variations in oxygen, carbon dioxide, pH, and temperature levels. Carotid body tumors (CBTs) characteristically splay the carotid bifurcation ("lyre" sign). As they grow, they encase but do not narrow the ICA and ECA. Due to their hypervascularity, CBTs show avid contrast enhancement. On CT, large tumors (> 1-2 cm) demonstrate hyperdense areas signifying enhancement or calcification ("salt"), and hypodense areas suggesting necrosis ("pepper"). On MR, there are T1-hyperintense foci representing hemorrhage or slow flow ("salt"), and T2-hypointense foci due to high-velocity arterial flow voids and calcification ("pepper"). Because glomus tumors are frequently multiple, somatostatin receptor scintigraphy with indium-111 octreotide can help confirm the diagnosis and detect additional lesions.

References:

Olsen WL, Dillon WP, Kelly WM, et al. MR imaging of paragangliomas. *AJR Am J Roentgenol.* 1987;148(1):201-204.

Rao AB, Koeller KK, Adair CF. From the archives of the AFIP. Paragangliomas of the head and neck: radiologic-pathologic correlation. Armed Forces Institute of Pathology. *Radiographics.* 1999;19(6):1605-1632.

MOLAR TOOTH

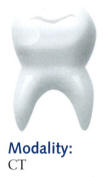

Modality:
CT

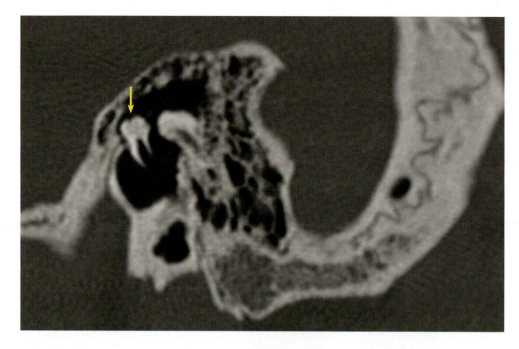

FINDINGS:

Temporal bone CT double-oblique sagittal MPR shows the incudomalleal joint (arrow), malleus manubrium anteriorly, and the long process of the incus posteriorly.

DIAGNOSIS:

Normal incus-malleus configuration

DISCUSSION:

In the early days of polytomography, lateral projections of the temporal bone depicted the combined outline of the incus and malleus, resembling a "molar tooth" with the head of the malleus and the body of the incus forming the "crown," the incudomalleal joint forming a central "saddle," the malleus manubrium forming the "anterior root," and the long process of the incus forming the "posterior root." On temporal bone CT, axial and coronal images do not optimally depict the long axes of the malleus and incus, which are oriented posteromedially. The double-oblique sagittal MPR recreates the polytomographic lateral view of the incudomalleal joint, while the double-oblique coronal MPR visualizes the malleus and incudostapedial joint. Loss of the normal "molar tooth" appearance can be caused by cholesteatoma with ossicular erosions, traumatic dislocation, and congenital anomalies.

References:

Lane JI, Lindell EP, Witte RJ, et al. Middle and inner ear: improved depiction with multiplanar reconstruction of volumetric CT data. *Radiographics.* 2006;26(1):115-124.

Potter GD. The lateral projection in tomography of the petrous pyramid. *Am J Roentgenol Radium Ther Nucl Med.* 1968;104(1):194-200.

MOUSTACHE

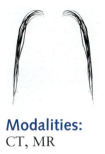

Modalities:
CT, MR

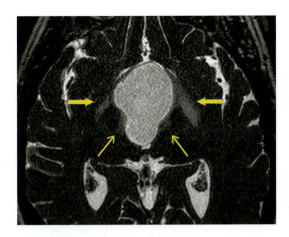
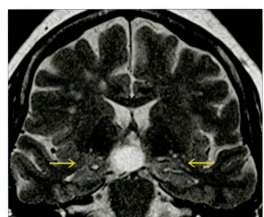

FINDINGS:

Axial and coronal T2-weighted MR show a complex sellar/suprasellar cystic mass with adjacent edema in the posterior limbs of the internal capsules (thick arrows) and optic tracts (thin arrows).

DIAGNOSIS:

Pituitary region mass (craniopharyngioma)

DISCUSSION:

Craniopharyngioma is a benign (WHO grade I) neoplasm, derived from the Rathke pouch epithelium that gives rise to the anterior pituitary gland. The adamantinomatous type usually occurs in children, and is the most common pediatric intracranial tumor of nonglial origin. At imaging, it appears as a mixed cystic and solid mass in the sellar/suprasellar region. Both the solid components and cyst walls enhance avidly. Cysts are intrinsically T1-hyperintense due to "machinery oil"-like cholesterol, protein, and blood contents. Dense calcifications are also common. The papillary type of craniopharyngioma, which is less frequent, occurs in adults and has a primarily solid composition. Craniopharyngiomas can grow to very large sizes, extending into the suprasellar region and cranial fossae. Mass effect on the diencephalon produces a characteristic "moustache" pattern of edema in the hypothalami, optic tracts, and posterior limbs of the internal capsules. White matter fibers in these structures are densely packed and fairly resistant to edema. However, large tumors can compress the Virchow-Robin spaces and block drainage of interstitial fluid. This phenomenon is most commonly described in craniopharyngioma, but can also occur with other sellar/suprasellar lesions including pituitary macroadenoma, germ cell tumor, meningioma, lymphoma, and metastases.

References:

Higashi S, Yamashita J, Fujisawa H, et al. "Moustache" appearance in craniopharyngiomas: unique magnetic resonance imaging and computed tomographic findings of perifocal edema. *Neurosurgery.* 1990;27(6):993-996.

Saeki N, Uchino Y, Murai H, et al. MR imaging study of edema-like change along the optic tract in patients with pituitary region tumors. *AJNR Am J Neuroradiol.* 2003;24(3):336-342.

OMEGA

Modalities:
CT, MR

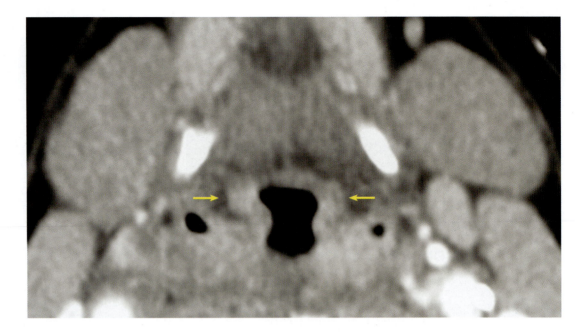

FINDINGS:

Axial contrast-enhanced CT shows a thickened and curled epiglottis (arrows).

DIAGNOSIS:

Laryngomalacia

DISCUSSION:

Laryngomalacia refers to inward collapse of the epiglottis during inhalation, due to cartilage deficiency and/or neuromuscular weakness. Shortening of the aryepiglottic folds results in tight curling of the epiglottis over the airway. Infantile laryngomalacia usually resolves as the child matures, but severe cases can be treated with supraglottoplasty, epiglottopexy, and/or tracheostomy.

Reference:

Prescott CA. The current status of corrective surgery for laryngomalacia. *Am J Otolaryngol.* 1991;12(4):230-235.

PANDA

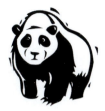

Modality:
NM

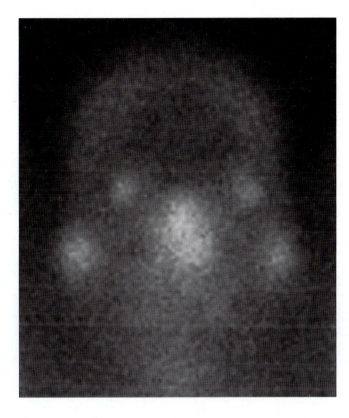

FINDINGS:

Anterior planar ^{67}Ga-citrate scan shows tracer uptake in the lacrimal glands, parotid glands, and nasopharynx.

DIFFERENTIAL DIAGNOSIS:

- Sarcoidosis
- Malignancy
- Collagen vascular disorder
- Renal disease
- AIDS

DISCUSSION:

Gallium-67 scanning is used to identify sites of inflammation and infection, and was the gold standard for cancer staging prior to the emergence of positron emission tomography (PET). A common application is in sarcoidosis, a systemic inflammatory disease characterized histologically by noncaseating granulomas. Within the face, symmetric uptake in the lacrimal and salivary glands is superimposed on normal nasopharyngeal uptake, giving the appearance of a "panda." In the chest, the "lambda" sign refers to uptake in right paratracheal and bilateral hilar lymph nodes. Less common causes of the "panda" sign include malignancy (lymphoma, leukemia, carcinoma); collagen vascular disorders (Sjögren syndrome, lupus, scleroderma, rheumatoid arthritis); renal disease; and AIDS.

References:

Kurdziel KA. The panda sign. *Radiology*. 2000;215(3):884-885.

Sulavik SB, Spencer RP, Weed DA, et al. Recognition of distinctive patterns of gallium-67 distribution in sarcoidosis. *J Nucl Med*. 1990;31(12):1909-1914.

PARALLEL LINES, TWO DASHES

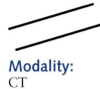

Modality:
CT

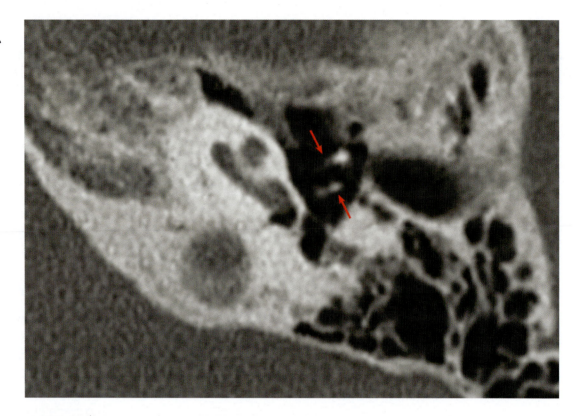

FINDINGS:

Axial temporal bone CT shows parallel orientation of the tensor tympani and malleus neck anteriorly; and the lenticular process of the incus, incudostapedial joint, and stapes superstructure posteriorly (arrows).

DIAGNOSIS:

Normal auditory ossicles

DISCUSSION:

Axial temporal bone CT normally demonstrates two parallel lines in the middle ear. The anterior line is formed by the tensor tympani and malleus neck. The posterior line is formed by the lenticular process of the incus, incudostapedial joint, and stapes superstructure. Defects in the posterior line may be observed in patients with cholesteatoma and ossicular erosions.

Reference:

Swartz JD, Loevner LA. *Imaging of the Temporal Bone.* 4th ed. New York: Thieme; 2008.

PATCHY, TUFT

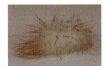

Modality:
MR

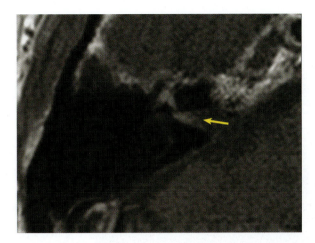

FINDINGS:

Axial contrast-enhanced T1-weighted MR shows patchy enhancement in the distal meatal (arrow), labyrinthine, and proximal tympanic segments of the right facial nerve.

DIFFERENTIAL DIAGNOSIS:

- Bell palsy
- Infection/inflammation
- Demyelination
- Lymphoma

DISCUSSION:

The facial nerve has seven segments, which from central to peripheral are the intraaxial (brainstem), cisternal (cerebellopontine angle), canalicular/meatal (internal auditory canal), labyrinthine (internal auditory canal to geniculate ganglion), tympanic (geniculate ganglion to pyramidal eminence), mastoid (pyramidal eminence to stylomastoid foramen), and extracranial (distal to stylomastoid foramen). The geniculate ganglion, tympanic, and mastoid segments can normally enhance because of their rich circumneural vascular plexus. However, enhancement of the distal intrameatal and labyrinthine segments is pathologic and presents clinically with facial nerve palsy. It has been theorized that the decreased caliber of the facial canal in the premeatal and midtympanic regions predisposes to inflammation between these segments ("bottleneck" theory of Fisch). The most common etiology is Bell palsy, which is idiopathic and self-limited. Imaging is unnecessary for diagnosis, but reveals patchy "tuftlike" enhancement. Other causes of facial nerve enhancement include infection (viral, bacterial, fungal); inflammation (sarcoid); demyelination; trauma; benign tumors (hemangioma, schwannoma); and malignant tumors (lymphoma, metastases, perineural spread).

References:

Fisch U, Esslen E. Total intratemporal exposure of the facial nerve. *Arch Otolaryngol.* 1972;95:335-341.

Kinoshita T, Ishii K, Okitsu T, et al. Facial nerve palsy: evaluation by contrast-enhanced MR imaging. *Clin Radiol.* 2001;56(11):926-932.

POSTERIOR PITUITARY BRIGHT SPOT

Modality:
MR

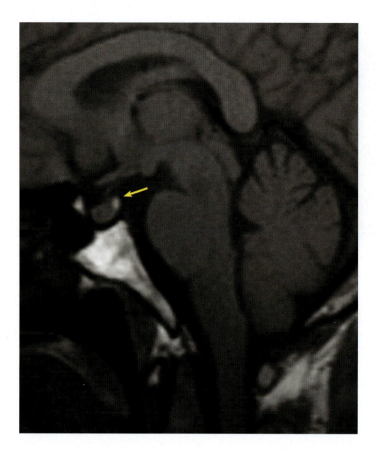

FINDINGS:

Sagittal T1-weighted MR shows normal hyperintensity of the posterior pituitary (arrow).

DIAGNOSIS:

Normal posterior pituitary

DISCUSSION:

The posterior pituitary gland (neurohypophysis) is connected to the hypothalamus via the pituitary stalk (infundibulum) and produces the hormones oxytocin and vasopressin (antidiuretic hormone). In the majority of normal individuals, the posterior pituitary demonstrates T1-hyperintense signal due to the presence of neurosecretory granules containing ADH, neurophysin/copeptin proteins, and phospholipid membranes. Absence of this finding should prompt a search for an ectopic posterior pituitary gland, an important cause of infundibuloneurohypophyseal dysfunction. Displacement or absence of the "bright spot" can also occur because of infiltration/compression by a sellar mass or enlarged CSF space (empty sella). Occasionally, the anterior pituitary (adenohypophysis) can also appear T1-hyperintense because of hormonal hypersecretion. This is typically seen in newborns and pregnant, postpartum, or lactating women.

References:

Bonneville F, Cattin F, Marsot-Dupuch K, et al. T1 signal hyperintensity in the sellar region: spectrum of findings. *Radiographics*. 2006;26(1):93-113.

Kurokawa H, Fujisawa I, Nakano Y, et al. Posterior lobe of the pituitary gland: correlation between signal intensity on T1-weighted MR images and vasopressin concentration. *Radiology*. 1998;207(1):79-83.

REVERSE CUPPING

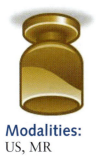

Modalities:
US, MR

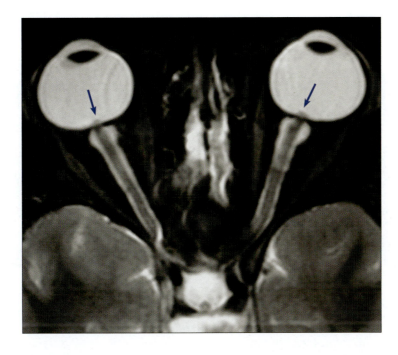

FINDINGS:

Axial T2-weighted MR shows bilateral tortuous and fluid-filled optic nerve sheaths, flattened posterior sclerae, and abnormal protrusion of the optic discs (arrows) into the globes.

DIAGNOSIS:

Papilledema

DISCUSSION:

Papilledema refers to optic disc swelling caused by increased intracranial pressure. The optic nerve sheaths are continuous with the intracranial subarachnoid space. When under increased pressure, they become dilated and tortuous. Severe cases produce edema of the optic nerve heads with reduced diffusion and/or enhancement, inversion/protrusion of the optic discs ("reverse cupping"), and flattening of the posterior sclerae. Unilateral papilledema suggests ipsilateral orbital pathology. In rare cases, a frontal lobe tumor can compress the adjacent optic nerve and raise intracranial pressure, producing ipsilateral optic nerve atrophy with contralateral papilledema (Foster-Kennedy syndrome). Bilateral papilledema indicates increased intracranial pressure, which may be idiopathic (pseudotumor cerebri) or secondary hemorrhage, tumor, infection, or arterial/venous ischemia. Prompt treatment of the underlying cause is crucial, as longstanding papilledema leads to denervation and permanent visual impairment.

Reference:

Passi N, Degnan AJ, Levy LM. MR imaging of papilledema and visual pathways: effects of increased intracranial pressure and pathophysiologic mechanisms. *AJNR Am J Neuroradiol.* 2012 Mar 15.

RICE KERNEL

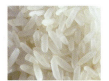

Modalities:
XR, CT

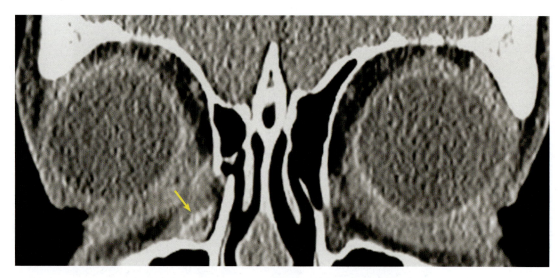

FINDINGS:

Coronal CT shows a calcified dacryolith (arrow) impacted in the right nasolacrimal duct, with surrounding edema.

DIAGNOSIS:

Dacryolithiasis

DISCUSSION:

Dacryolithiasis is a complication of chronic dacryocystitis, usually with fungal colonization. Over time, mineralized proteins and debris accumulate in the lacrimal sac and/or nasolacrimal duct. This is difficult to identify on conventional radiographs, and much better seen on CT with a calcified "rice kernel" appearance. Dacryocystography identifies round or oval filling defects within the nasolacrimal duct. Treatment involves surgical removal, often with balloon dacryocystoplasty or dacryocystorhinostomy.

Reference:

Asheim J, Spickler E. CT demonstration of dacryolithiasis complicated by dacryocystitis. *AJNR Am J Neuroradiol.* 2005;26(10):2640-2641.

ROSE THORN

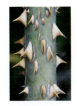

Modalities:
CT, MR

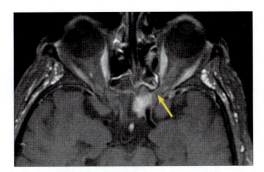 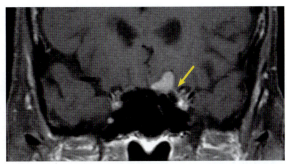

FINDINGS:

Axial and coronal contrast-enhanced T1-weighted MR with fat saturation show an enhancing left parasellar mass that extends along the left sulcus chiasmaticus into the optic nerve canal (arrows).

DIAGNOSIS:

Intracanalicular optic nerve meningioma

DISCUSSION:

Perioptic (optic nerve sheath) meningiomas are benign tumors arising from the arachnoid cap cells in the optic nerve sheath. They may arise within the orbit (optic nerve sheath meningioma), optic nerve canal (intracanalicular meningioma), or optic foramen (foraminal meningioma). Intracanalicular meningiomas can demonstrate a "rose-thorn" appearance with proximal nodular component and en plaque extension along the optic groove (sulcus chiasmaticus), orbital apex, and optic nerve canal. Distinction from optic neuritis (inflammation of the optic nerve) is key, as patients present with early visual loss due to nerve compression in the anatomically limited orbital apex.

Reference:

Jackson A, Patankar T, Laitt RD. Intracanalicular optic nerve meningioma: a serious diagnostic pitfall. *AJNR Am J Neuroradiol.* 2003;24(6):1167-1170.

SAIL

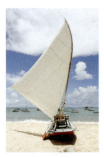

Modalities:
CT, MR

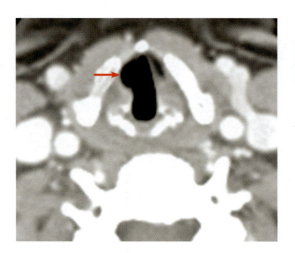

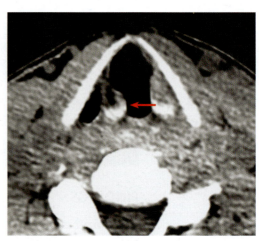

FINDINGS:

- Axial contrast-enhanced CT shows enlargement of the right laryngeal ventricle (arrow).
- Axial contrast-enhanced CT in a different patient shows enlargement of the right laryngeal ventricle and piriform sinus, with medialization of the aryepiglottic fold (arrow).

DIAGNOSIS:

Vocal cord paralysis

DISCUSSION:

Vocal cord paralysis results from injury or compression of the vagus nerve (CN X) anywhere between the medulla and the recurrent laryngeal branches. CN X originates from the medulla, traverses the jugular foramen, and descends down the neck within the carotid sheath. On the right, it extends to the clavicle and recurs around the right subclavian artery; on the left, it extends into the mediastinum and recurs via the aortopulmonary window. The recurrent laryngeal nerves then ascend to the larynx within the tracheoesophageal grooves. In cases of suspected vocal cord paralysis, contrast-enhanced CT with coverage from skull base to carina is the imaging examination of choice. The paralyzed cord is flaccid and may be fixed in a medial or lateral position. Imaging signs include ballooning of the laryngeal ventricle ("sail" sign), enlargement of the pyriform sinus, medial displacement and thickening of the aryepiglottic fold, anteromedial rotation of the arytenoid cartilage, and atrophy of the posterior cricoarytenoid muscle. On PET, the denervated cord shows absent uptake compared to the normal contralateral cord. Therapeutic options include voice therapy, vocal cord augmentation with temporary or permanent injectables, and laryngeal framework surgery (medialization thyroplasty, arytenoid adduction, and laryngeal re-innervation).

References:

Chin SC, Edelstein S, Chen CY, et al. Using CT to localize side and level of vocal cord paralysis. *AJR Am J Roentgenol.* 2003;180(4):1165-1170.

Kumar VA, Lewin JS, Ginsberg LE. CT assessment of vocal cord medialization. *AJNR Am J Neuroradiol.* 2006;27(8):1643-1646.

SALT AND PEPPER

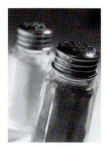

Modalities:
CT, MR

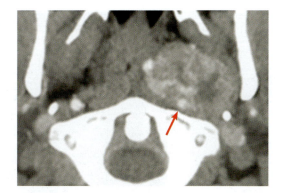
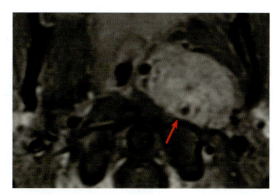

FINDINGS:

Axial contrast-enhanced CT and contrast-enhanced T1-weighted MR with fat saturation show a heterogeneous and avidly enhancing mass in the left carotid space (arrows).

DIAGNOSIS:

Glomus vagale

DISCUSSION:

Glomus tumors (paragangliomas, chemodectomas, glomangiomas) are neuroendocrine neoplasms in the head and neck region originating from paraganglia. Lesions are frequently multiple and occur in characteristic locations: carotid body (glomus caroticum or carotid body tumor), middle ear (glomus tympanicum), jugular foramen (glomus jugulare), vagus nerve (glomus vagale), and facial nerve canal (glomus faciale). Because of their hypervascularity, glomus tumors show avid contrast enhancement. On CT, large tumors (>1-2 cm) demonstrate hyperdense areas signifying enhancement or calcification ("salt"), and hypodense areas suggesting necrosis ("pepper"). On MR, there are T1-hyperintense foci representing hemorrhage or slow flow ("salt"), and T2-hypointense foci due to high-velocity arterial flow voids and calcification ("pepper"). Permeative and destructive changes may be present in the surrounding bone. Other vascular lesions, such as hypervascular schwannomas and metastases, can occasionally have a similar appearance. Because glomus tumors are frequently multiple, somatostatin receptor scintigraphy with indium-111 octreotide can help confirm the diagnosis and detect additional lesions.

References:

Eldevik OP, Gabrielsen TO, Jacobsen EA. Imaging findings in schwannomas of the jugular foramen. *AJNR Am J Neuroradiol.* 2000;21(6):1139-1144.

Olsen WL, Dillon WP, Kelly WM, et al. MR imaging of paragangliomas. *AJR Am J Roentgenol.* 1987;148(1):201-204.

Rao AB, Koeller KK, Adair CF. From the archives of the AFIP. Paragangliomas of the head and neck: radiologic-pathologic correlation. Armed Forces Institute of Pathology. *Radiographics.* 1999;19(6):1605-1632.

SANDWICH, TRAM TRACK

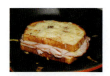
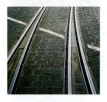

Modalities:
US, CT, MR

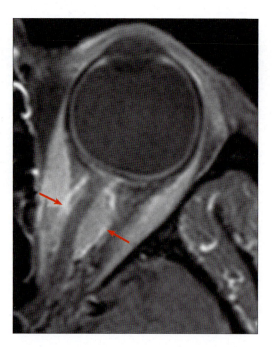
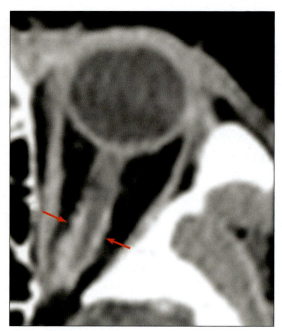

FINDINGS:

- Axial contrast-enhanced T1-weighted MR with fat saturation shows an enhancing mass (arrows) encasing the optic nerve.
- Axial noncontrast CT in a different patient shows linear calcifications along the optic nerve sheath (arrows).

DIAGNOSIS:

Perioptic meningioma

DISCUSSION:

Perioptic meningiomas are benign tumors arising from the arachnoid cap cells in the optic nerve sheath. These may arise within the orbit (optic nerve sheath meningioma), optic nerve canal (intracanalicular meningioma), or optic foramen (foraminal meningioma). Three distinct morphologies have been described: tubular, exophytic, and fusiform. The tubular form symmetrically surrounds and compresses the optic nerve, with associated enhancement and/or calcification. This gives rise to the "doughnut" sign en face and the "tram-track" sign in long axis. In contrast, optic gliomas are infiltrative tumors that are intimately associated with the optic nerve. Other causes of perioptic enhancement include orbital pseudotumor, infection, sarcoidosis, leukemia/lymphoma, and metastases.

References:

Jackson A, Patankar T, Laitt RD. Intracanalicular optic nerve meningioma: a serious diagnostic pitfall. *AJNR Am J Neuroradiol.* 2003;24(6):1167-1170.

Kanamalla US. The optic nerve tram-track sign. *Radiology.* 2003;227(3):718-719.

SITTING DUCK

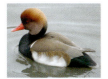

Modalities:
CT, MR

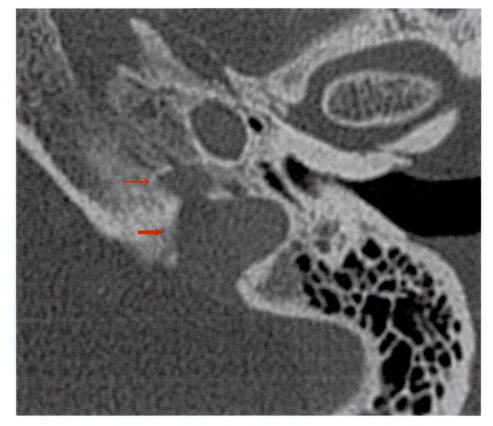

FINDINGS:

Axial temporal bone CT shows the normal jugular foramen with smaller anteromedial pars nervosa (thin arrow) and larger posterolateral pars vascularis (thick arrow).

DIAGNOSIS:

Normal jugular foramen

DISCUSSION:

The jugular foramen is located on the medial and inferior surface of the petrous pyramid, which is formed by the temporal and occipital bones. It consists of two divisions that are separated by a fibrous or bony septum ("sitting duck" appearance). The smaller pars nervosa is located anteromedially, and houses the inferior petrosal sinus and glossopharyngeal nerve (CN IX). The larger pars vascularis is located posterolaterally and contains the jugular bulb, as well as the vagus and spinal accessory nerves (CN X and XI). The wall of the jugular fossa is smooth and well corticated, with small dehiscences for the tympanic branch of the glossopharyngeal nerve (Jacobson nerve) and auricular branch of the vagus nerve (Arnold nerve).

Reference:

Caldemeyer KS, Mathews VP, Azzarelli B, et al. The jugular foramen: a review of anatomy, masses, and imaging characteristics. *Radiographics.* 1997;17(5):1123-1139.

SNAKE EYES

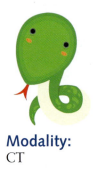

Modality:
CT

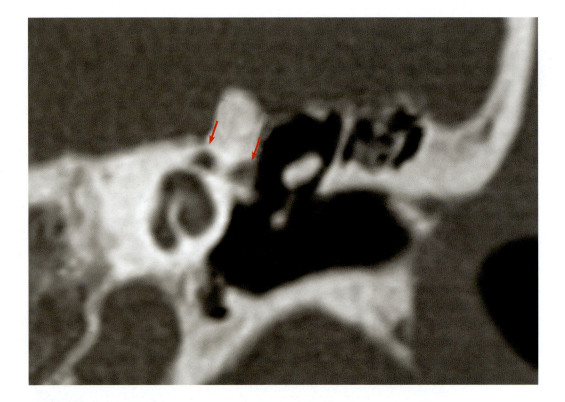

FINDINGS:

Coronal temporal bone CT intersects the facial nerve at the labyrinthine segment superomedially and the tympanic segment inferolaterally (arrows).

DIAGNOSIS:

Normal facial nerve

DISCUSSION:

The facial nerve is a mixed cranial nerve with motor, parasympathetic, and sensory branches. It originates in the brainstem nuclei, courses through the temporal bone and parotid gland, and innervates the face. The major segments are intraaxial, cisternal (cerebellopontine angle), canalicular/meatal (internal auditory canal), labyrinthine (internal auditory canal to geniculate ganglion), tympanic (geniculate ganglion to pyramidal eminence), mastoid (pyramidal eminence to stylomastoid foramen), and extracranial (distal to stylomastoid foramen). Coronal CT through the cochlea, just anterior to the internal auditory canal, intersects the facial nerve in two areas. This produces the characteristic "snake eyes" appearance, with the labyrinthine segment superomedially and the tympanic segment inferolaterally. More anteriorly, these two segments converge to the geniculate ganglion.

Reference:

Swartz JD, Loevner LA. *Imaging of the Temporal Bone*. 4th ed. New York: Thieme; 2008.

TEARDROP

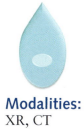

Modalities:
XR, CT

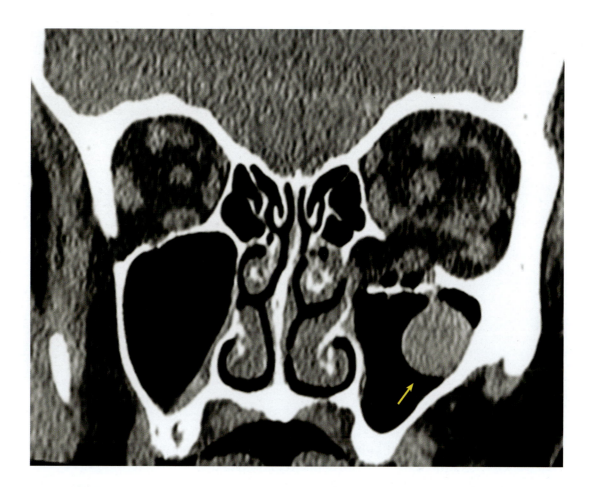

FINDINGS:

Coronal CT shows a left orbital blowout fracture with herniation of inferior rectus and periorbital fat (arrow) into the maxillary sinus.

DIAGNOSIS:

Orbital blowout fracture

DISCUSSION:

Blowout fractures, the most common fractures of the orbit, are caused by direct trauma to the globe or upper eyelid. The orbital floor is most commonly fractured, followed by the medial wall. The "teardrop" sign refers to prolapse of periorbital fat and/or orbital contents into the maxillary sinus. Complications to identify at imaging include extraocular muscle herniation and entrapment, hemorrhage, globe injury, and infraorbital nerve injury.

Reference:

Winegar BA, Murillo H, Tantiwongkosi B. Spectrum of critical imaging findings in complex facial skeletal trauma. *Radiographics*. 2013;33(1):3-19.

THIRD WINDOW

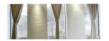

Modality:
CT

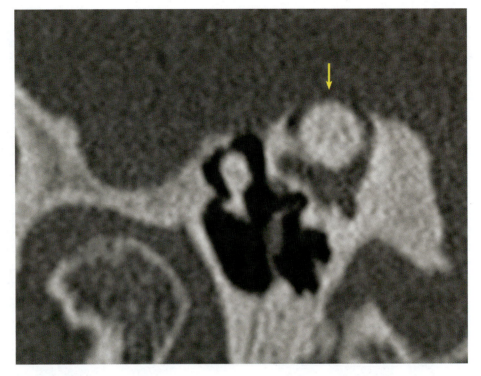

FINDINGS:

Temporal bone CT MPR, Pöschl plane, shows a large defect (arrow) in the roof of the right superior semicircular canal.

DIAGNOSIS:

Superior semicircular canal dehiscence

DISCUSSION:

Third window abnormalities are defects in the bony structure of the inner ear, forming a superfluous communication with the middle ear in addition to the physiologic oval and round windows. Classic clinical findings including sound/pressure-induced vertigo (Tullio/Hennebert signs), a low-frequency air-bone gap at audiometry, and decreased thresholds for vestibular evoked myogenic potentials (VEMPs). Superior semicircular canal dehiscence, or loss of the bony roof of the semicircular canal, is the prototypical example of third window pathology. This is best identified on temporal bone CT with multiplanar reconstruction in the Pöschl plane, parallel to the superior semicircular canal. The third window phenomenon has also been described in posterior semicircular canal dehiscence, carotid-cochlear dehiscence, perilabyrinthine fistula, enlarged vestibular aqueduct, and X-linked stapes gusher.

References:

Merchant SN, Rosowski JJ. Conductive hearing loss caused by third-window lesions of the inner ear. *Otol Neurotol.* 2008;29(3):282-289.

Minor LB, Solomon D, Zinreich JS, et al. Sound- and/or pressure-induced vertigo due to bone dehiscence of the superior semicircular canal. *Arch Otolaryngol Head Neck Surg.* 1998;124:249-258.

THUMB

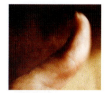

Modalities:
CT, MR

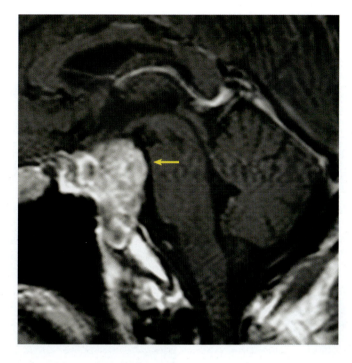

FINDINGS:

Sagittal contrast-enhanced T1-weighted MR shows an exophytic enhancing clival mass that indents the pons (arrow).

DIFFERENTIAL DIAGNOSIS:

- Notochordal lesion
- Chondrosarcoma

DISCUSSION:

Notochordal remnants are present in the midline spheno-occipital synchondrosis and may proliferate along the dorsal wall of the clivus into the prepontine cistern. From least to most aggressive, the spectrum of notochordal retroclival lesions includes ecchordosis physaliphora (EP), benign notochordal cell tumor (BNCT), and malignant chordoma. EP is classically small and T2-hyperintense with a bony pedicle, no enhancement, and no mass effect. BNCT has an intermediate appearance, with variable enhancement and mass effect. Chordomas are large and expansile with soft tissue components, heterogeneous "honeycomb" enhancement, and bone destruction. Classic chordomas are T2-hyperintense with reduced diffusion due to myxoid stroma. Poorly differentiated chordomas may be T2-hypointense and show even more reduced diffusion. In contrast to notochordal lesions, chondrosarcoma is a malignant mesenchymal tumor that tends to occur off midline at the petro-occipital (petroclival) synchondrosis. This tumor also appears T2-hyperintense with heterogeneous enhancement. However, "arc and ring" mineralization on CT and increased (rather than reduced) diffusion on MR may be identified, because of the cartilaginous stroma.

References:

Golden LD, Small JE. Benign notochordal lesions of the posterior clivus: retrospective review of prevalence and imaging characteristics. *J Neuroimaging.* 2013 Mar 6.

Mehnert F, Beschorner R, Küker W, et al. Retroclival ecchordosis physaliphora: MR imaging and review of the literature. *AJNR Am J Neuroradiol.* 2004;25(10):1851-1855.

Yeom KW, Lober RM, Mobley BC, et al. Diffusion-weighted MRI: distinction of skull base chordoma from chondrosarcoma. *AJNR Am J Neuroradiol.* 2012 Nov 1.

THUMB(PRINT), VALLECULA

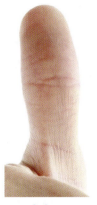

Modalities:
XR, CT

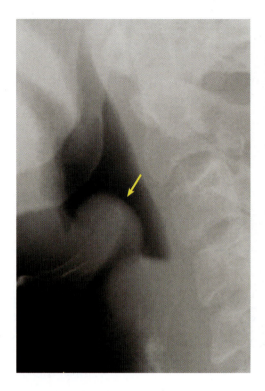

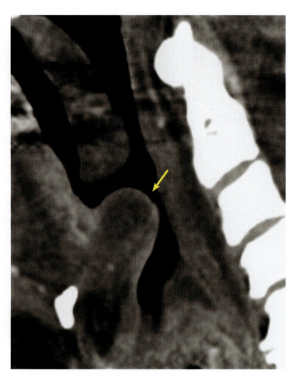

FINDINGS:

Lateral radiograph and sagittal CT show epiglottic enlargement and edema (arrows), with obscuration of the vallecula.

DIAGNOSIS:

Epiglottitis

DISCUSSION:

The epiglottis is a small flap of cartilage that projects over the glottis (vocal folds) and closes over the trachea during swallowing to prevent aspiration. On lateral radiographs, the normal epiglottis has a thin appearance likened to a "little finger." Acute epiglottitis can be caused by infection with *Haemophilus influenzae* or *Streptococci*. The epiglottis becomes severely swollen and edematous, resembling a "thumb." In addition, there is loss of definition of the epiglottic vallecula behind the root of tongue.

References:

Ducic Y, Hébert PC, MacLachlan L, et al. Description and evaluation of the vallecula sign: a new radiologic sign in the diagnosis of adult epiglottitis. *Ann Emerg Med.* 1997;30(1):1-6.

Podgore JK, Bass JW. Letter: The "thumb sign" and "little finger sign" in acute epiglottitis. *J Pediatr.* 1976;88(1):154-155.

ABSENCE OF FLOW VOIDS

Modality:
MR

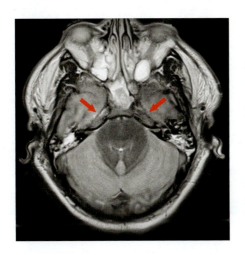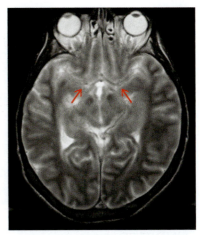

FINDINGS:

Axial T2-weighted MR shows absent flow voids and abnormal hyperintense intraluminal signal in the ICAs (thick arrows), ACAs, and MCAs (thin arrows).

DIAGNOSIS:

Brain death

DISCUSSION:

Accurate diagnosis of brain death is necessary prior to discontinuing life support in a comatose patient, particularly when organ donation is being considered. Clinical examination is only reliable in the absence of hypothermia, barbiturates, sedatives, and hypnotics. If the diagnosis is unclear, imaging examinations such as nuclear medicine, CT, MR, or angiography may be helpful. Contrast-enhanced imaging reveals absence of intracranial perfusion above the level of the skull base. On T2-weighted MR, intermediate-signal intraluminal thrombus replaces the normal signal voids seen with high-velocity arterial flow ("absence of flow voids"). Care must be taken to distinguish absent flow from very slow flow within the cerebral arteries and/or veins. Additional imaging signs include diffuse cerebral edema with obscuration of gray-white differentiation, as well as downward transtentorial and tonsillar herniation. Increased collateral flow to the ECA may result in nasal and scalp enhancement ("MR hot nose" sign).

Reference:

Ishii K, Onuma T, Kinoshita T, et al. Brain death: MR and MR angiography. *AJNR Am J Neuroradiol.* 1996;17(4):731-735.

ARROW

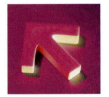

Modality:
CT

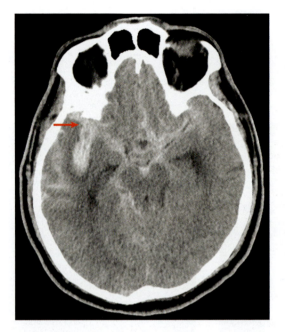
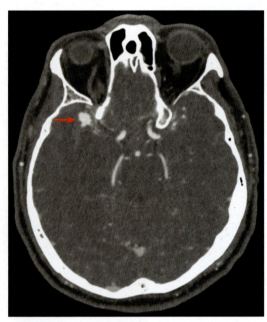

FINDINGS:

- Axial CT shows diffuse subarachnoid hemorrhage concentrated in the right sylvian fissure (arrow).
- Axial CTA shows a ruptured right MCA bifurcation aneurysm (arrow).

DIAGNOSIS:

Ruptured MCA bifurcation aneurysm

DISCUSSION:

The middle cerebral artery is divided into four major segments. The M1 (sphenoidal or horizontal) segment originates from the ICA and bifurcates into superior and inferior divisions. The M2 (insular) segment begins at the MCA bifurcation, coursing laterally and anteriorly to the margin of the insula. The M3 (opercular) segment begins at the circular sulcus of the insula, then loops and curves over the frontal and temporal opercula to reach the surface of the sylvian fissure. The M4 (cortical or terminal) segment consists of various branches that course over the cerebral convexity and supply the cortex. When MCA bifurcation aneurysms rupture, the resulting subarachnoid hemorrhage can track along the ipsilateral sylvian fissure and outline the frontotemporal operculum, producing an "arrow" sign.

References:

Fossett DT, Caputy AJ, eds. *Operative Neurosurgical Anatomy*. New York: Thieme; 2002.

Maramattom BV, Wijdicks EF. Arrow sign in MCA trifurcation aneurysm. *Neurology*. 2004;63(7):1323.

ARTERIAL HYPERINTENSITY, (CENTRAL) DOT, (HYPER) DENSE ARTERY, HYPERINTENSE VESSEL, SUSCEPTIBILITY

Modalities:
CT, MR

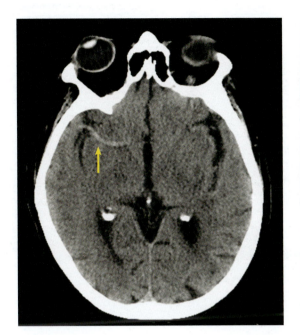
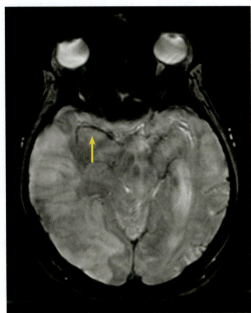

FINDINGS:

- Axial noncontrast CT shows a hyperdense right MCA (arrow).
- Axial SWI MR shows intraluminal susceptibility (arrow), compatible with thrombus. There is cytotoxic edema in the right temporal and occipital lobes.

DIAGNOSIS:

Arterial infarct

DISCUSSION:

Cerebral arterial slow flow and occlusion produce increased attenuation within the arterial lumen, yielding a "hyperdense artery" sign in long axis or "central dot" en face. This is the earliest CT sign of arterial ischemia and is best appreciated in the MCA, with a lower detection rate in the vertebrobasilar arteries, ICA, ACA, and PCA. On MR, arterial thrombus produces intraluminal hyperintensity on FLAIR and T2-weighted sequences ("hyperintense vessel" sign), as well as hypointensity on SWI ("susceptibility" sign). Mimics include elevated hematocrit ("diffuse hyperdense intracranial circulation"), mural calcifications in atherosclerosis, and cerebral edema or atrophy with relatively hypodense brain parenchyma.

References:

Koo CK, Teasdale E, Muir KW. What constitutes a true hyperdense middle cerebral artery sign? *Cerebrovasc Dis.* 2000;10(6):419-423.

Makkat S, Vandevenne JE, Verswijvel G, et al. Signs of acute stroke seen on fluid-attenuated inversion recovery MR imaging. *AJR Am J Roentgenol.* 2002;179(1):237-243.

Shinohara Y, Kinoshita T, Kinoshita F. Changes in susceptibility signs on serial T2*-weighted single-shot echo-planar gradient-echo images in acute embolic infarction: comparison with recanalization status on 3D time-of-flight magnetic resonance angiography. *Neuroradiology.* 2012;54(5):427-434.

ATTENUATED/DENSE SINUS/VEIN, CORD, TRAM TRACK

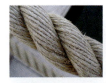

Modalities:
CT, MR

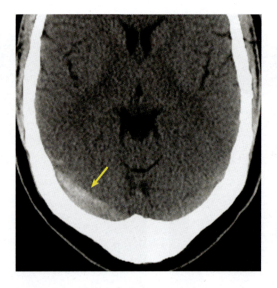

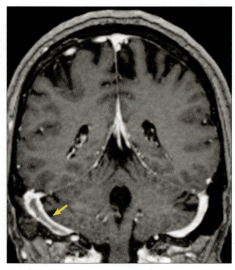

FINDINGS:

- Axial noncontrast CT shows a curvilinear hyperdensity in the expected region of the right transverse sinus (arrow).
- Coronal contrast-enhanced T1-weighted MR shows nonocclusive centralized thrombus outlined by contrast in the right transverse sinus (arrow).

DIAGNOSIS:

Cerebral venous thrombosis

DISCUSSION:

Cerebral venous thrombosis is a rare and frequently misdiagnosed condition that can affect the dural venous sinuses, deep veins, and superficial veins. Risk factors include young age, dehydration, sinusitis, pregnancy, various medications (oral contraceptives, steroids), trauma or surgery, intracranial hypotension or hypertension, hematologic and autoimmune disorders, malignancy, and other hypercoagulable states. Newly formed thrombus may be appreciated on noncontrast CT as a "cordlike" hyperdensity in the expected region of the sinus or vein. Subacute thrombus demonstrates variable hyperintensity on T1-weighted MR and hypointensity on T2-weighted and SWI MR. Contrast-enhanced images may demonstrate a "tram track" sign with contrast outlining a centralized filling defect. Dedicated CTV or MRV should be performed to confirm the diagnosis and evaluate the extent of disease. In the acute setting, prompt correction of the underlying cause is indicated with consideration for anticoagulation, as untreated cerebral venous thrombosis can progress to venous infarction and hemorrhage. In addition, chronic venous thrombosis can be complicated by dural arteriovenous fistula (dAVF) formation.

Reference:

Rizzo L, Crasto SG, Rudà R, et al. Cerebral venous thrombosis: role of CT, MRI and MRA in the emergency setting. *Radiol Med.* 2010;115(2):313-325.

BAG OF WORMS, HONEYCOMB, SERPENTINE, SOAP BUBBLE, TANGLE

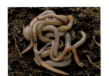

Modalities:
XA, CT, MR

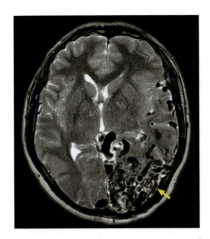
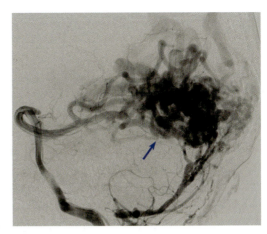

FINDINGS:

- Axial T2-weighted MR shows multiple serpiginous flow voids centered in the left temporal and occipital lobes (arrow), with associated mass effect.
- Left vertebral artery angiogram, lateral projection, identifies the large nidus (arrow), with early arterial enhancement and superficial venous drainage.

DIAGNOSIS:

Arteriovenous malformation

DISCUSSION:

Arteriovenous malformation (AVM) is a high-flow vascular malformation characterized by abnormal arteriovenous shunting without an intervening capillary bed. Communication can occur through either a nidus (tangle of abnormal vessels) or a direct fistulous communication (forming a pial arteriovenous fistula). The nidus can be glomerular (compact) or diffuse (proliferative) with interspersed brain parenchyma. At imaging, the nidus has a tortuous "bag of worms" appearance, with early arterial enhancement and venous drainage. Characteristics that increase the risk of rupture include feeding artery or intranidal aneurysms, venous ectasias, and venous stenoses. Complications include hemorrhage, infarction, seizures, and hydrocephalus. Treatment options include radiation, transcatheter embolization, and surgical resection. Operative outcome correlates with the Spetzler-Martin grading system, which evaluates nidus size (1 point: < 3 cm, 2 points: 3-6 cm, 3 points: > 6 cm); venous drainage (0 points: superficial, 1 point: deep); and eloquence of adjacent brain (0 points: non-eloquent, 1 point: eloquent). Spetzler-Martin grades range from 1 to 5, with 6 being reserved for non-operative candidates. Multiple AVMs can be seen in cerebrofacial arteriovenous metameric syndrome (Wyburn-Mason syndrome, Bonnet-Dechaume-Blanc disease) and hereditary hemorrhagic telangiectasia (Osler-Weber-Rendu syndrome).

Reference:

Geibprasert S, Pongpech S, Jiarakongmun P, et al. Radiologic assessment of brain arteriovenous malformations: what clinicians need to know. *Radiographics*. 2010;30(2):483-501.

BERRY

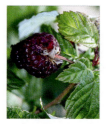

Modalities:
XA, CT, MR

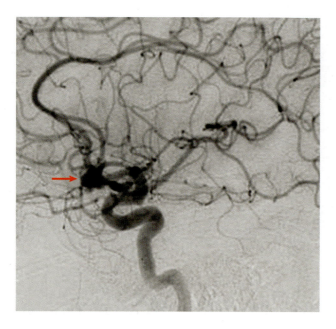

FINDINGS:

ICA angiogram, lateral projection, shows an anteriorly directed ACOM aneurysm (arrow).

DIAGNOSIS:

Berry aneurysm

DISCUSSION:

The majority of intracranial aneurysms are small saccular ("berry") aneurysms that develop at major arterial branch points, where there is thinning of the internal elastic lamina and tunica media. Characteristic locations include the distal ICA, ACOM, PCOM, MCA bifurcation, basilar tip, SCA, and PICA. Multiple cerebral aneurysms are seen in association with various acquired and congenital disorders including hypertension, hyperlipidemia, vasculitis, drug abuse, connective tissue disorders, autosomal dominant polycystic kidney disease, neurofibromatosis type I, tuberous sclerosis, hereditary hemorrhagic telangiectasia (Osler-Weber Rendu syndrome), Klippel-Trenaunay-Weber syndrome, and alpha-1-antitrypsin (AAT_1) deficiency. The main cause of morbidity and mortality is aneurysm rupture, which depends on several factors including aneurysm size, morphology, and location; underlying etiology; and patient comorbidities. Ruptured aneurysms should be treated emergently. For unruptured aneurysms, definitive therapy (endovascular therapy or surgical clipping) should be considered for sizes exceeding 7 mm and location within the posterior fossa, because of the significantly increased risk of rupture.

Reference:

Hacein-Bey L, Provenzale JM. Current imaging assessment and treatment of intracranial aneurysms. *AJR Am J Roentgenol.* 2011;196(1):32-44.

BERRY, MULBERRY, POPCORN (BALL), STONE

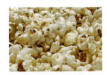

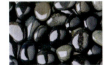

Modalities:
CT, MR

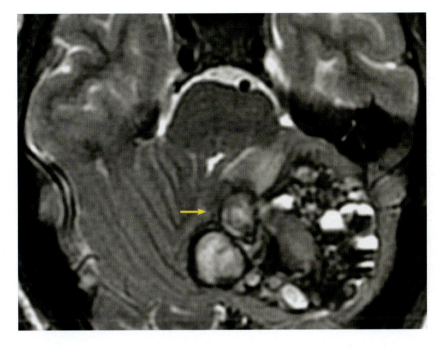

FINDINGS:

Axial T2-weighted MR shows a multiloculated left cerebellar lesion (arrow) with associated fluid-blood levels, peripheral hemosiderin, and vasogenic edema. Superficial siderosis is also noted along the cerebellar folia and pons.

DIAGNOSIS:

Giant cavernoma

DISCUSSION:

Cavernous malformations (angiomas, cavernomas, cavernous hemangiomas) are slow-flow vascular malformations consisting of capillary/cavernous spaces and vascular sinusoids without intervening brain parenchyma. They are angiographically occult or "cryptic" lesions, due to their slow flow. Repeated episodes of hemorrhage produce blood products of various ages, which can be associated with vasogenic edema, fluid-blood levels, and calcification. Over time, hemosiderin is cleared from the center of the lesion and deposited around the periphery, producing a "dark halo" on T2-weighted and SWI MR. Large multiloculated lesions demonstrate a "popcorn ball" appearance, also known as "hemangioma calcificans" or "brain stone." Multiple cavernomas are seen in familial multiple cavernous malformation syndrome, and also occur following cranial irradiation.

References:

Hegde AN, Mohan S, Lim CC. CNS cavernous haemangioma: "popcorn" in the brain and spinal cord. *Clin Radiol.* 2012;67(4):380-388.

Vilanova JC, Barceló J, Smirniotopoulos JG, et al. Hemangioma from head to toe: MR imaging with pathologic correlation. *Radiographics.* 2004;24(2):367-385.

BLACK/DARK HALO, IRON RIM/RING

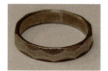

Modality:
MR

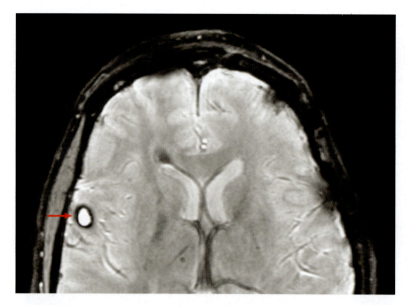

FINDINGS:

Axial SWI MR shows a right perirolandic lesion with peripheral rim of susceptibility (arrow).

DIFFERENTIAL DIAGNOSIS:

- Cavernoma
- Hematoma
- Abscess

DISCUSSION:

Cavernous malformations (angiomas, cavernomas, cavernous hemangiomas) are developmental vascular malformations consisting of capillary/cavernous vascular spaces and sinusoids without intervening brain parenchyma. These are angiographically occult, because of their slow flow. Repeated episodes of microhemorrhage produce blood products of various ages, which can be associated with fluid-blood levels and calcification. Over time, hemosiderin is cleared from the center of the lesion and deposited around the periphery, producing a "dark halo" on T2-weighted and SWI MR. Rarely, other hemorrhagic lesions (hematoma, primary and metastatic tumors, granulomatous disease) may demonstrate a hemosiderin rim, but this tends to be more discontinuous and irregular. Abscesses can also demonstrate a dark rim, which is thought to relate to free radical formation and macrophage activity.

References:

Haimes AB, Zimmerman RD, Morgello S, et al. MR imaging of brain abscesses. *AJR Am J Roentgenol.* 1989;152(5):1073-1085.

Vilanova JC, Barceló J, Smirniotopoulos JG, et al. Hemangioma from head to toe: MR imaging with pathologic correlation. *Radiographics.* 2004;24(2):367-385.

BORDER ZONE

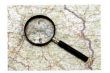

Modalities:
CT, MR

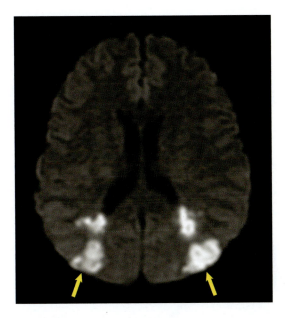
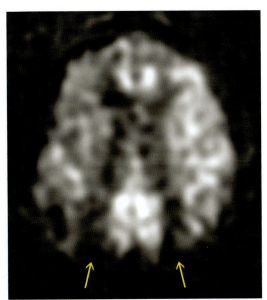

FINDINGS:

- Axial DWI MR shows wedge-shaped areas of reduced diffusion along the bilateral MCA/PCA border zones (thick arrows).
- Axial ASL MR shows signal dropout along the bilateral MCA/PCA border zones (thin arrows), with high signal in the surrounding cortex.

DIAGNOSIS:

External watershed infarct

DISCUSSION:

Watershed (borderland, border zone, boundary zone, end zone, terminal zone) infarcts are caused by decreased perfusion at the boundaries between arterial territories. External (cortical) border zones are located at the junctions of the anterior, middle, and posterior cerebral artery territories. Strokes in these locations are associated with atherosclerosis and microembolism, with or without global hypoperfusion. On DWI MR, multiple ovoid or wedge-shaped areas of reduced diffusion are seen in a watershed distribution. Arterial spin labeling (ASL), a noncontrast MR technique for measuring cerebral perfusion, shows signal dropout in watershed areas. Often, there is high signal in the surrounding cortex, which is thought to represent labeled blood in feeding arteries that has not yet reached the capillary bed ("arterial transit artifact").

Reference:

Zaharchuk G, Bammer R, Straka M, et al. Arterial spin-label imaging in patients with normal bolus perfusion-weighted MR imaging findings: pilot identification of the borderzone sign. *Radiology.* 2009;252(3):797-807.

BOWTIE

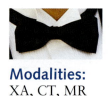

Modalities:
XA, CT, MR

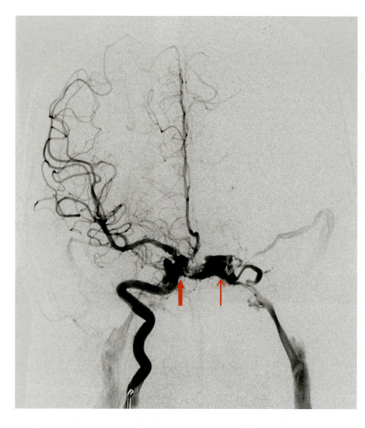

FINDINGS:

Right ICA angiogram, AP projection, shows early opacification of the right cavernous sinus (thick arrow). This communicates across midline with the left cavernous sinus (thin arrow). There is early drainage into the bilateral superior/inferior petrosal sinuses, sigmoid sinuses, and internal jugular veins.

DIAGNOSIS:

Carotid-cavernous fistula

DISCUSSION:

Carotid-cavernous fistula (CCF) is an abnormal communication between the arteries and veins within the cavernous sinus. Predisposing factors include trauma, surgery, pregnancy, aneurysm rupture, connective tissue disorders, atherosclerosis, and infection. Direct CCF refers to a single-hole, high-flow direct communication between the ICA and cavernous sinus. Indirect CCF is a low-flow dural arteriovenous fistula (dAVF) that involves multiple ECA and/or ICA branches. The Barrow classification separates CCF into four types: A = direct CCF, B = indirect CCF with ICA supply, C = indirect CCF with ECA supply, D = indirect CCF with ICA and ECA supply. Angiography is the most sensitive imaging examination and shows early opacification of the ipsilateral cavernous sinus in the arterial phase. Due to communication through anterior and posterior intercavernous sinuses, the contralateral cavernous sinus also enhances, creating a "bowtie" pattern. There is early venous drainage, often through the ipsilateral superior ophthalmic vein. This appears dilated and tortuous with accompanying proptosis, extraocular muscle enlargement, and periorbital edema. Treatment options include conservative management, carotid compression therapy, transcatheter embolization, and surgical repair.

References:

Chen CC, Chang PC, Shy CG, et al. CT angiography and MR angiography in the evaluation of carotid cavernous sinus fistula prior to embolization: a comparison of techniques. *AJNR Am J Neuroradiol.* 2005;26(9):2349-2356.

Ducruet AF, Albuquerque FC, Crowley RW, et al. The evolution of endovascular treatment of carotid cavernous fistulas: a single-center experience. *World Neurosurg.* 2013.

BRUSH

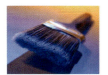

Modalities:
XA, CT, MR

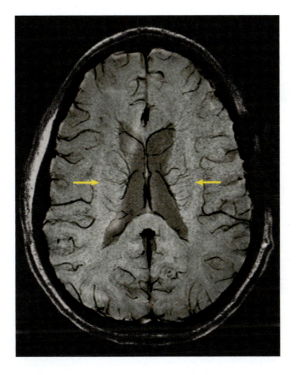

FINDINGS:

Axial SWI MR shows increased size and number of deep medullary veins (arrows).

DIAGNOSIS:

Moyamoya disease

DISCUSSION:

Moyamoya, the Japanese term for "puff of smoke," refers to progressive stenosis/ occlusion of the distal ICAs and proximal ACAs/MCAs with relative sparing of the posterior circulation. The etiology may be idiopathic (moyamoya disease) or secondary (moyamoya syndrome) to various conditions including atherosclerosis, Down syndrome, neurofibromatosis, sickle cell anemia, and connective tissue disorders. Collateral circulation is supplied by basal parenchymal perforators, leptomeningeal branches from the PCA, and transdural vessels from the ECA. Hypertrophy of the deep medullary veins produces the "brush" sign, with multiple parallel vessels that are best seen on SWI MR. Pediatric patients tend to present with cerebral ischemia or infarction, whereas adults can develop infarction or hemorrhage due to rupture of small aneurysms. Surgical procedures are aimed at revascularization and include direct (STA-MCA bypass) or indirect (encephalo-duro-arterio-synangiosis, encephalo-myo-synangiosis, pial synangiosis, omental transplantation) techniques.

Reference:

Horie N, Morikawa M, Nozaki A, et al. "Brush sign" on susceptibility-weighted MR imaging indicates the severity of moyamoya disease. *AJNR Am J Neuroradiol.* 2011;32(9):1697-1702.

BRUSH, DOT, LACE, LATTICE, PAINT, SPECKLED, STIPPLED

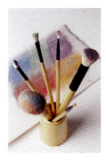

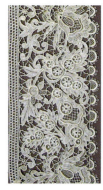

Modality:
MR

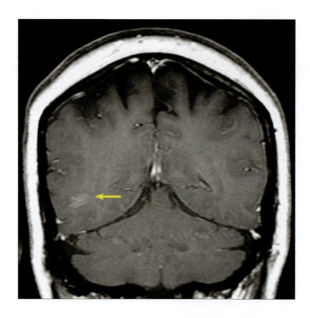

FINDINGS:

Coronal contrast-enhanced T1-weighted MR shows patchy enhancement in the right temporal lobe (arrow).

DIAGNOSIS:

Capillary telangiectasia

DISCUSSION:

Capillary telangiectasia is the second most common vascular anomaly of the central nervous system, following developmental venous anomaly. This is a slow-flow malformation consisting histologically of dilated capillaries with a thin endothelial lining, sometimes accompanied by a dilated draining vein ("dot in the spot" appearance). The intervening brain parenchyma is normal, without mass effect. Lesions are iso- to hypointense on T1-weighted MR, iso- to hyperintense on T2-weighted MR, and hypointense on SWI MR due to the presence of deoxyhemoglobin. On contrast-enhanced T1-weighted MR, there is ill-defined "lattice"-like enhancement. Small capillary telangiectasias are generally asymptomatic and occult on CT or angiography. Larger lesions (over 1 cm) may be symptomatic and complicated by hemorrhage. The majority of capillary telangiectasias occur in the pons, but can also be seen in the cerebrum, cerebellum, and spinal cord. Lesions may be accompanied by other vascular anomalies including DVA, cavernoma, and AVM. Syndromic associations include Osler-Weber-Rendu (hereditary hemorrhagic telangiectasia), Louis-Bar (ataxia-telangiectasia), and Sturge-Weber (encephalotrigeminal angiomatosis).

References:

Lee RR, Becher MW, Benson ML, et al. Brain capillary telangiectasia: MR imaging appearance and clinicohistopathologic findings. *Radiology.* 1997;205(3):797-805.

Sayama CM, Osborn AG, Chin SS, et al. Capillary telangiectasias: clinical, radiographic, and histopathological features. *J Neurosurg.* 2010;113(4):709-714.

CANDELABRA, SYLVIAN POINT, SYLVIAN TRIANGLE

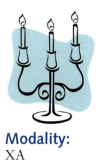

Modality:
XA

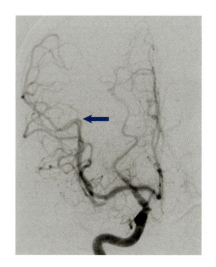

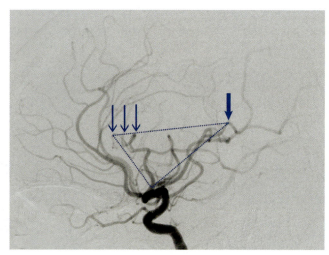

FINDINGS:

Right ICA angiogram, AP and lateral projections, show the angular artery curving to exit the sylvian fissure (thick arrows). The sylvian triangle (dotted lines) is formed by prefrontal arteries (thin arrows), insular loops, and the MCA trunk.

DIAGNOSIS:

Normal MCA

DISCUSSION:

On AP angiography, the "sylvian point" represents the most medial aspect of the highest cortical MCA branch (usually the angular artery). Here, the artery turns anteriorly and inferiorly to exit the sylvian fissure, demarcating the posterior margin of the insula. On lateral angiography, the tops of multiple insular loops form a relatively straight line. This is known as the "superior insular line," and terminates posteriorly at the sylvian point. The operculofrontal (ascending frontal) complex arises from the superior division of the MCA and consists of prefrontal and central sulcus arteries. On lateral angiography, the prefrontal arteries fan out over the frontal operculum, creating a "candelabra" appearance. These supply the middle and inferior frontal gyri, including the Broca area. The inferior insular line connects the base of the most anterior branch of the candelabra to the sylvian point, paralleling the MCA trunk. The "sylvian triangle" is formed superiorly by the superior insular line, anteriorly by the candelabra, and posteroinferiorly by the inferior insular line. Displacements of the sylvian point and triangle are important signs of supratentorial mass effect or volume loss.

References:

Lee SH, Goldberg HI. The normal angiographic sylvian point on the lateral cerebral angiogram. *Neuroradiology.* 1979;17(2):101-103.

Rowbotham GF, Little E. The candelabra arteries and the circulation of the cerebral cortex. *Br J Surg.* 1963;50:694-697.

CAPUT MEDUSAE, CROWN, FAN, (INVERSE) UMBRELLA, MEDUSA HEAD, PALM TREE, SPOKE WHEEL, WEDGE

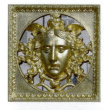

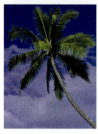

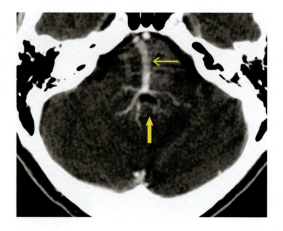

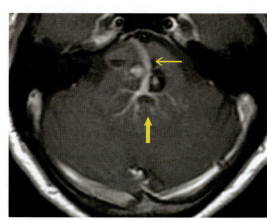

Modalities:
XA, CT, MR

FINDINGS:

Axial contrast-enhanced CT and contrast-enhanced T1-weighted MR show anomalous cerebellar draining veins (thick arrows) that converge toward a common pontine venous trunk (thin arrows). Several associated pontine cavernomas are present, with fluid-blood levels and susceptibility.

DIAGNOSIS:

Developmental venous anomaly

DISCUSSION:

Developmental venous anomaly (DVA), formerly known as venous angioma, is the most common vascular malformation of the central nervous system. This is a slow-flow malformation consisting histologically of dilated and thin-walled veins separated by intervening brain. On venous phase imaging, dilated and radially arranged collecting veins converge toward a common trunk ("Medusa head" or "palm tree" appearance), which drains to either the superficial or deep venous network. Deoxyhemoglobin also produces susceptibility artifact on T2-weighted and SWI MR. The most common locations are the frontal lobe, parietal lobe, and posterior fossa. DVA is usually asymptomatic and should not be resected, as this represents the primary venous drainage pathway for involved brain. There is an association with other vascular malformations including cavernoma, cervicofacial venous malformations, and blue rubber bleb nevus syndrome.

References:

Lee C, Pennington MA, Kenney CM 3rd. MR evaluation of developmental venous anomalies: medullary venous anatomy of venous angiomas. *AJNR Am J Neuroradiol.* 1996;17(1):61-70.

Saba PR. The caput medusae sign. *Radiology.* 1998;207(3):599-600.

CARTWHEEL, LINEAR, RADIAL, SPOKE WHEEL, SUNBURST, TREE ROOT

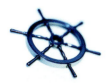

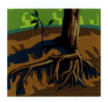

Modalities:
XA, CT, MR

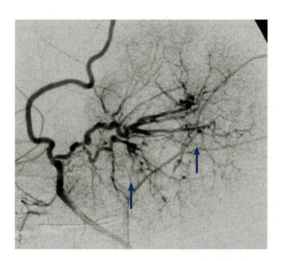

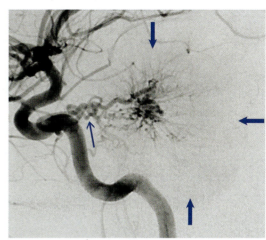

FINDINGS:

- ECA angiography with selective MMA injection, lateral projection, shows arterial tumor blush with radiating feeding vessels (arrows).
- ICA angiography, lateral projection, in a different patient shows tumor blush (thick arrows) with feeding vessels radiating from a central vascular pedicle. Arterial supply is from meningohypophyseal and inferolateral branches of the cavernous ICA (thin arrow).

DIFFERENTIAL DIAGNOSIS:

- Meningioma
- Hemangiopericytoma
- Metastasis

DISCUSSION:

Meningioma is a usually benign extra-axial tumor arising from the arachnoid cap cells of the meninges. Tumors are hypervascular and often derive blood supply from branches of the ECA (particularly the MMA), which course into the center of the lesion. As tumors gradually enlarge, a "sunburst" of hypertrophied arterial branches is seen radiating from the central vascular pedicle. Ultimately, lesions outgrow this blood supply and recruit ICA branches to supply the periphery. In tumors with dual blood supply, ECA angiography classically shows "spoke-wheel" enhancement within the tumor, whereas ICA angiography yields a "doughnut" appearance along the periphery. This angiographic appearance is characteristic of meningioma, but can be seen in other vascular neoplasms such as hemangiopericytoma or metastasis.

Reference:

Manelfe C, Lasjaunias P, Ruscalleda J. Preoperative embolization of intracranial meningiomas. *AJNR Am J Neuroradiol.* 1986;7(5):963-972.

CIGAR, ROSARY, STRING OF PEARLS

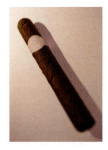

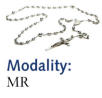

Modality:
MR

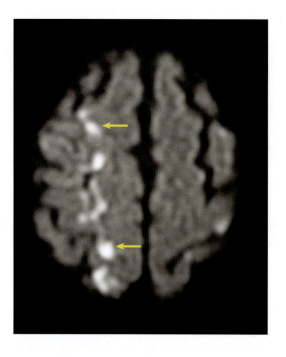

FINDINGS:

Axial DWI MR shows bilateral foci of reduced diffusion, right greater than left. Linearly arranged microinfarcts are seen in the right centrum semiovale (arrows).

DIAGNOSIS:

Internal watershed infarcts

DISCUSSION:

Watershed (borderland, border zone, boundary zone, end zone, terminal zone) infarcts are caused by decreased perfusion at the boundaries between arterial territories. External (cortical) border zones are located at the junctions of the anterior, middle, and posterior cerebral artery territories. Strokes in these locations are associated with atherosclerosis and microembolism, with or without global hypoperfusion. At imaging, they have an ovoid or wedge-shaped appearance. Internal (subcortical) border zones are located at the junctions of the cerebral artery territories with the medial striate, lenticulostriate, and anterior choroidal artery territories. Infarcts in these locations are caused by arterial stenosis/occlusion or hemodynamic compromise, and have a poorer prognosis. At imaging, these are classified as partial or confluent. Partial infarcts appear linearly arranged with a "cigar" or "rosary" appearance, paralleling the lateral ventricle in the centrum semiovale or corona radiata.

References:

Mangla R, Kolar B, Almast J, et al. Border zone infarcts: pathophysiologic and imaging characteristics. *Radiographics.* 2011;31(5):1201-1214.

Moustafa RR, Momjian-Mayor I, Jones PS, et al. Microembolism versus hemodynamic impairment in rosary-like deep watershed infarcts: a combined positron emission tomography and transcranial Doppler study. *Stroke.* 2011;42(11):3138-3143.

CORKSCREW, PSEUDOPHLEBITIC

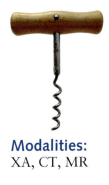

Modalities:
XA, CT, MR

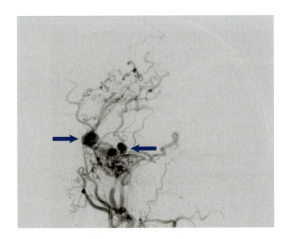
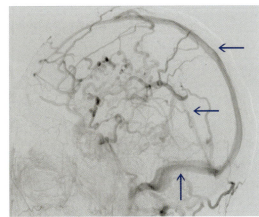

FINDINGS:

- ECA angiogram, arterial phase in the lateral projection, shows early opacification of tortuous collaterals with multifocal dilations (thick arrows).
- Venous phase shows direct shunting into superficial and deep veins, with delayed drainage to the cerebral venous sinuses (thin arrows).

DIAGNOSIS:

Dural arteriovenous fistula

DISCUSSION:

Dural arteriovenous fistula (dAVF) is a pathologic, high-flow shunt between dural arteries and venous sinuses, meningeal veins, and/or cortical veins. The majority are idiopathic, but there is an association with dural venous thrombosis, venous hypertension, prior craniotomy, trauma, and infection. At imaging, tortuous feeding arteries and draining veins produce a "corkscrew" or "pseudophlebitic" pattern. Flow-related aneurysms, venous stenosis, and thrombosis increase the risk of complications, including venous infarction and hemorrhage. Treatment options include radiation, transcatheter embolization, venous angioplasty/stenting, and surgical resection. Prognosis correlates with the Merland-Cognard or Borden classifications. The Merland-Cognard classification consists of 5 categories (I: antegrade drainage into venous sinus, IIa: drainage into and reflux within sinus, IIb: drainage into sinus with reflux into cortical veins, III: cortical venous drainage, IV: cortical venous drainage with ectasia, V: spinal perimedullary venous drainage). The Borden classification includes types of venous drainage (I: anterograde, II: anterograde and retrograde, III: retrograde) and number of fistulae (a: single, b: multiple).

References:

Gandhi D, Chen J, Pearl M, et al. Intracranial dural arteriovenous fistulas: classification, imaging findings, and treatment. *AJNR Am J Neuroradiol.* 2012;33(6):1007-1013.

Gomez J, Amin AG, Gregg L, et al. Classification schemes of cranial dural arteriovenous fistulas. *Neurosurg Clin N Am.* 2012;23(1):55-62.

CORTICAL/INSULAR RIBBON, DISAPPEARING BASAL GANGLIA, LENTIFORM NUCLEUS EDEMA, OBSCURATION OF LENTIFORM NUCLEUS

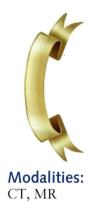

Modalities:
CT, MR

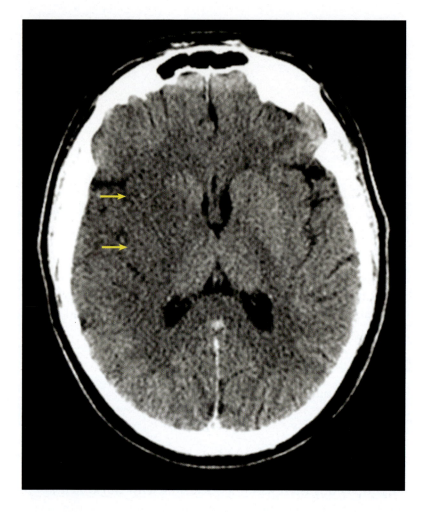

FINDINGS:

Axial CT shows edema of the right insula (arrows), obscuring the adjacent putamen.

DIAGNOSIS:

MCA infarct

DISCUSSION:

The insular cortex is supplied by the insular branches of the middle cerebral artery. When the MCA circulation is occluded, this area effectively becomes a watershed arterial zone distal to the ACA and PCA circulations. Acute insular edema ("insular ribbon") obscures the adjacent basal ganglia and is an early finding of MCA infarction, along with the "dense artery" sign.

Reference:

Truwit CL, Barkovich AJ, Gean-Marton A, et al. Loss of the insular ribbon: another early CT sign of acute middle cerebral artery infarction. *Radiology*. 1990;176(3):801-806.

CRESCENT

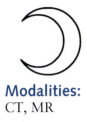

Modalities:
CT, MR

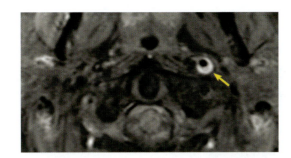 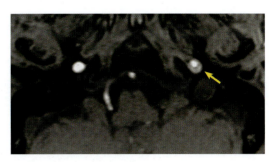

FINDINGS:

- Axial T1-weighted MR with fat saturation shows a hyperintense crescent of hemorrhage (arrow) surrounding the left ICA.
- Axial contrast-enhanced T1-weighted MR with fat saturation shows intermediate-signal thrombus (arrow) surrounding and narrowing the left ICA lumen.

DIAGNOSIS:

ICA dissection

DISCUSSION:

Carotid artery dissection results from a primary intramural hematoma or intimal tear, enabling penetration of blood into the arterial wall. The extracranial portion of the ICA is most commonly affected, due to its greater mobility and proximity to the cervical spine and styloid process. Predisposing conditions include trauma, atherosclerosis, connective tissue disorders, fibromuscular dysplasia, and vasculitis. When thrombosed, the false lumen can compress the true lumen and serve as a nidus for distal embolization. Subacute hemorrhage appears hyperintense on T1-weighted MR with fat saturation, and may produce an eccentric ("crescent") or concentric ("target") morphology. Bilateral ICA dissections have been described with a "puppy eyes" appearance. Patients can present with head or neck pain, Horner syndrome, and anterior circulation ischemia. Treatment options include anticoagulation or antiplatelet therapy, thrombolysis, endovascular angioplasty/ stenting, and surgical reconstruction.

References:

Feddersen B, Linn J, Klopstock T. Neurological picture. "Puppy sign" indicating bilateral dissection of internal carotid artery. *J Neurol Neurosurg Psychiatry*. 2007;78(10):1055.

Rodallec MH, Marteau V, Gerber S, et al. Craniocervical arterial dissection: spectrum of imaging findings and differential diagnosis. *Radiographics*. 2008;28(6):1711-1728.

CUTOFF, MENISCUS

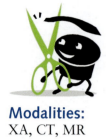

Modalities:
XA, CT, MR

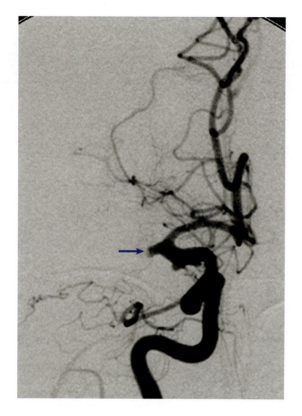

FINDINGS:

Right ICA angiogram, LAO Townes projection, shows abrupt truncation of the proximal right M1 (arrow) with absence of distal MCA opacification.

DIAGNOSIS:

Acute arterial occlusion

DISCUSSION:

Stroke is a leading cause of morbidity and mortality in developed countries. Imaging workup is performed to assess for hemorrhage, identify etiology, and determine appropriate therapy. Ischemic stroke can be embolic or thrombotic in nature. At imaging, arterial occlusion manifests as a sharp vessel cutoff with failure of distal opacification. Acute occlusive emboli appear as convex filling defects outlined by a "meniscus" of contrast. Therapeutic options include intravenous or intraarterial thrombolysis and mechanical thrombectomy.

References:

Hunter GJ, Hamberg LM, Ponzo JA, et al. Assessment of cerebral perfusion and arterial anatomy in hyperacute stroke with three-dimensional functional CT: early clinical results. *AJNR Am J Neuroradiol.* 1998;19(1):29-37.

Srinivasan A, Goyal M, Al Azri F, et al. State-of-the-art imaging of acute stroke. *Radiographics.* 2006;26(Suppl 1):S75-S95.

DAUGHTER SAC, MURPHY

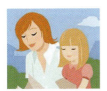

Modalities:
XA, CT, MR

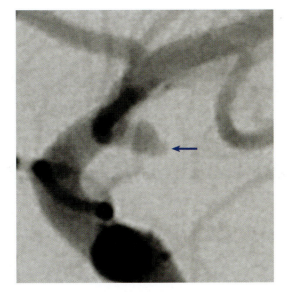
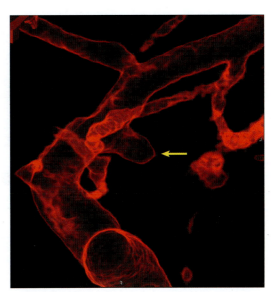

FINDINGS:

Left ICA angiogram, LAO Townes projection, and 3D reconstruction show a ruptured PCOM aneurysm with irregularity at the apex (arrows).

DIAGNOSIS:

Ruptured aneurysm

DISCUSSION:

The majority of intracranial aneurysms are small saccular ("berry") aneurysms that develop at major arterial branch points, where there is thinning of the internal elastic lamina and tunica media. Weakening of an artery wall causes focal outpouching of the vessel. According to the law of Laplace, wall tension increases with vessel radius for a given blood pressure. The aneurysm continues to expand until wall tension exceeds wall strength, at which point the aneurysm ruptures. Irregularly shaped aneurysms have a higher risk of rupture, due to unbalanced mechanical stresses. The apex of an aneurysm is located farthest from the blood supply within the lumen, and is most prone to ischemia. The Murphy sign or "daughter sac" refers to a focal outpouching at the apex. This represents the site of prior or impending aneurysm rupture, and should be urgently treated.

Reference:

Hacein-Bey L, Provenzale JM. Current imaging assessment and treatment of intracranial aneurysms. *AJR Am J Roentgenol.* 2011;196(1):32-44.

DENSE TRIANGLE, EMPTY DELTA

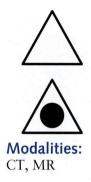

Modalities:
CT, MR

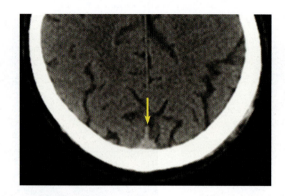 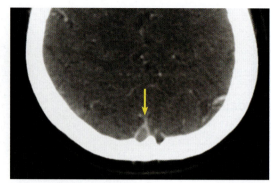

FINDINGS:

- Axial noncontrast CT shows triangular hyperdensity in the superior sagittal sinus (arrow).
- Axial contrast-enhanced CT shows a central filling defect outlined by contrast in the superior sagittal sinus (arrow).

DIAGNOSIS:

Sagittal sinus thrombosis

DISCUSSION:

Cerebral venous thrombosis is a rare and frequently misdiagnosed condition that can affect the dural venous sinuses, deep veins, and superficial veins. Risk factors include young age, dehydration, sinusitis, pregnancy, various medications (oral contraceptives, steroids), trauma or surgery, intracranial hypotension or hypertension, hematologic and autoimmune disorders, malignancy, and other hypercoagulable states. Newly formed thrombus may be appreciated on noncontrast CT as hyperdensity in the expected region of the sinus or vein. The "dense triangle" sign is seen on axial images when the superior sagittal sinus is involved. Care must be taken to distinguish this from the "pseudo-delta" sign due to adjacent cerebral edema or atrophy, hyperdense dura in children, or interhemispheric subdural hemorrhage. Contrast-enhanced images demonstrate an "empty delta" appearance, with central filling defect surrounded by contrast. Dedicated CTV or MRV should be performed to confirm the diagnosis and evaluate the extent of disease. In the acute setting, prompt correction of the underlying cause is indicated with consideration for anticoagulation, as untreated cerebral venous thrombosis can progress to venous infarction and hemorrhage. In addition, chronic venous thrombosis can be complicated by dural arteriovenous fistula (dAVF) formation.

References:

Daif A, Kolawole TM, Ogunniyi A, et al. The pseudo-delta sign is unreliable in differentiating between aneurysmal SAH and sinus thrombosis in unenhanced brain CT. *Eur J Radiol.* 1998;28(1):95-97.

Renowden S. Cerebral venous sinus thrombosis. *Eur Radiol.* 2004;14(2):215-226.

DIFFUSE HYPERDENSE INTRACRANIAL CIRCULATION

Modality:
CT

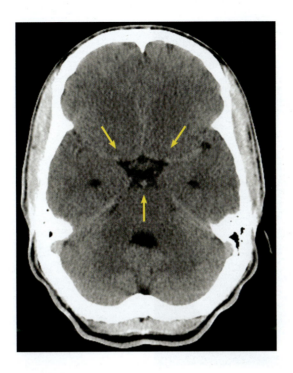

FINDINGS:

Axial noncontrast CT shows mildly increased density of the intracranial arteries (arrows).

DIFFERENTIAL DIAGNOSIS:

- Elevated hematocrit
- Physiologic hyperdensity

DISCUSSION:

Elevated hematocrit can produce diffuse hyperdensity throughout the intracranial arterial circulation. Causes include dehydration, chronic hypoxia, polycythemia vera, malignancy, and medications. In addition, diffuse cerebral hypodensity caused by edema or atrophy can cause normal vessels to appear relatively hyperdense. With severe edema, crowding of the subarachnoid spaces also mimics subarachnoid hemorrhage ("pseudo-SAH"). In newborns, the cerebral arteries and dural venous sinuses are normally hyperdense relative to the unmyelinated and relatively edematous brain parenchyma. Care must be taken to distinguish diffuse hyperdense intracranial circulation from the "dense artery" sign of early infarction, which is focal and unilateral.

References:

Morita S, Ueno E, Masukawa A, et al. Hyperattenuating signs at unenhanced CT indicating acute vascular disease. *Radiographics.* 2010;30(1):111-125.

Rancier R, Woessner H, Freeman WD. The diffuse hyperdense intracranial circulation sign. *Neurohospitalist.* 2011;1(3):137.

DOT, SPOT, TAIL

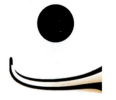

Modality:
CT

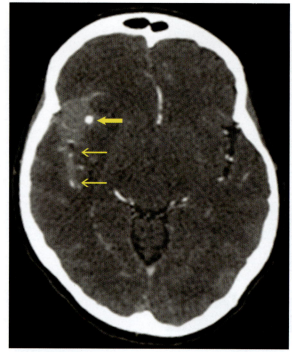

FINDINGS:

Axial CTA shows right insular hemorrhage with a large arterially enhancing focus (thick arrow) and multiple small enhancing arteries (thin arrows).

DIAGNOSIS:

Actively bleeding hematoma

DISCUSSION:

In patients with acute intracranial hematomas, CT is the imaging examination of choice to identify the cause of bleeding. The CTA or CTP "spot" sign has been defined as a focal area of enhancement greater than 1.5 mm, with attenuation at least twice that of the background hematoma. The presence of arterial enhancement indicates active extravasation within the hematoma. Occasionally, the bleeding artery can be identified as a linear density or "tail" extending into the collection. More numerous, larger, and denser spots indicate a higher risk of hematoma expansion and poorer prognosis. Aggressive blood pressure control with emergent endovascular or surgical therapy is necessary to minimize patient morbidity and mortality.

References:

Koculym A, Huynh TJ, Jakubovic R, et al. CT perfusion spot sign improves sensitivity for prediction of outcome compared with CTA and postcontrast CT. *AJNR Am J Neuroradiol*. 2012.

Thompson AL, Kosior JC, Gladstone DJ, et al. Defining the CT angiography 'spot sign' in primary intracerebral hemorrhage. *Can J Neurol Sci*. 2009;36(4):456-461.

DOUBLE BARREL/LUMEN, INTIMAL FLAP

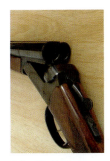

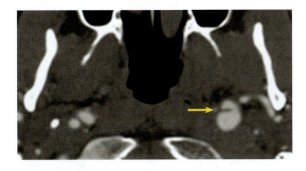 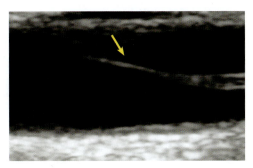

Modalities:
US, CT, MR

FINDINGS:

- Axial CTA shows left cervical ICA dissection with intimal flap (arrow).
- Sagittal US shows the intimal flap (arrow) separating the true and false lumens.

DIAGNOSIS:

ICA dissection

DISCUSSION:

Carotid artery dissection results from a primary intramural hematoma or intimal tear, enabling penetration of blood into the arterial wall. The extracranial portion of the ICA is most commonly affected, due to its greater mobility and proximity to the cervical spine and styloid process. Predisposing conditions include trauma, atherosclerosis, connective tissue disorders, fibromuscular dysplasia, and vasculitis. At imaging, the displaced intimal flap may be identified as a linear intraluminal filling defect. Flow through both true and false lumens creates a "double barrel" appearance en face. The true lumen opacifies earlier, while slower flow in the false lumen predisposes to thrombosis and can serve as a nidus for distal embolization. Treatment options include anticoagulation or antiplatelet therapy, thrombolysis, endovascular angioplasty/stenting, and surgical reconstruction.

Reference:

Rodallec MH, Marteau V, Gerber S, et al. Craniocervical arterial dissection: spectrum of imaging findings and differential diagnosis. *Radiographics*. 2008;28(6):1711-1728.

DOUBLE DENSITY

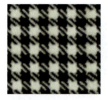

Modality:
XA

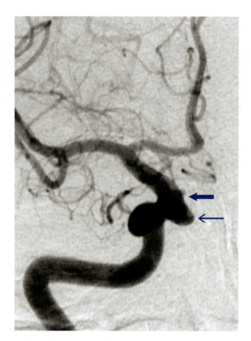
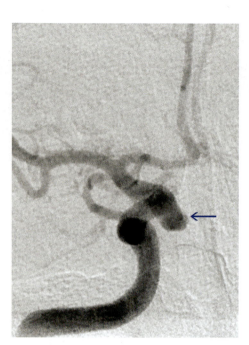

FINDINGS:

Right ICA angiogram, LAO Townes projections, show a clinoid ICA aneurysm (thin arrows) that is partially superimposed on the ICA lumen (thick arrow) in the initial projection, and better delineated on the subsequent view.

DIAGNOSIS:

Aneurysm

DISCUSSION:

The majority of intracranial aneurysms are small saccular ("berry") aneurysms that develop at major arterial branch points, where there is thinning of the internal elastic lamina and tunica media. Characteristic locations include the distal ICA, ACOM, PCOM, MCA bifurcation, basilar tip, SCA, and PICA. On angiography, small aneurysms may be overlooked if they project in front of or behind a vessel of similar caliber. The "double density" sign refers to an area of focally increased density in a vessel that cannot be attributed to tortuosity or branching. This raises concern for a superimposed aneurysm, and requires oblique views for confirmation. The main cause of morbidity and mortality is aneurysm rupture, which depends on several factors including aneurysm size, morphology, and location; underlying etiology; and patient comorbidities. Ruptured aneurysms should be treated emergently. For unruptured aneurysms, definitive therapy (endovascular coiling or surgical clipping) should be considered for sizes exceeding 7 mm and location within the posterior fossa, because of the significantly increased risk of rupture.

Reference:

Hacein-Bey L, Provenzale JM. Current imaging assessment and treatment of intracranial aneurysms. *AJR Am J Roentgenol.* 2011;196(1):32-44.

FLAME, RADISH, RAT TAIL

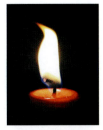

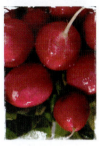

Modalities:
XA, US, CT, MR

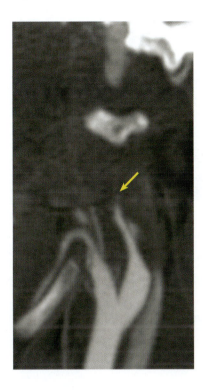

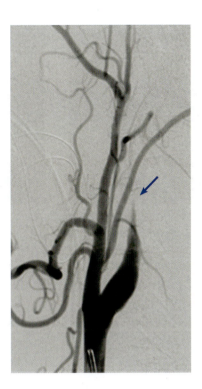

FINDINGS:

Sagittal CTA and CCA angiogram, lateral projection, show abrupt tapering of the ICA (arrows) just above the carotid bifurcation. The ECA branches are normally opacified.

DIAGNOSIS:

ICA dissection

DISCUSSION:

Carotid artery dissection results from a primary intramural hematoma or intimal tear, enabling penetration of blood into the arterial wall. The extracranial portion of the ICA is most commonly affected, due to its greater mobility and proximity to the cervical spine and styloid process. Predisposing conditions include trauma, atherosclerosis, connective tissue disorders, fibromuscular dysplasia, and vasculitis. The true lumen opacifies earlier, while slower flow within the false lumen predisposes to thrombosis. This can compress the true lumen and serve as a nidus for distal embolization. In severe cases, apposition of the intimal flap with the opposite wall causes complete occlusion of the true lumen, with a tapered "flame" appearance. Patients can present with head or neck pain, Horner syndrome, and anterior circulation ischemia. Treatment options include anticoagulation or antiplatelet therapy, thrombolysis, endovascular angioplasty/stenting, and surgical reconstruction.

Reference:

Rodallec MH, Marteau V, Gerber S, et al. Craniocervical arterial dissection: spectrum of imaging findings and differential diagnosis. *Radiographics*. 2008;28(6):1711-1728.

FLIP-FLOP

Modality:
NM

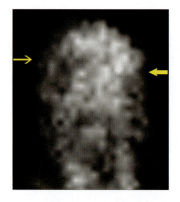 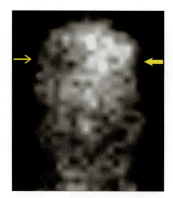

FINDINGS:

- Anterior planar images from a ^{99m}Tc-HMPAO scan in the arterial phase show decreased tracer uptake in the right (thin arrow) and left (thick arrow) MCA territories.
- Venous phase image shows persistently decreased activity on the right and slightly increased uptake on the left.

DIAGNOSIS:

Cerebral ischemia

DISCUSSION:

Planar radionuclide brain imaging is an infrequently performed study, with the most common application being evaluation of brain death. Nuclear medicine agents include technetium-99m ethyl cysteinate dimer (^{99m}Tc-ECD), hexamethylpropylene amine oxime (^{99m}Tc-HMPAO), and diethylene triamine pentaacetic acid (^{99m}Tc-DTPA). HMPAO and ECD are preferred, being lipophilic agents that selectively cross the blood-brain barrier and are taken up by the brain parenchyma. Initial dynamic flow images are acquired in the anterior projection, followed by delayed static blood pool images in anterior, posterior, and lateral projections. Acute arterial ischemia (<3 days) can demonstrate the "flip-flop" sign: decreased perfusion in arterial phase, equalization of activity in capillary phase, and increased activity in venous phase relative to normal brain. This sign identifies ischemic penumbra ("tissue at risk"), in which limited collateral vascular supply results in delayed arrival and slow washout of blood. Emergent neurologic consultation is advised to determine whether the patient is a candidate for intravenous or intraarterial thrombolysis. Further imaging with SPECT, CT, or MR can be performed as appropriate. In the subacute period (1-3 weeks), irreversible brain damage has occurred, with reactive "luxury" perfusion producing normal to increased tracer uptake in all phases. Chronic infarction (>1 month) results in encephalomalacia with decreased uptake in all phases.

References:

Gado MH, Coleman RE, Merlis AL, et al. Comparison of computerized tomography and radionuclide imaging in "stroke." *Stroke.* 1976;7(2):109-113.

MacDonald A, Burrell S. Infrequently performed studies in nuclear medicine: part 2. *J Nucl Med Technol.* 2009;37(1):1-13.

HAIRPIN

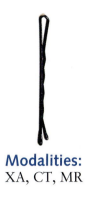

Modalities:
XA, CT, MR

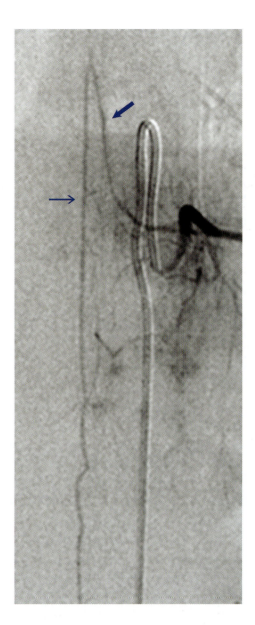

FINDINGS:

Selective injection of a left intercostal artery, AP projection, shows the artery of Adamkiewicz (thick arrow) ascending across midline, then taking an abrupt downward turn to join the anterior spinal artery (thin arrow).

DIAGNOSIS:

Artery of Adamkiewicz

DISCUSSION:

The thoracolumbar spinal cord receives its vascular supply from intercostal and lumbar branches of the aorta, which divide into anterior and posterior branches. The posterior branch subdivides into a radiculomedullary artery, muscular branch, and dorsal somatic branch. The radiculomedullary artery further divides into anterior and posterior radiculomedullary arteries. The artery of Adamkiewicz (great anterior radiculomedullary artery) is the largest anterior radiculomedullary artery and supplies the lower third of the spinal cord. It usually arises from a lower intercostal or upper lumbar artery on the left. The artery enters the spinal canal through a left-sided neural foramen and briefly ascends before making an abrupt downward "hairpin" turn to join the anterior spinal artery. This configuration reflects faster growth of vertebrae relative to the spinal cord during development, resulting in relative ascent of the cord. Angiography is the gold standard for identifying the artery of Adamkiewicz, but CTA and MRA can also be utilized. An important mimic is the relationship of the anterior radiculomedullary vein and anterior spinal vein, which demonstrate a wider ("coat hook") angle. These vessels are also larger, opacify later, and are not continuous with the aorta. Identification of the artery of Adamkiewicz prior to endovascular and surgical procedures is essential to minimize the risk of spinal cord ischemia and paraplegia.

References:

Murthy NS, Maus TP, Behrns CL. Intraforaminal location of the great anterior radiculomedullary artery (artery of Adamkiewicz): a retrospective review. *Pain Med.* 2010;11(12):1756-1764.

Yoshioka K, Niinuma H, Ehara S, et al. MR angiography and CT angiography of the artery of Adamkiewicz: state of the art. *Radiographics.* 2006;26(Suppl 1):S63-S73.

IVY

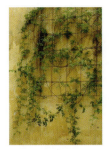

Modalities:
XA, CT, MR

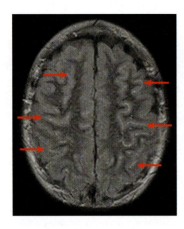 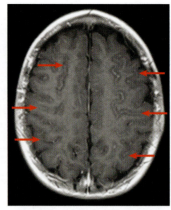 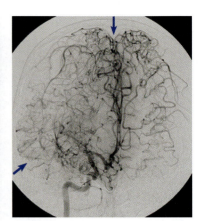

FINDINGS:

- Axial FLAIR MR shows multifocal subarachnoid hyperintensities (arrows).
- Axial contrast-enhanced T1-weighted MR shows corresponding leptomeningeal enhancement (arrows).
- Right ICA angiogram, AP projection, shows stenosis of the supraclinoid ICA, ACA, and MCA, with diffuse leptomeningeal collaterals (arrows).

DIAGNOSIS:

Moyamoya disease

DISCUSSION:

Moyamoya, the Japanese term for "puff of smoke," refers to progressive stenosis/occlusion of the distal ICAs and proximal ACAs/MCAs with relative sparing of the posterior circulation. The etiology may be idiopathic (moyamoya disease) or secondary (moyamoya syndrome) to various conditions including atherosclerosis, Down syndrome, neurofibromatosis, sickle cell anemia, and connective tissue disorders. Collateral circulation is supplied by basal parenchymal perforators, leptomeningeal branches from the PCA, and transdural vessels from the ECA. Engorgement and congestion of superficial pial vessels produces the "ivy" sign, with subarachnoid hyperintensities on FLAIR MR and leptomeningeal enhancement on contrast-enhanced images. Pediatric patients tend to present with cerebral ischemia or infarction, whereas adults can develop infarcts or hemorrhage due to rupture of small aneurysms. Surgical procedures are aimed at revascularization and include direct (STA-MCA bypass) or indirect (encephalo-duro-arterio-synangiosis, encephalo-myo-synangiosis, pial synangiosis, omental transplantation) techniques.

Reference:

Yoon HK, Shin HJ, Chang YW. "Ivy sign" in childhood moyamoya disease: depiction on fluid-attenuated inversion recovery (FLAIR) and contrast-enhanced T1-weighted MR images. *Radiology.* 2002;223(2):384-389.

KISSING CAROTIDS

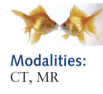

Modalities:
CT, MR

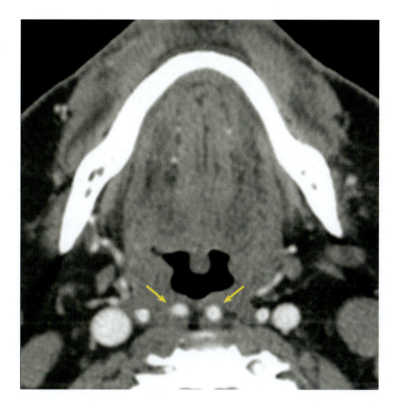

FINDINGS:

Axial CTA shows medial deviation of both ICAs (arrows) into the retropharyngeal region.

DIAGNOSIS:

Retropharyngeal ICAs

DISCUSSION:

The internal carotid arteries form in utero from the third branchial arches and cranial portion of the dorsal aorta. There is wide variation in morphology and course, which can be straight, curved, kinked, and/or coiled. Variations are more common in patients with craniofacial syndromes, atherosclerosis, connective tissue disorders, and fibromuscular dysplasia. The carotid sheath is located at the lateral boundary of the retropharyngeal space. Therefore, medial transposition of the cervical ICA brings the vessel directly behind the posterior pharyngeal wall. When bilateral, this yields a "kissing carotids" appearance. Patients can present with globus sensation and a pulsatile retrotonsillar mass on examination. Biopsy or surgical manipulation should be avoided at all costs.

References:

Paulsen F, Tillmann B, Christofides C, et al. Curving and looping of the ICA in relation to the pharynx: frequency, embryology and clinical implications. *J Anat.* 2000;197(pt 3):373-381.

Pfeiffer J, Ridder GJ. A clinical classification system for aberrant internal carotid arteries. *Laryngoscope.* 2008;118(11):1931-1936.

MERCEDES-BENZ

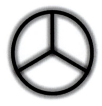

Modalities:
XA, CT, MR

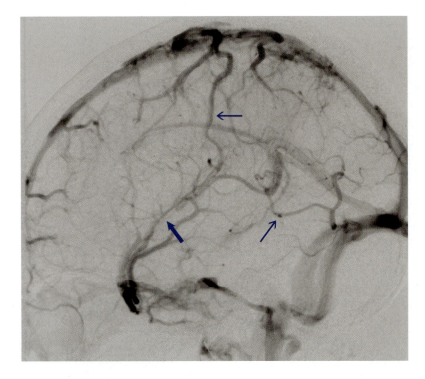

FINDINGS:

Venous phase of ICA angiogram, lateral projection, shows the superficial sylvian vein (thick arrow) connecting to the veins of Trolard and Labbé (thin arrows), which subsequently drain into the superior sagittal and transverse sinuses.

DIAGNOSIS:

Normal superficial cerebral veins

DISCUSSION:

The cerebral venous system consists of deep cerebral veins, which drain the white matter and deep gray structures; and superficial cerebral veins, which drain the cerebral cortex. The superficial system includes superior, middle, and inferior cerebral veins. The superficial middle cerebral vein (of Sylvius) runs along the lateral cerebral hemisphere to the sphenoparietal sinus, coursing posteriorly within the sylvian fissure. The superior anastomotic vein (of Trolard) connects the superficial sylvian vein to the superior sagittal sinus, coursing superiorly with the central sulcus. The inferior anastomotic vein (of Labbé) connects the superficial sylvian vein to the transverse or sigmoid sinus, crossing inferiorly over the temporal lobe. These three veins have overlapping drainage territories and form an anastomotic network that, when balanced, gives the appearance of a "Mercedes-Benz" sign. This is best visualized by catheter angiography, but may be appreciated on CTV and MRV reconstructions.

Reference:

Kiliç T, Akakin A. Anatomy of cerebral veins and sinuses. *Front Neurol Neurosci.* 2008;23:4-15.

MOTHER-IN-LAW

Modality:
XA

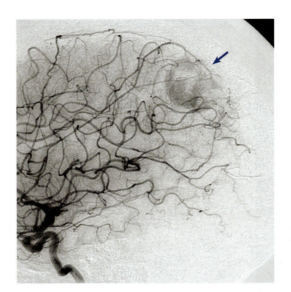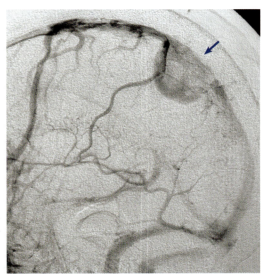

FINDINGS:

ICA angiogram, lateral projection, shows a rounded parietal mass (arrows) supplied by branches of the MCA. There is peripheral contrast blush in the arterial phase and persistent enhancement during the venous phase.

DIFFERENTIAL DIAGNOSIS:

- Meningioma
- Hemangiopericytoma
- Metastasis

DISCUSSION:

Meningioma is a usually benign extra-axial tumor arising from the arachnoid cap cells of the meninges. Tumors are hypervascular and often derive blood supply from branches of the ECA (particularly the MMA), which course into the center of the lesion. As tumors enlarge, a "sunburst" of hypertrophied arterial branches is seen radiating from the central vascular pedicle. Ultimately, lesions outgrow this blood supply and recruit ICA branches to supply the periphery. In tumors with dual blood supply, ECA angiography classically shows "spoke-wheel" enhancement within the tumor, whereas ICA angiography yields a "doughnut" appearance along the periphery. The angiographoc "mother-in-law" sign refers to early and intense contrast blush that persists into the venous phase ("comes early and stays late"). This appearance is characteristic of meningioma, but can be seen in other vascular neoplasms such as hemangiopericytoma and metastasis.

Reference:

Buetow MP, Buetow PC, Smirniotopoulos JG. Typical, atypical, and misleading features in meningioma. *Radiographics.* 1991;11(6):1087-1106.

PENETRATING NICHE

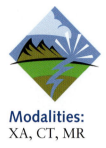

Modalities:
XA, CT, MR

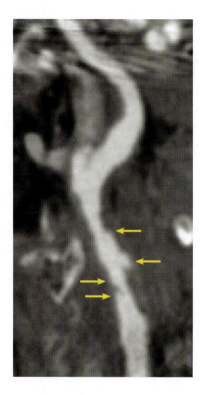 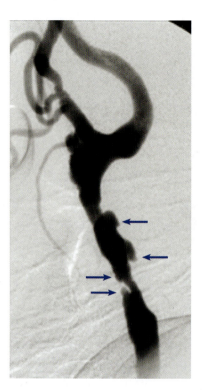

FINDINGS:

CTA, sagittal curved MPR, and CCA angiogram, lateral view, show severe atherosclerosis with multiple ulcerations (arrows) that are outlined by contrast.

DIAGNOSIS:

Ulcerated plaque

DISCUSSION:

Carotid artery atherosclerosis is an important risk factor for stroke. The likelihood of complications depends on the degree and length of stenosis as well as plaque volume, composition, and morphology. Plaques may consist of varying amounts of atheroma (macrophages and cholesterol crystals), fibrous tissue (extracellular matrix and smooth muscle), and calcification. Plaque ulceration is caused by rupture of the fibrous cap, exposing the necrotic lipid core to the circulation. This creates an unstable lesion with increased risk of stenosis, thrombosis, and embolism. On contrast-enhanced imaging, the vessel lumen appears irregular with contrast tracking into the plaque.

References:

Etesami M, Hoi Y, Steinman DA, et al. Comparison of carotid plaque ulcer detection using contrast-enhanced and time-of-flight MRA techniques. *AJNR Am J Neuroradiol.* 2013;34(1):177-184.

Saba L, Caddeo G, Sanfilippo R, et al. CT and ultrasound in the study of ulcerated carotid plaque compared with surgical results: potentialities and advantages of multidetector row CT angiography. *AJNR Am J Neuroradiol.* 2007;28(6):1061-1066.

PSEUDOPHLEBITIC

Modalities:
XA, US, CT, MR

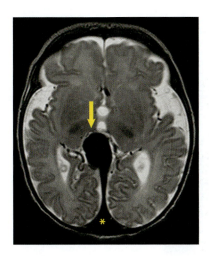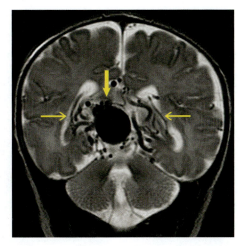

FINDINGS:

Axial and coronal T2-weighted MR show a dilated midline vein (thick arrows) with surrounding tortuous vessels (thin arrows) and drainage into a persistent embryonic falcine sinus (asterisk).

DIAGNOSIS:

Vein of Galen malformation

DISCUSSION:

Vein of Galen malformation (VGAM) is the most common vascular malformation in fetuses and infants. This represents an abnormal communication between intracranial arteries and a persistent embryonic median prosencephalic vein of Markowski (MPV). High flow in the MPV prevents it from regressing to form the normal internal cerebral veins and vein of Galen. Under high pressures, the MPV balloons out and appears as a rounded midline mass with turbulent internal flow, centered in the cistern of velum interpositum and quadrigeminal plate cistern. Drainage is into the straight sinus or a persistent embryonic falcine sinus. Severe VGAM can be complicated by hydrocephalus, cerebral ischemia, and high-output cardiac failure. Surrounding tortuous "pseudophlebitic" collaterals are seen in the subarachnoid space. The imaging differential includes vein of Galen aneurysmal dilatation (VGAD), in which a pial or dural AVM drains into a normally formed vein of Galen. Patients present later in life with increased risk of hemorrhage. Classification schemes include the Lasjaunias (choroidal: multiple feeders converge on MPV, mural: fistulae in wall of MPV) and Yasargil (I: pure fistula, II: multiple communications, III: mixed, type IV: VGAD) systems. Treatment options include transarterial and/or transvenous embolization, microsurgery, and radiation.

References:

Alvarez H, Garcia Monaco R, Rodesch G, et al. Vein of Galen aneurysmal malformations. *Neuroimaging Clin N Am*. 2007;17(2):189-206.

Horowitz MB, Jungreis CA, Quisling RG, et al. Vein of Galen aneurysms: a review and current perspective. In: Horowitz MB, Levy EI, eds. Neuroendovascular Surgery. *Prog Neurol Surg*. Vol 17. Basel: Karger; 2005:216-231.

PSEUDOSTENOSIS, VENOUS COLLAPSE

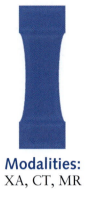

Modalities:
XA, CT, MR

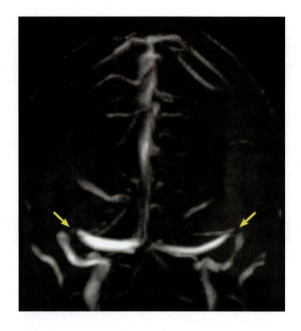

FINDINGS:

Coronal MRV MIP shows focal thinning at the junctions of the transverse and sigmoid sinuses (arrows).

DIFFERENTIAL DIAGNOSIS:

- Idiopathic intracranial hypertension
- Normal variant

DISCUSSION:

Idiopathic intracranial hypertension (pseudotumor cerebri) is a condition of increased intracranial pressure without an identifiable cause, and preferentially affects young obese females. Symptoms include nausea/vomiting, headache, tinnitus, and vision changes. Symmetric thinning or "collapse" of the venous sinuses, particularly at the junction of the transverse and sigmoid sinuses, has been described. Other imaging signs of intracranial hypertension (either idiopathic or secondary) include effacement of the subarachnoid spaces, slit ventricles, empty sella, papilledema, and calvarial remodeling. The cavernous sinuses, Meckel caves, and cranial nerve meati may be narrowed in the acute phase, with expansion in the chronic phase due to transmitted CSF pulsations. In some patients with pseudotumor cerebri, aggressive weight loss leads to complete resolution of symptoms and imaging findings (hence the term "pseudostenosis"). Other treatment options include medical therapy (particularly acetazolamide), CSF drainage, optic nerve sheath fenestration, and venous sinus angioplasty/stenting (controversial).

References:

Rohr A, Dörner L, Stingele R, et al. Reversibility of venous sinus obstruction in idiopathic intracranial hypertension. *AJNR Am J Neuroradiol*. 2007;28(4):656-659.

Saindane AM, Bruce BB, Riggeal BD, et al. Association of MRI findings and visual outcome in idiopathic intracranial hypertension. *AJR Am J Roentgenol*. 2013;201(2):412-418.

PUFF OF SMOKE

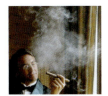

Modalities:
XA, CT, MR

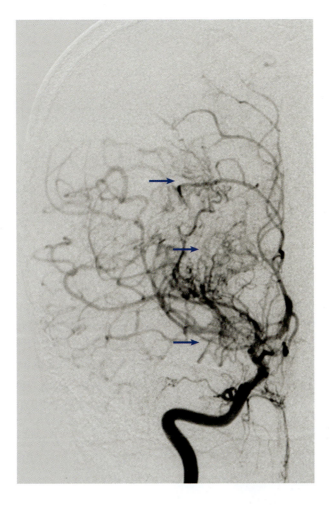

FINDINGS:

Right ICA angiogram, AP projection, shows stenoses of the supraclinoid ICA, A1, and M1 segments with multiple lenticulostriate collaterals (arrows).

DIAGNOSIS:

Moyamoya disease

DISCUSSION:

Moyamoya, the Japanese term for "puff of smoke," refers to progressive stenosis/occlusion of the distal ICAs and proximal ACAs/MCAs with relative sparing of the posterior circulation. The etiology may be idiopathic (moyamoya disease) or secondary (moyamoya syndrome) to various conditions including atherosclerosis, Down syndrome, neurofibromatosis, sickle cell anemia, and connective tissue disorders. Collateral circulation is supplied by basal parenchymal perforators, leptomeningeal branches from the PCA, and transdural branches from the ECA. The "puff of smoke" sign is formed by hazy enlargement of collateral vessels including lenticulostriate, anterior choroidal, and posterior choroidal arteries. Pediatric patients tend to present with cerebral ischemia or infarction, whereas adults can develop infarcts or hemorrhage due to rupture of small aneurysms. Surgical procedures are aimed at revascularization and include direct (STA-MCA bypass) or indirect (encephalo-duro-arterio-synangiosis, encephalo-myo-synangiosis, pial synangiosis, omental transplantation) techniques.

Reference:

Ortiz-Neira CL. The puff of smoke sign. *Radiology*. 2008;247(3):910-911.

RIBBON, RIPPLE, SLIM, STRING (AND PEARL)

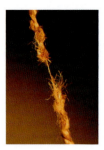

Modalities:
XA, US, CT, MR

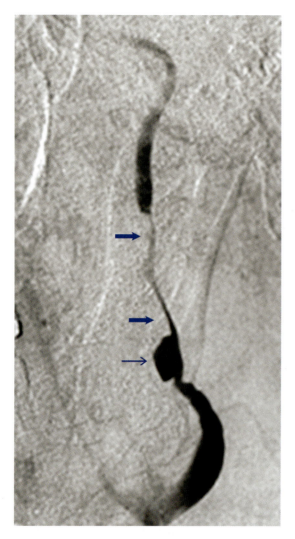

FINDINGS:

Left ICA angiogram, LAO projection, shows severe long-segment stenosis of the cervical ICA (thick arrows), with proximal pseudoaneurysm (thin arrow).

DIFFERENTIAL DIAGNOSIS:

- Dissection
- Atherosclerosis
- Thrombosis
- Stenosis

DISCUSSION:

The "string" sign refers to long-segment severe luminal narrowing within an artery. In the ICA, this can be seen with dissection, preocclusive atherosclerosis, partially occlusive or recanalized thrombus, and long-segment stenosis due to radiation. In carotid dissection, the "string" represents residual true lumen compressed by thrombosed false lumen. There may be associated vessel dilation or pseudoaneurysm (dissecting aneurysm), creating the "string and pearl" sign. With severe atherosclerosis at the carotid bifurcation, reduced perfusion pressures lead to collapse of the distal ICA (even if the ICA is nondiseased). Angiography is the gold standard for evaluation, with other options including carotid US, CTA, and MRA. The North American Symptomatic Carotid Endarterectomy Trial (NASCET) classified carotid stenosis according to the ratio of diameters of the stenotic segment and normal distal ICA. Stenosis is graded as mild (less than 50%), moderate (50% to 69%), or severe (70% to 99%). Endovascular angioplasty/stenting or surgical endartectomy are highly beneficial for severe stenoses, and fairly beneficial in moderate stenoses. Patients with complete occlusions receive little benefit from intervention and are managed medically.

References:

North American Symptomatic Carotid Endarterectomy Trial Collaborators. Beneficial effect of carotid endarterectomy in symptomatic patients with high-grade stenosis. *N Engl J Med*. 1991;325: 445-453.

Pappas JN. The angiographic string sign. *Radiology*. 2002;222(1):237-238.

SAUSAGE STRING, THREAD

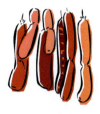

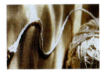

Modalities:
XA, US, CT, MR

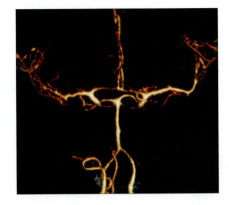

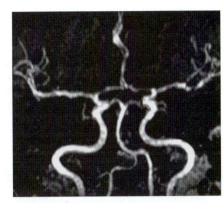

FINDINGS:

CTA and MRA 3D reconstructions show irregular narrowing of the intracranial arteries.

DIFFERENTIAL DIAGNOSIS:

- Vasculitis
- Vasospasm

DISCUSSION:

Diffuse "threadlike" narrowing of the intracranial arteries can be seen in the setting of vasculitis or vasospasm. This can be appreciated with a variety of imaging techniques including transcranial Doppler, CTA, MRA, and angiography. The vasculitides are a heterogeneous group of inflammatory disorders that may affect large, medium, or small vessels. Vasculitis may be primary (primary angiitis of the CNS) or secondary to connective tissue disorders, systemic disease, medications/drugs, infection, and malignancy. Imaging findings include vessel wall thickening and luminal irregularity/stenosis. Treatment involves steroids, other immunosuppressants, and correction of the underlying cause. Cerebral vasospasm is a well-known complication of subarachnoid hemorrhage. Reversible cerebral vasoconstriction syndrome (RCVS), or Call-Fleming syndrome, is a self-limited form of vasospasm with a monophasic course that resolves spontaneously within 3 months. There is an association with migraine, serotonergic and adrenergic drugs, postpartum or postcoital state, and posterior reversible encephalopathy syndrome. At imaging, vasospasm appears as segmental concentric narrowing that can be focal, multifocal, or diffuse. Alternation with normal-caliber or dilated vessels produces the characteristic "sausage string" appearance. Prompt correction of the underlying cause is indicated to prevent ischemia and/or hemorrhage. Treatment options include hypervolemic hypertensive therapy; oral, intravenous, or intraarterial calcium channel blockers; and balloon angioplasty.

Reference:

Marder CP, Donohue MM, Weinstein JR, et al. Multimodal imaging of reversible cerebral vasoconstriction syndrome: a series of 6 cases. *AJNR Am J Neuroradiol.* 2012;33(7):1403-1410.

SHAGGY SINUS, SHAGGY TENTORIUM

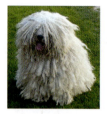

Modalities:
XA, CT, MR

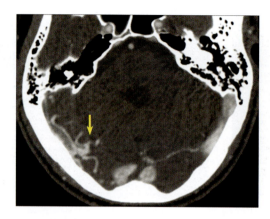

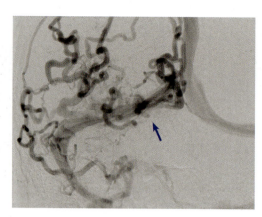

FINDINGS:

- Axial CTA MIP shows multiple serpiginous vessels (arrow) draining into the right transverse sinus.
- Right ECA angiogram, venous phase in LAO projection, shows multiple tortuous veins draining into the right transverse sinus (arrow).

DIAGNOSIS:

Intracranial dural arteriovenous fistula

DISCUSSION:

Dural arteriovenous fistula (dAVF) is a pathologic high-flow shunt between dural arteries and venous sinuses, meningeal veins, and/or cortical veins. The majority are idiopathic, but there is an association with dural venous thrombosis, venous hypertension, prior craniotomy, trauma, and infection. At imaging, dAVF appears as a collection of tortuous feeding arteries and draining veins. The recipient dural venous sinus loses its normally smooth contour and appears "shaggy." This may reflect enlargement of dural venous channels, intimal thickening and stenosis, venous hypertension, and/or reflux into cortical veins. Treatment options include radiation, transcatheter embolization, venous angioplasty/stenting, and surgical resection. Prognosis correlates with the Merland-Cognard or Borden classifications. The Merland-Cognard classification consists of 5 categories (I: antegrade drainage into venous sinus, IIa: drainage into and reflux within sinus, IIb: drainage into sinus with reflux into cortical veins, III: cortical venous drainage, IV: cortical venous drainage with ectasia, V: spinal perimedullary venous drainage). The Borden classification includes types of venous drainage (I: anterograde, II: anterograde and retrograde, III: retrograde) and number of fistulae (a: single, b: multiple).

References:

Gandhi D, Chen J, Pearl M, et al. Intracranial dural arteriovenous fistulas: classification, imaging findings, and treatment. *AJNR Am J Neuroradiol.* 2012;33(6):1007-1013.

Narvid J, Do HM, Blevins NH, et al. CT angiography as a screening tool for dural arteriovenous fistula in patients with pulsatile tinnitus: feasibility and test characteristics. *AJNR Am J Neuroradiol.* 2011;32(3):446-453.

SIGNET

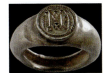

Modalities:
CT, MR

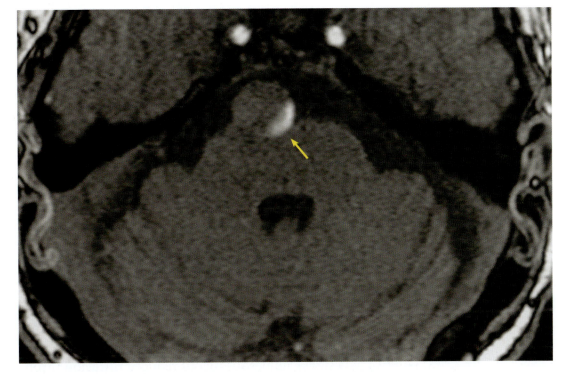

FINDINGS:

Axial 3D TOF MRA shows a partially thrombosed basilar artery aneurysm, with eccentric residual flow (arrow).

DIAGNOSIS:

Partially thrombosed aneurysm

DISCUSSION:

Partially thrombosed aneurysms are a complex group of aneurysms with organized intraluminal thrombus. The majority are large (16 to 25 mm) or giant (25 to 50 mm), and present with symptoms of mass effect on the brainstem and cranial nerves. Near-complete thrombosis with a small eccentric residual lumen produces a "signet" appearance at imaging. Endovascular treatment is usually preferred, while neurosurgical approaches are complex and require advanced techniques such as thrombectomy, bypass, and reconstruction.

References:

Ferns SP, van Rooij WJ, Sluzewski M, et al. Partially thrombosed intracranial aneurysms presenting with mass effect: long-term clinical and imaging follow-up after endovascular treatment. *AJNR Am J Neuroradiol.* 2010;31(7):1197-1205.

Martin AJ, Hetts SW, Dillon WP, et al. MR imaging of partially thrombosed cerebral aneurysms: characteristics and evolution. *AJNR Am J Neuroradiol.* 2011;32(2):346-351.

STAR FIELD

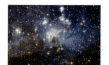

Modality:
MR

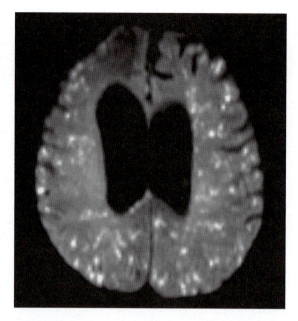

FINDINGS:

Axial DWI MR shows numerous foci of reduced diffusion throughout the gray and white matter of both cerebral hemispheres.

DIAGNOSIS:

Fat emboli

DISCUSSION:

Fat embolism syndrome (FES) is a rare and potentially lethal complication of long bone and pelvic fractures, occurring in 0.5%-3.5% of cases. This tends to present between 24-72 hours, but can occur anywhere from 12 hours to 2 weeks after the initial injury. It is theorized that fat globules from the marrow and/or toxic intermediaries in the blood can embolize to various organs, including the brain. The clinical triad consists of acute-onset respiratory distress, altered mental status, and petechial rash. At CT, large fat emboli may occasionally be visible as focal hypodensities in an arterial distribution ("hypodense artery" sign), which can be confirmed with CTA. On DWI MR, innumerable punctate foci of reduced diffusion are present in both gray and white matter ("star field" pattern). Bilateral microinfarcts can also be seen following central embolization from a cardiovascular source, but are not typically as numerous and diffuse. Treatment is supportive, and the majority of cases are reversible as the fat globules are reabsorbed from the circulation.

References:

Parizel PM, Demey HE, Veeckmans G, et al. Early diagnosis of cerebral fat embolism syndrome by diffusion-weighted MRI (starfield pattern). *Stroke*. 2001;32(12):2942-2944.

Simon AD, Ulmer JL, Strottmann JM. Contrast-enhanced MR imaging of cerebral fat embolism: case report and review of the literature. *AJNR Am J Neuroradiol*. 2003;24(1):97-101.

STRING OF BEADS/PEARLS

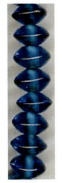

Modalities:
XA, US, CT, MR

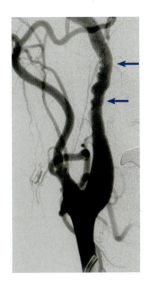

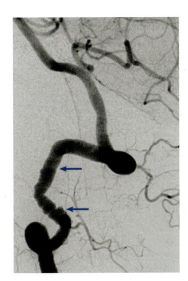

FINDINGS:

- Right CCA angiogram, AP projection, shows beading of the cervical ICA (arrows).
- Vertebral artery angiogram, lateral projection, shows beading of the distal cervical vertebral artery (arrows).

DIFFERENTIAL DIAGNOSIS:

- Fibromuscular dysplasia
- Vasospasm
- Standing waves

DISCUSSION:

Fibromuscular dysplasia (FMD) is a vasculitis of medium-sized arteries that is most prevalent in middle-aged females. Pathologically, there is fibroplasia or hyperplasia of the intimal, medial, perimedial (subadventitial), or periarterial (adventitial) layers. Medial fibroplasia is most common and produces the classic "string of beads" appearance, with fixed asymmetric stenoses and dilations. The extracranial ICA and main renal arteries are most commonly affected, followed by the vertebral, mesenteric, and iliac arteries. Dominant stenoses can be treated with angioplasty, but stenting should be avoided because of the probability of disease recurrence. Complications include dissection, aneurysm, and hemorrhage. The imaging differential includes vasospasm and standing waves. Vasospasm of the extracranial arteries is rare and may be provoked by mechanical manipulation, drugs, migraine, or sympathetic dysfunction. Segmental concentric narrowing is present and can be focal, multifocal, or diffuse. Alternation with normal-caliber or dilated vessels produces the characteristic "sausage string" appearance. Standing (stationary) waves are transient spastic contractions thought to be induced by mechanical contrast injection. These appear as regular periodic constrictions with a "corrugated" appearance. Unlike FMD, both vasospasm and standing waves resolve over time and with administration of vasodilatory agents.

Reference:

Lassiter FD. The string-of-beads sign. *Radiology.* 1998;206(2):437-438.

SUBCLAVIAN STEAL

Modalities:
XA, US, CT, MR

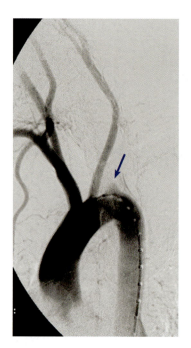 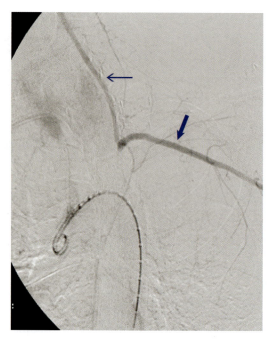

FINDINGS:

- Aortic angiogram, RAO projection in the arterial phase, shows severe left subclavian artery stenosis with failure of opacification beyond the proximal stump (arrow).
- Delayed phase image shows retrograde flow from the left vertebral artery (thin arrow) into the distal left subclavian artery (thick arrow).

DIAGNOSIS:

Subclavian steal

DISCUSSION:

Subclavian steal phenomenon refers to severe stenosis of the proximal subclavian artery, necessitating retrograde flow in the vertebral artery to supply the distal subclavian artery. This effectively "steals" blood from the posterior fossa, and may cause neurologic symptoms (subclavian steal syndrome) if there is inadequate intracranial collateral circulation. Subclavian steal is more common on the left than right, and usually occurs in older males. US or angiography are preferred to evaluate flow direction and dynamics, but the diagnosis can sometimes be made on multiphasic CTA or MRA. Treatment options include endovascular angioplasty/stenting and surgical bypass.

References:

Osiro S, Zurada A, Gielecki J, Shoja et al. A review of subclavian steal syndrome with clinical correlation. *Med Sci Monit.* 2012;18(5):RA57-RA63.

Sheehy N, MacNally S, Smith CS, et al. Contrast-enhanced MR angiography of subclavian steal syndrome: value of the 2D time-of-flight "localizer" sign. *AJR Am J Roentgenol.* 2005;185(4): 1069-1073.

SWIRL

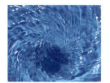

Modality:
CT

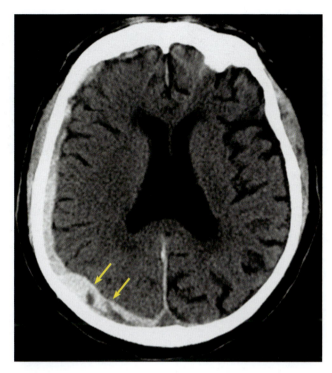

FINDINGS:

Axial CT shows a right holohemispheric subdural hematoma with internal curvilinear hypodensities (arrows).

DIAGNOSIS:

Actively bleeding hematoma

DISCUSSION:

The density of blood products on CT varies with age. Hyperacute blood (<24 hours), which has not yet coagulated, can appear hypodense. Following coagulation, acute blood (1-3 days) appears hyperdense, subacute blood (3-14 days) can be isodense, and chronic blood (>14 days) appears hypodense relative to gray matter. On noncontrast CT, the "swirl" sign refers to areas of low attenuation or irregular density within an acute hematoma, raising concern for hyperacute bleeding with a mix of unclotted and clotted blood. Subsequent CTA/CTV in these patients can confirm active extravasation, which may be arterial or venous in origin. This finding merits immediate surgical attention and is a poor prognostic sign. The "swirl" sign should not be confused with the normally heterogeneous appearance of subacute hematomas due to clot retraction, in which an active bleeding source is not identified.

References:

Al-Nakshabandi NA. The swirl sign. *Radiology.* 2001;218(2):433.

Selariu E, Zia E, Brizzi M, et al. Swirl sign in intracerebral haemorrhage: definition, prevalence, reliability and prognostic value. *BMC Neurol.* 2012;12:109.

TARGET

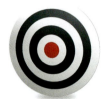

Modalities:
CT, MR

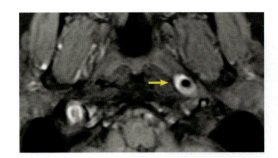
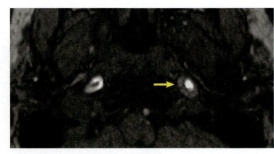

FINDINGS:

- Axial T1-weighted MR with fat saturation shows a hyperintense ring of hemorrhage (arrow) surrounding the left ICA.
- Axial 3D TOF MRA shows a circumferential ring of intermediate-signal thrombus (arrow) surrounding and narrowing the left ICA lumen.

DIAGNOSIS:

ICA dissection

DISCUSSION:

Carotid artery dissection results from a primary intramural hematoma or intimal tear, enabling penetration of blood into the arterial wall. The extracranial portion of the ICA is most commonly affected, due to its greater mobility and proximity to the cervical spine and styloid process. Predisposing conditions include trauma, atherosclerosis, connective tissue disorders, fibromuscular dysplasia, and vasculitis. When thrombosed, the false lumen can compress the true lumen and serve as a nidus for distal embolization. Subacute hemorrhage appears hyperintense on T1-weighted MR with fat saturation, and may produce an eccentric ("crescent") or concentric ("target") morphology. Bilateral ICA dissections have been described with a "puppy eyes" appearance. Patients can present with head or neck pain, Horner syndrome, and anterior circulation ischemia. Treatment options include anticoagulation or antiplatelet therapy, thrombolysis, endovascular angioplasty/ stenting, and surgical reconstruction.

References:

Feddersen B, Linn J, Klopstock T. Neurological picture. "Puppy sign" indicating bilateral dissection of internal carotid artery. *J Neurol Neurosurg Psychiatry*. 2007;78(10):1055.

Rodallec MH, Marteau V, Gerber S, et al. Craniocervical arterial dissection: spectrum of imaging findings and differential diagnosis. *Radiographics*. 2008;28(6):1711-1728.

TAU

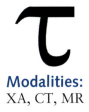

Modalities:
XA, CT, MR

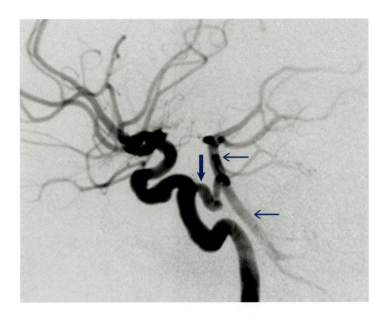

FINDINGS:

ICA angiogram, lateral projection, shows a persistent trigeminal artery (thick arrow) coursing posteriorly from the cavernous ICA. There is antegrade and retrograde opacification of the basilar artery (thin arrows), PCAs, and cerebellar arteries.

DIAGNOSIS:

Persistent trigeminal artery

DISCUSSION:

Persistent carotid-vertebrobasilar anastomoses are formed when the embryologic connections between the dorsal aortic arches and longitudinal neural arteries fail to regress. Persistent trigeminal artery is the most common and the most superiorly located anastomosis, connecting the cavernous ICA and basilar artery. The combination of the posteriorly directed trigeminal artery and the vertical/horizontal turns of the cavernous ICA forms the "tau" sign. A lateral-type trigeminal artery courses posterolaterally with the trigeminal nerve, whereas a medial-type runs posteromedially in an intrasellar or suprasellar position. In Saltzman type I anatomy, the ipsilateral PCOM is absent, and the trigeminal artery supplies the entire vertebrobasilar system distal to the anastomosis. In Saltzman type II anatomy, the ipsilateral PCOM supplies the PCA (fetal configuration). There is a significant association of persistent trigeminal artery with vascular anomalies and intracranial aneurysms. Other carotid-vertebrobasilar anastomoses include primitive hypoglossal artery, proatlantal intersegmental artery, and persistent otic artery.

References:

Dimmick SJ, Faulder KC. Normal variants of the cerebral circulation at multidetector CT angiography. *Radiographics*. 2009;29(4):1027-1043.

Goyal M. The tau sign. *Radiology*. 2001;220(3):618-619.

TRIDENT

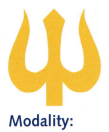

Modality:
NM

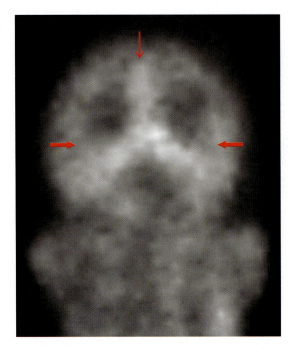

FINDINGS:

Anterior planar ^{99m}Tc-HMPAO scan in the arterial phase shows normal intracranial tracer uptake, with the paired ACAs in the midline (thin arrow) and the MCAs coursing laterally (thick arrows).

DIAGNOSIS:

Normal cerebral perfusion

DISCUSSION:

Planar radionuclide brain imaging is an infrequently performed study, with the most common application being evaluation of brain death. Nuclear medicine agents include technetium-99m ethyl cysteinate dimer (^{99m}Tc-ECD), hexamethylpropylene amine oxime (^{99m}Tc-HMPAO), and diethylene triamine pentaacetic acid (^{99m}Tc-DTPA). HMPAO and ECD are preferred, being lipophilic agents that selectively cross the blood-brain barrier and are taken up by the brain parenchyma. Initial dynamic flow images are acquired in the anterior projection, followed by delayed static blood pool images in anterior, posterior, and lateral projections. A normal dynamic arterial phase scan shows the classic "trident" pattern of the paired ACAs in the midline and the MCAs coursing laterally. Tracer uptake should be symmetric and extend to the cerebral convexities.

References:

MacDonald A, Burrell S. Infrequently performed studies in nuclear medicine: part 2. *J Nucl Med Technol.* 2009;37(1):1-13.

Mettler FA, Guiberteau MJ. *Essentials of Nuclear Medicine Imaging.* Philadelphia: Elsevier; 2012.

VENOUS DISTENSION

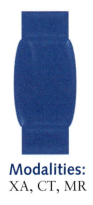

Modalities:
XA, CT, MR

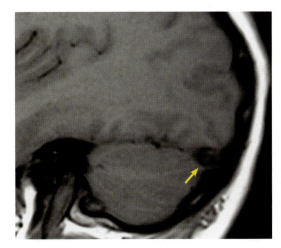
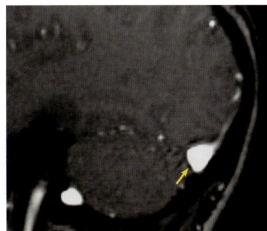

FINDINGS:

Sagittal noncontrast and contrast-enhanced T1-weighted MR show enlargement of the dominant transverse sinus with a convex inferior margin (arrows).

DIAGNOSIS:

Intracranial hypotension

DISCUSSION:

Intracranial hypotension can be caused by idiopathic, degenerative, traumatic, and iatrogenic etiologies. Dural tears in the brain or spine cause continuous loss of fluid, resulting in CSF hypovolemia. The Monro-Kellie doctrine states that in a closed compartment, the total volume of brain, blood, and CSF must remain constant. As a result, the high-capacitance venous system becomes engorged with blood. The "venous distension" sign refers to enlargement of the dominant transverse sinus. On sagittal images, there is convex rounding of the midportion of the sinus, which normally has a straight or slightly concave lower margin. Associated findings include pituitary and midbrain edema; low-lying brainstem, cerebellar tonsils, third ventricle, optic chiasm, mammillary bodies, and splenium; pachymeningeal enhancement; and subdural effusions. Patients may present with orthostatic headaches, cranial neuropathies, nausea/vomiting, and fatigue. Strategies for identifying the site of leakage include radionuclide cisternography and conventional, CT, or MR myelography. Once identified, the leak can be repaired by epidural blood patch, percutaneous fibrin glue injection, or surgery.

Reference:

Farb RI, Forghani R, Lee SK, et al. The venous distension sign: a diagnostic sign of intracranial hypotension at MR imaging of the brain. *AJNR Am J Neuroradiol.* 2007;28(8):1489-1493.

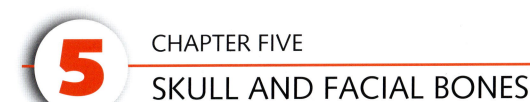

SKULL AND FACIAL BONES

ARC AND RING, CURVILINEAR, POPCORN, SPECKLED, STIPPLED

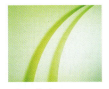

Modalities:
XR, CT

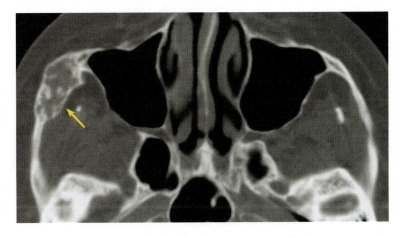

FINDINGS:

Axial CT shows an expansile right zygomatic arch lesion (arrow) with curvilinear calcifications.

DIAGNOSIS:

Chondroid tumor

DISCUSSION:

Bone tumors may be composed of osseous, cartilaginous, and/or fibrous tissue. The pattern of calcification may provide clues to the underlying tumor matrix. Osseous tumors demonstrate dense "cloudlike" calcification, chondroid tumors show curvilinear "arc and ring" calcification, and fibrous tumors have a "ground glass" appearance without calcification. Benign chondroid neoplasms include osteochondroma, enchondroma, chondroblastoma, juxtacortical chondroma, and chondromyxoid fibroma. Malignant chondroid tumors are known as chondrosarcomas and include conventional intramedullary, clear cell, juxtacortical, myxoid, mesenchymal, extraskeletal, and dedifferentiated subtypes. At imaging, features concerning for an aggressive lesion include a wide zone of transition, deep endosteal scalloping or cortical breakthrough, irregular periosteal reaction, and soft tissue extension.

References:

Murphey MD, Walker EA, Wilson AJ, et al. From the archives of the AFIP: imaging of primary chondrosarcoma: radiologic-pathologic correlation. *Radiographics*. 2003;23(5):1245-1278.

Robbin MR, Murphey MD. Benign chondroid neoplasms of bone. *Semin Musculoskelet Radiol*. 2000;4(1):45-58.

ASTERION, LAMBDOID

Modalities:
XR, CT, MR

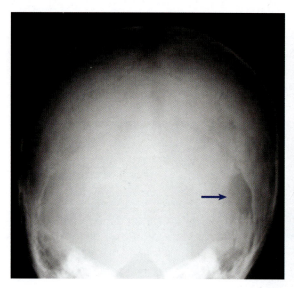

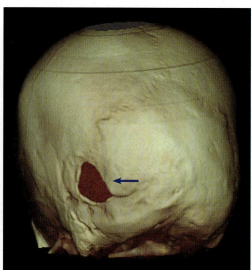

FINDINGS:

- PA Townes radiograph shows a focal lucency adjacent to the left lambdoid suture (arrow).
- 3D CT reconstruction shows a defect at the junction of the left lambdoid, parieto-mastoid, and occipitomastoid sutures (arrow).

DIAGNOSIS:

Neurofibromatosis type I

DISCUSSION:

The asterion ("star" in Greek) represents the point of confluence of the parietal bone, occipital bone, and mastoid portion of the temporal bone. It is located at the confluence of the lambdoid, parietomastoid, and occipitomastoid sutures. Calvarial underdevelopment with a sutural defect in this region is pathognomonic for neurofibromatosis type I (NF1). This defect is more common on the left than right, and is associated with hypoplasia and underpneumatization of the ipsilateral mastoid process.

Reference:

Mann H, Kozic Z, Medinilla OR. Computed tomography of lambdoid calvarial defect in neurofibromatosis. A case report. *Neuroradiology.* 1983;25(3):175-176.

ASYMMETRIC SELLA, DOUBLE FLOOR

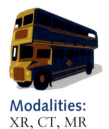

Modalities:
XR, CT, MR

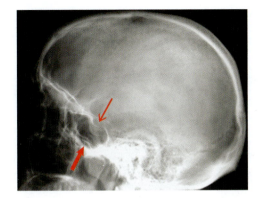

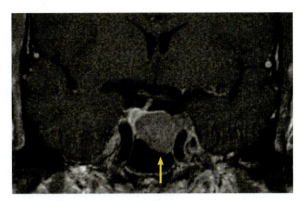

FINDINGS:

- Lateral skull radiograph shows unilateral expansion and depression of the sella (thick arrow), superimposed on normal contralateral sella (thin arrow).
- Coronal contrast-enhanced T1-weighted MR shows a hypoenhancing left pituitary mass (arrow) with rightward displacement of the infundibulum and partial encasement of the cavernous ICA.

DIFFERENTIAL DIAGNOSIS:

- Sellar mass
- Parasellar mass
- Normal variant

DISCUSSION:

Pituitary adenomas tend to grow asymmetrically, resulting in uneven enlargement of the bony sella. This can be appreciated as a "double contour" of the sellar floor on lateral skull radiographs, and asymmetric osseous erosion on cross-sectional imaging. In the days of skull radiography, the combination of asymmetric ballooned sella with ipsilateral elevated anterior clinoid process and thinned, posteriorly bowed dorsum sellae were used to diagnose an intrasellar mass. However, this finding can also be seen in parasellar lesions, such as meningiomas and aneurysms; as well as with normal variations in sellar anatomy ("pseudodouble sellar floor").

Reference:

Feiz-Erfan I, Lanzino G, White WL. Double sellar floor: radiographic sign for a pituitary adenoma. *Barrow Q.* 2002;18(3).

AX, BEAK AND NOTCH, KEEL, PEAR, QUIZZICAL EYE

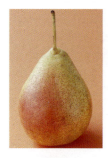

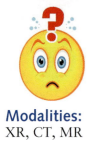

Modalities:
XR, CT, MR

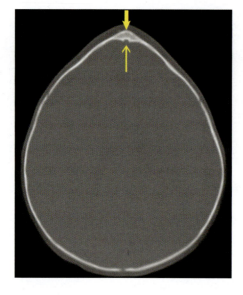

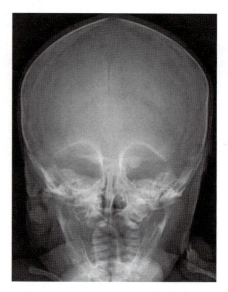

FINDINGS:

- Axial CT shows premature fusion of the metopic suture with hypoplastic frontal bone, ectocranial beak (thick arrow), and endocranial notch (thin arrow).
- PA skull radiograph shows hypotelorism with elevation of the medial orbital rims.

DIAGNOSIS:

Metopic synostosis

DISCUSSION:

The fibrous sutures of the infant skull serve to absorb mechanical forces and allow for cranial expansion during brain growth. Normally, the frontal suture closes between 3 and 9 months; the sagittal, coronal, and lambdoid sutures fuse between 20-40 years; and the squamosal suture closes after 60 years of age. Craniosynostosis refers to the premature fusion of one or more sutures as a result of genetic, metabolic, mechanical, and/or environmental factors. This prevents bone growth perpendicular to the fused suture, necessitating compensatory expansion parallel and distal to the involved suture. Metopic synostosis, or trigonocephaly (Greek for "triangle head"), represents 15%-20% of all craniosynostoses. Premature fusion of the frontal (metopic) suture produces a hypoplastic and triangular-shaped frontal bone ("ax" or "pear" shape), with prominent ectocranial ridge and endocranial notch ("beak and notch"). Hypotelorism with elevation of the medial orbital rims gives the eyes a "quizzical" appearance. Trigonocephaly can be seen sporadically; following in utero exposure to valproic acid; secondary to various endocrine and metabolic disorders; and as part of various syndromes (Baller-Gerold, Christian, Jacobsen, Opitz, Say-Meyer).

References:

Nagaraja S, Anslow P, Winter B. Craniosynostosis. *Clin Radiol.* 2013;68(3):284-292.

Rice DP. *Craniofacial Sutures: Development, Disease, and Treatment.* Basel: Karger; 2008.

BARE/EMPTY ORBIT

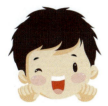

Modalities:
XR, CT

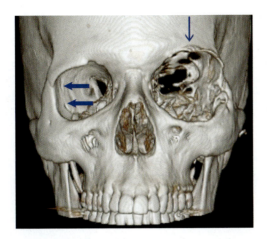

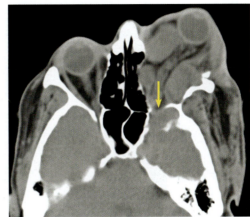

FINDINGS:

- 3D CT reconstruction shows an enlarged and dysplastic left orbit with loss of the normal innominate line (thick arrows) and elevation of the pars orbitalis (thin arrow).
- Axial CT shows left sphenoid wing dysplasia (arrow). Numerous neurofibromas are seen involving the left orbit and orbital apex, cavernous sinus, and scalp. There is associated proptosis and bone remodeling.

DIAGNOSIS:

Neurofibromatosis type I, orbitotemporal subtype

DISCUSSION:

Neurofibromatosis type I (NF1), or von Recklinghausen disease, is the most common phakomatosis. Caused by a mutation in the *NF1* gene on the long arm of chromosome 17, it is transmitted with autosomal dominant inheritance. At least two of the following diagnostic criteria must be present to make the diagnosis: café-au-lait spots, multiple or plexiform neurofibromas, axillary or inguinal freckling, optic gliomas, Lisch nodules (iris hamartomas), osseous abnormalities (sphenoid dysplasia, long bone thinning, and pseudoarthrosis), and first-degree relative with NF1. Orbitotemporal (orbitopalpebral, orbitofacial, cranio-orbital, cranio-orbital-temporal) neurofibromatosis is a rare subtype of NF1 that is characterized by buphthalmos/proptosis, periorbital neurofibromas, sphenoid wing dysplasia, and temporal meningoencephalocele. The "bare orbit" sign refers to loss of the innominate line, which is the radiographic projection of the greater wing of the sphenoid. The pars orbitalis of the frontal bone may also be thinned and enlarged. Occasionally, the "bare orbit" sign can be seen in other processes that destroy the sphenoid wing, such as meningioma, Langerhans cell histiocytosis, neuroblastoma, and rhabdomyosarcoma.

Reference:

Chung EM, Murphey MD, Specht CS, et al. From the Archives of the AFIP. Pediatric orbit tumors and tumorlike lesions: osseous lesions of the orbit. *Radiographics*. 2008;28(4):1193-1214.

BEATEN/HAMMERED BRASS/COPPER/SILVER, CLOUDY

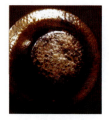

Modalities:
XR, CT, MR

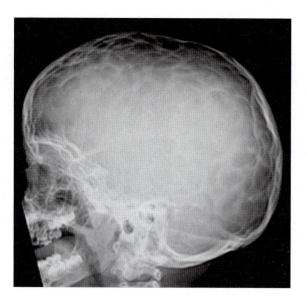

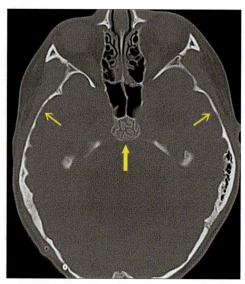

FINDINGS:

- Lateral radiograph shows smooth rounded lucencies throughout the skull, separated by nonbranching lines.
- Axial CT shows multifocal scalloping of the inner table (thin arrows) and linear lucencies in the clivus (thick arrow).

DIAGNOSIS:

Increased intracranial pressure

DISCUSSION:

The "beaten brass" skull is an acquired abnormality in patients with craniosynostosis, space-occupying masses, aqueductal stenosis, or other causes of chronic increased intracranial pressure. This deformity is thought to represent pressure erosions or "negative casts" of cerebral gyri plastered against the calvarium. At imaging, multifocal scalloping of the inner table is separated by thin nonbranching linear markings. The anterior and inferior portions of the calvarium are preferentially affected. This finding is not present at birth and only becomes prominent after several months of age. Additional imaging signs of increased intracranial pressure include erosion of the dorsum sella ("empty sella"), sutural diastasis, and papilledema. In contrast, convolutional (digital) markings are mild gyral impressions on the posterior calvarium, normally seen during periods of rapid brain growth (3-7 years). Luckenschädel (German for "lacunar skull") is a membranous skull dysplasia associated with Chiari II malformation. Multiple islands of nonossified fibrous bone are separated by dense branching strips of ossified bone. The upper calvarium is most frequently affected. Luckenschädel skull is typically evident at birth, and disappears by 1 year of age.

Reference:

Glass RB, Fernbach SK, Norton KI, et al. The infant skull: a vault of information. *Radiographics*. 2004;24(2):507-522.

BEVELED EDGE

Modalities:
XR, CT

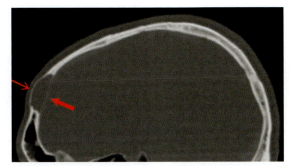

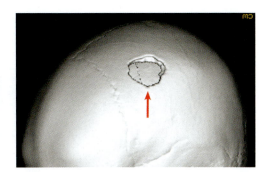

FINDINGS:

- Sagittal CT shows an expansile lytic frontal bone lesion with scalloping of the outer table (thin arrow) and cortical breakthrough along the inner table (thick arrow).
- 3D CT reconstruction in a different patient shows a lytic left parietal skull lesion (arrow) with asymmetric erosion of the inner and outer tables.

DIFFERENTIAL DIAGNOSIS:

- Langerhans cell histiocytosis
- Dermoid/epidermoid cyst
- Hemangioma
- Metastasis
- Osteomyelitis

DISCUSSION:

Langerhans cell histiocytosis (LCH), previously known as histiocytosis X, is a proliferative disorder of Langerhans cells in the bone marrow, skin, and/or lymph nodes. Unifocal LCH (eosinophilic granuloma) affects the skeletal and/or pulmonary systems. Multifocal unisystem LCH (Hand-Schüller-Christian disease) is characterized by exophthalmos, diabetes insipidus, and lytic skull lesions. Multifocal multisystem LCH (Letterer-Siwe disease) is an acute disseminated disease affecting multiple organs. Bone involvement is lytic with ill-defined margins and periosteal reaction in the acute phase, and well-defined with sclerotic margins in the chronic phase. Asymmetric erosion of the inner and outer tables of the skull produces a "beveled edge" sign in tangential views and a "bullseye" appearance en face. There may be a central fragment of devascularized bone, known as a "button sequestrum." Multiple confluent lesions may produce a "geographic" skull, with large lytic areas surrounded by normal bone. Lesions within the maxilla and mandible can result in "floating teeth." Lytic skull lesions that can mimic LCH include dermoid/epidermoid cyst, hemangioma, fibrous dysplasia, early Paget disease, hyperparathyroidism, multiple myeloma, metastasis, infection, and surgical burr hole. Clinical history and time course aid in diagnosis.

Reference:

David R, Oria RA, Kumar R, et al. Radiologic features of eosinophilic granuloma of bone. *AJR Am J Roentgenol.* 1989;153(5):1021-1026.

BLACKBEARD, LINCOLN

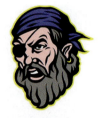

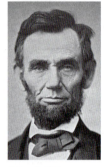

Modality:
NM

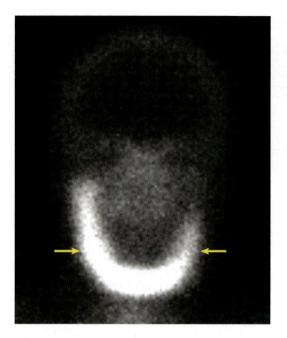 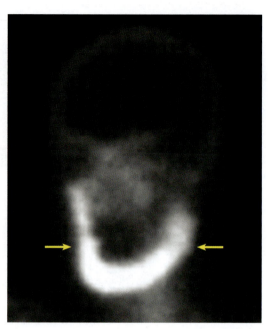

FINDINGS:

Anterior planar and LAO images from ^{99m}Tc-MDP scan show avid tracer uptake throughout the mandible (arrows).

DIFFERENTIAL DIAGNOSIS:

- Paget disease
- Metastasis
- Osteomyelitis

DISCUSSION:

Diffusely increased mandibular uptake on technetium-99m methylene diphosphonate bone scan ("Blackbeard" or "Lincoln" sign) has been described in active Paget disease. The differential includes metastasis, infection, and bisphosphonate-related osteonecrosis of the jaw, but these entitics are more commonly unifocal or multifocal. Clinical history and anatomic imaging aid in diagnosis.

References:

Mailander JC. The "black beard" sign of monostotic Paget's disease of the mandible. *Clin Nucl Med.* 1986;11(5):325-327.

Nahum E, Chandramouly B, Thornhill B. Paget's disease of the mandible. Lincoln sign on bone scintigraphy. *Clin Nucl Med.* 1996;21(3):246-247.

BLISTER

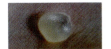

Modalities:
XR, CT, MR

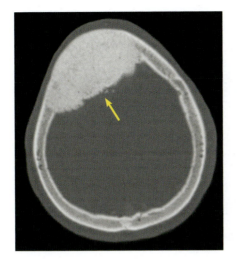
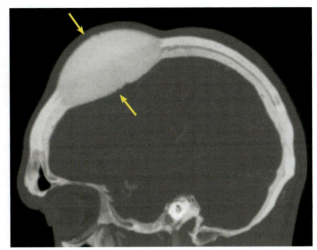

FINDINGS:

Axial CT and sagittal CT MIP show an expansile right frontal calvarial lesion (arrows).

DIAGNOSIS:

Calvarial meningioma

DISCUSSION:

Meningioma is a usually benign tumor arising from the arachnoid cap cells of the meninges. Extracranial meningothelial cells that become trapped in sutures or fracture lines can give rise to meningiomas of the calvarium and/or extracalvarial soft tissues. These represent 1%-2% of all meningiomas and are variably known as ectopic, extradural, epidural, calvarial, cutaneous, extracranial, extraneuraxial, or intraosseous meningiomas. Calvarial meningiomas expand the diploic space and tend to be lytic, with variable soft tissue components and "blistered" hyperostosis. There is a greater risk of malignant degeneration as compared to intracranial meningiomas. If atypical or aggressive features are present, biopsy should be performed to exclude primary (plasmacytoma, sarcoma) and metastatic malignant tumors. Other benign lytic calvarial lesions include hemangioma, fibrous dysplasia, epidermoid, eosinophilic granuloma, early Paget disease, giant cell tumor, and aneurysmal bone cyst. Clinical history and time course aid in diagnosis.

Reference:

Tokgoz N, Oner YA, Kaymaz M, et al. Primary intraosseous meningioma: CT and MRI appearance. *AJNR Am J Neuroradiol.* 2005;26(8):2053-2056.

BOAT, CANOE

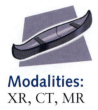

Modalities:
XR, CT, MR

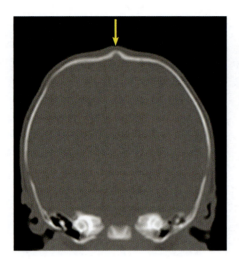
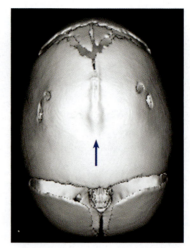

FINDINGS:

- Coronal CT shows fusion of the sagittal suture with a prominent ectocranial ridge (arrow).
- 3D CT reconstruction shows fused sagittal suture (arrow) with dolichocephaly.

DIAGNOSIS:

Sagittal synostosis

DISCUSSION:

The fibrous sutures of the infant skull serve to absorb mechanical forces and allow for cranial expansion during brain growth. Normally, the frontal suture closes between 3 and 9 months; the sagittal, coronal, and lambdoid sutures fuse between 20-40 years; and the squamosal suture closes after 60 years of age. Craniosynostosis refers to the premature fusion of one or more sutures due to genetic, metabolic, mechanical, and/or environmental factors. This prevents bone growth perpendicular to the fused suture, necessitating compensatory expansion parallel and distal to the involved suture. Sagittal synostosis represents 40%-60% of all craniosynostoses. Premature fusion of the sagittal suture produces a skull that is elongated in the anteroposterior direction, known as dolichocephaly (Greek for "long head"). When a prominent ectocranial ridge is present, the defect can be termed scaphocephaly ("boat head"). Compensatory growth of the coronal suture anteriorly and lambdoid sutures posteriorly causes frontal bossing, hypertelorism, and occipital coning. The skull base is not involved. Scaphocephaly has a male preponderance and is usually seen as a sporadic defect. Associations include maternal smoking, endocrine and metabolic disorders, and various syndromes (Marfan, Sensenbrenner, Sotos).

Reference:

Nagaraja S, Anslow P, Winter B. Craniosynostosis. *Clin Radiol.* 2013;68(3):284-292.

BOMBAY DOOR, OPEN DOOR, TRAPDOOR

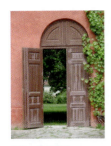

Modalities:
XR, CT

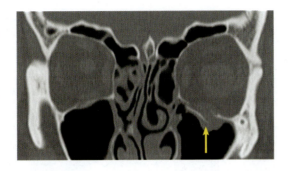

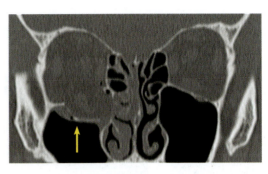

FINDINGS:

- Coronal CT shows a left orbital blowout fracture with single displaced bony fragment (arrow). There is displacement of the inferior rectus and herniation of periorbital fat.
- Coronal CT in a different patient shows a right orbital blowout fracture with two displaced bony fragments (arrow). There is displacement of the inferior rectus and herniation of periorbital fat.

DIAGNOSIS:

Orbital blowout fracture

DISCUSSION:

Blowout fractures are the most common fractures of the orbit. It is theorized that direct trauma to the globe or upper eyelid results in preferential transmission of force to the orbital floor, followed by the medial wall. Bone fragments from the orbital floor can be displaced into the maxillary sinus, and are best evaluated on coronal CT images. The "trapdoor" deformity is most common in children, and comprises over 40% of pediatric orbital fractures. There is herniation of the inferior rectus muscle with entrapment by flexible bone fragments returning to normal position. This is a surgical emergency requiring prompt extraocular muscle release and orbital reconstruction. Additional complications to identify at imaging include globe trauma, hemorrhage, foreign bodies, and infraorbital nerve disruption.

References:

Hopper RA, Salemy S, Sze RW. Diagnosis of midface fractures with CT: what the surgeon needs to know. *Radiographics.* 2006;26(3):783-793.

Winegar BA, Murillo H, Tantiwongkosi B. Spectrum of critical imaging findings in complex facial skeletal trauma. *Radiographics.* 2013;33(1):3-19.

BOXER/PUG/SADDLE NOSE

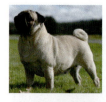

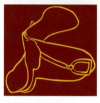

Modalities:
XR, CT, MR

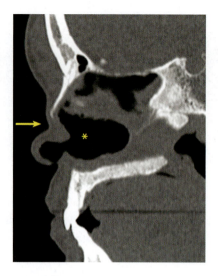

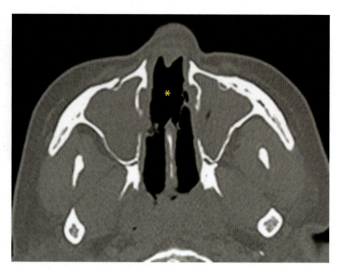

FINDINGS:

Sagittal and axial CT show collapse of the nasal dorsum (arrow) with absence of the cartilaginous and anterior bony nasal septum (asterisks).

DIFFERENTIAL DIAGNOSIS:

- Trauma/surgery
- Drug inhalation
- Granulomatous disease
- Infection/inflammation
- Malignancy
- Congenital disorders

DISCUSSION:

The "saddle nose" deformity refers to collapse of the nasal bridge (dorsum) following loss of the bony and/or cartilaginous nasal septum. The differential diagnosis is wide, including both acquired septal defects and congenital disorders. Causes include trauma; surgery; drug inhalation (cocaine, heroin); granulomatous disease (Wegener granulomatosis, sarcoidosis); infection (congenital syphilis, leprosy); inflammatory/autoimmune disorders (relapsing polychondritis); malignancy (lethal midline granuloma or ulcerating midline lymphoma); and congenital disorders (achondroplasia, thanatophoric dysplasia, ectodermal dysplasia). Clinical history, physical examination, and systemic imaging findings aid in diagnosis. Cosmetic deformity can be corrected with augmentation rhinoplasty using bone, cartilage, or synthetic graft material.

Reference:

Pribitkin EA, Ezzat WH. Classification and treatment of the saddle nose deformity. *Otolaryngol Clin North Am.* 2009;42(3):437-461.

BUBBLY, HONEYCOMB, SOAP BUBBLE

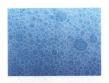

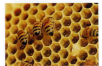

Modalities:
XR, CT, MR

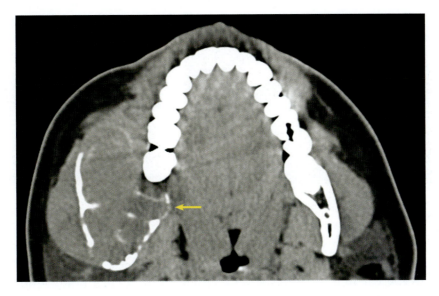

FINDINGS:

Axial CT shows an expansile septated lesion of the right mandibular angle (arrow).

DIFFERENTIAL DIAGNOSIS:

- Ameloblastoma
- Odontogenic myxoma
- Nonodontogenic bone tumor

DISCUSSION:

Ameloblastoma is a usually benign, locally aggressive tumor composed of ameloblasts, the enamel-forming cells of the odontogenic epithelium. The multicystic type is most common and affects patients between the third and fifth decades. It usually involves the posterior mandible and appears as an expansile lytic lesion with "soap bubble" appearance consisting of well-circumscribed corticated margins, coarse curved septations, and solid components. Associated tooth impaction, "knife edge" root erosion, and follicular cysts are common. Other forms of ameloblastoma include the unicystic (mural) type, which is seen in children and occurs in pericoronal locations; and peripheral (extraosseous) type, which affects the gingiva. Odontogenic myxoma is a rare tumor arising from odontogenic connective tissue. It typically affects patients in the second or third decades. At imaging, this has similar characteristics to ameloblastoma, but may be smaller and contain thin straight septations with a "tennis racket" appearance. Odontogenic carcinoma can have internal septations, but demonstrates an aggressive growth pattern with wide zone of transition and cortical destruction. Nonodontogenic bone lesions (aneurysmal bone cyst, giant cell granuloma, fibrous dysplasia) can have a lytic septated appearance on radiography.

Reference:

Dunfee BL, Sakai O, Pistey R, et al. Radiologic and pathologic characteristics of benign and malignant lesions of the mandible. *Radiographics*. 2006;26(6):1751-1768.

BULLSEYE, BUTTON SEQUESTRUM, DOUBLE CONTOUR, HOLE WITHIN HOLE

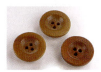

Modalities:
XR, CT

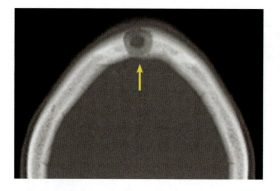

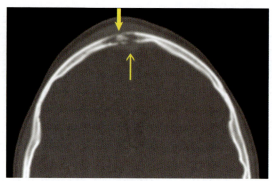

FINDINGS:

- Axial CT shows a well-circumscribed lytic frontal bone lesion (arrow) with concentric erosions of the inner and outer tables.
- Axial CT in a different patient shows an ill-defined lytic frontal bone lesion with central sclerotic fragment (thick arrow). There is complete destruction of the inner table with intracranial soft tissue extension (thin arrow).

DIAGNOSIS:

Langerhans cell histiocytosis

DISCUSSION:

Langerhans cell histiocytosis (LCH), previously known as histiocytosis X, is a proliferative disorder of Langerhans cells in the bone marrow, skin, and/or lymph nodes. Unifocal LCH (eosinophilic granuloma) affects the skeletal and/or pulmonary systems. Multifocal unisystem LCH (Hand-Schüller-Christian disease) is characterized by exophthalmos, diabetes insipidus, and lytic calvarial lesions. Multifocal multisystem LCH (Letterer-Siwe disease) is an acute disseminated disease affecting multiple organs. Bone involvement is lytic with ill-defined margins and periosteal reaction in the acute phase, and well-defined with sclerotic margins in the chronic phase. Asymmetric erosion of the inner and outer tables of the skull produces a "beveled edge" sign in tangential views and a "bullseye" appearance en face. There may be a central fragment of devascularized bone, known as a "button sequestrum." Multiple confluent lesions may produce a "geographic" skull, with large lytic areas surrounded by normal bone. Lesions within the maxilla and mandible can result in "floating teeth." Other lytic skull lesions include dermoid/epidermoid cyst, hemangioma, fibrous dysplasia, early Paget disease, hyperparathyroidism, multiple myeloma, metastasis, and infection. Clinical history and time course aid in diagnosis.

Reference:

David R, Oria RA, Kumar R, et al. Radiologic features of eosinophilic granuloma of bone. *AJR Am J Roentgenol.* 1989;153(5):1021-1026.

CHERUB, LION

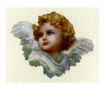

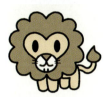

Modalities:
XR, CT, MR

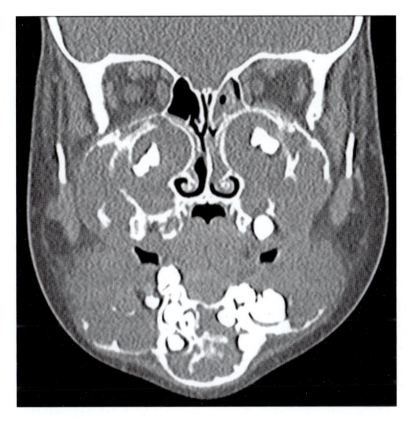

FINDINGS:

Coronal CT shows expanded multicystic maxilla and mandible, with crowded and unerupted teeth.

DIFFERENTIAL DIAGNOSIS:

- Fibrous dysplasia
- Other metabolic disorders

DISCUSSION:

Cherubism is an autosomal dominant form of polyostotic fibrous dysplasia that affects the maxilla and mandible. Increased osteoclastic and osteoblastic activity produces disorganized woven bone with enlarged cystic spaces. This results in early dental loss and permanent eruption problems. The face appears deformed with prominent jaw and upturned eyes ("eyes raised to heaven"), which tend to regress or improve with age. Leontiasis ossea (Greek for "lion face") refers to generalized overgrowth of the face and calvarium. This can be seen in polyostotic fibrous dysplasia as well as acromegaly, Paget disease, hyperparathyroidism, renal osteodystrophy, leprosy, and syphilis.

Reference:

Jain V, Sharma R. Radiographic, CT and MRI features of cherubism. *Pediatr Radiol.* 2006;36(10): 1099-1104.

CLOUDY

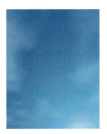

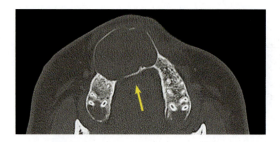

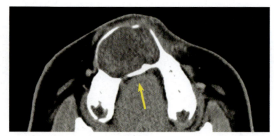

Modalities:
XR, CT

FINDINGS:

Axial CT shows a unilocular expansile lesion with internal soft tissue in the right maxilla (arrows).

DIFFERENTIAL DIAGNOSIS:

- Keratocystic odontogenic tumor
- Dentigerous cyst
- Radicular cyst
- Simple bone cyst

DISCUSSION:

Keratocystic odontogenic tumor (KCOT), formerly known as odontogenic keratocyst, is a benign and locally aggressive tumor arising from the dental lamina. It appears as an expansile cystic lesion in the mandibular body or ramus, often in association with an impacted and dysplastic tooth. Small lesions are unilocular, while larger lesions are multilocular with daughter cysts and osseous erosions. There is internal keratinaceous debris with a "cloudy" appearance. Multiple KCOTs can be seen in Gorlin-Goltz (basal cell nevus) syndrome, orofaciodigital syndrome, and connective tissue disorders. Rare malignant transformation to squamous cell carcinoma can occur. Dentigerous (follicular) cyst is the most common developmental odontogenic cyst and consists of fluid surrounding the crown of an unerupted or impacted tooth. When an erupting tooth is involved, the lesion is known as an eruption cyst. Multiple dentigerous cysts are seen in cleidocranial dysplasia, Gorlin syndrome, and mucopolysaccharidosis type VI (Maroteaux-Lamy). Rarely, these can develop into ameloblastoma, squamous cell carcinoma, or mucoepidermoid carcinoma. Radicular (periapical) cyst is the most common odontogenic cyst and occurs at the root of an infected tooth, usually measuring less than 1 cm in size. Simple bone cyst, which results from trauma with intramedullary hemorrhage, can also have a unilocular cystic appearance.

Reference:

Dunfee BL, Sakai O, Pistey R, et al. Radiologic and pathologic characteristics of benign and malignant lesions of the mandible. *Radiographics*. 2006;26(6):1751-1768.

CLOVERLEAF, KLEEBLATTSCHÄDEL, TRILOBAR

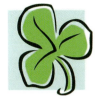

Modalities:
XR, US, CT, MR

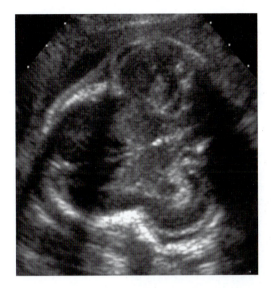

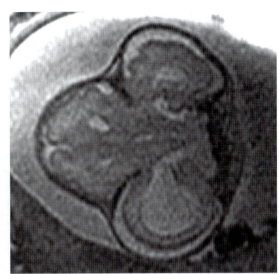

FINDINGS:

Fetal US and MR, coronal plane, show a trilobar skull with bulging forehead and temporal bones.

DIAGNOSIS:

Pansynostosis

DISCUSSION:

The fibrous sutures of the infant skull serve to absorb mechanical forces and allow for cranial expansion during brain growth. Normally, the frontal suture closes between 3 and 9 months; the sagittal, coronal, and lambdoid sutures fuse between 20-40 years; and the squamosal suture closes after 60 years of age. Craniosynostosis refers to the premature fusion of one or more sutures due to genetic, metabolic, mechanical, and/or environmental factors. Pansynostosis of all cranial sutures, which occurs in 5% of all craniosynostoses, causes marked restriction of cranial growth. This can present as microcephaly, in which the skull and brain remain diffusely small; or as Kleeblattschädel (German for "cloverleaf skull"), in which there is outward bulging of the skull distal to the fused sutures. This produces a "trilobar" configuration with towering forehead, shallow orbits, bulging temporal bones, and flattened occiput. Kleeblattschädel has a high association with thanatophoric dysplasia and Pfeiffer, Crouzon, Apert, Carpenter, and amniotic band syndromes. The prognosis is extremely poor because of severe hydrocephalus and mental deficiency.

References:

Rice DP. *Craniofacial Sutures: Development, Disease, and Treatment.* Basel: Karger; 2008.

Tubbs RS, Sharma A, Griessenauer C, et al. Kleeblattschädel skull: a review of its history, diagnosis, associations, and treatment. *Childs Nerv Syst.* 2013;29(5):745-748.

CORTICAL RING

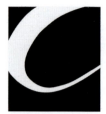

Modalities:
XR, CT

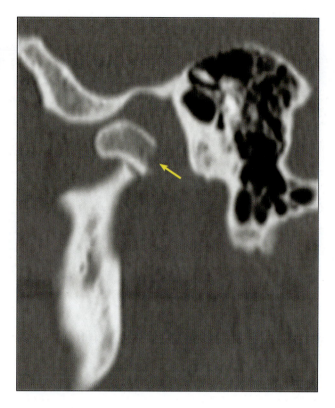

FINDINGS:

Sagittal CT shows a transverse mandibular neck fracture, with dislocation and anterior rotation of the condyle (arrow).

DIAGNOSIS:

Mandibular subcondylar fracture

DISCUSSION:

The mandible is a U-shaped bone that articulates with the cranium at the temporomandibular joints, forming a mechanical ring. As a result, trauma to the mandible usually produces at least two discrete fractures. Isolated fractures of the mandibular condyle can occur as part of a fracture-dislocation complex, with anteromedial rotation of the fracture fragment and dislocation from the glenoid fossa. On lateral radiographs or CT, the dislocated condylar process is oriented horizontally and appears as a dense "cortical ring." Surgical options include conservative management for minor fractures; closed external (maxillomandibular) fixation for moderate fractures; and open reduction with internal fixation for severe injuries.

References:

Cacciarelli AA, Tabor HD. The cortical ring: a sign of anteromedial fracture dislocation of the mandibular condylar neck. *AJR Am J Roentgenol.* 1982;138(2):355-356.

Winegar BA, Murillo H, Tantiwongkosi B. Spectrum of critical imaging findings in complex facial skeletal trauma. *Radiographics.* 2013;33(1):3-19.

COTTON WOOL

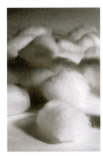

Modalities:
XR, CT

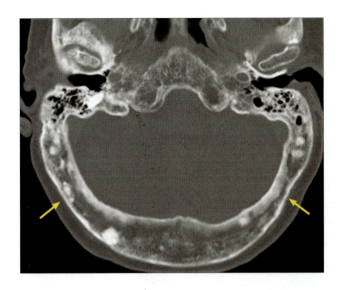

FINDINGS:

Axial CT shows a diffusely thickened calvarium with multiple patchy areas of sclerosis (arrows).

DIAGNOSIS:

Paget disease, sclerotic phase

DISCUSSION:

Paget disease, also known as osteodystrophia deformans, is a chronic metabolic disorder characterized by increased bone turnover and remodeling. The cause is unknown, but has been linked to chronic paramyxovirus infection and mutations in bone remodeling proteins. Disease progresses in three stages: lytic (incipient active), in which osteoclasts predominate; mixed lytic/sclerotic (active), in which osteoblast repair and osteoclast resorption occur simultaneously; and sclerotic (late inactive), in which osteoblasts predominate. Paget disease involves the skull in 25%-65% of cases. The lytic phase is known as osteoporosis circumscripta and manifests as sharply marginated, lucent lesions favoring the frontal and occipital bones. The intermediate phase yields a "jigsaw" or "mosaic" pattern with thickened cortex, trabecular disorganization, and alternating islands of lysis/sclerosis. The sclerotic phase produces a "cotton-wool" appearance with fluffy areas of sclerosis that can cross sutures. Advanced disease produces the "Tam o' Shanter" (Scottish bonnet) appearance with a broad and flattened calvarium. Late complications of Paget disease include hydrocephalus, cranial neuropathies, syringohydromyelia, and sarcomatous transformation.

References:

Smith SE, Murphey MD, Motamedi K, et al. From the archives of the AFIP. Radiologic spectrum of Paget disease of bone and its complications with pathologic correlation. *Radiographics*. 2002;22(5):1191-1216.

Theodorou DJ, Theodorou SJ, Kakitsubata Y. Imaging of Paget disease of bone and its musculoskeletal complications: review. *AJR Am J Roentgenol*. 2011;196(6 Suppl):S64-S75.

CRANIUM BIFIDUM, CRANIOSCHISIS, SPLIT CRANIUM

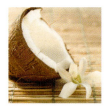

Modalities:
XR, US, CT, MR

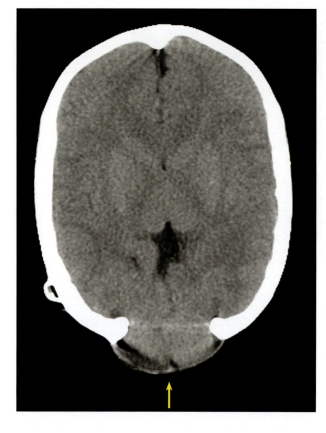

FINDINGS:

Axial CT shows a midline occipital skull defect with herniation of brain parenchyma and meninges (arrow).

DIAGNOSIS:

Encephalocele

DISCUSSION:

Encephalocele (cephalocele) refers to protrusion of intracranial contents through a calvarial or skull base defect. This is known as a meningocele when the defect includes meninges and CSF; meningoencephalocele when brain parenchyma is present; and meningoencephalocystocele when ventricles are involved. The etiology may reflect disruptions in neural tube closure, dura formation, or bone induction/fusion. The most common locations are occipital, frontoethmoidal (sincipital), and basal. Occipital encephaloceles are commonly seen in North America/Europe and are associated with callosal/migrational anomalies, Chiari III, Dandy-Walker, and Meckel-Gruber syndrome. Sincipital encephaloceles predominate in Southeast Asia and Africa. The majority of encephaloceles are clinically apparent at birth ("cleft skull" appearance) and can be surgically corrected. Small or atretic encephaloceles may go undetected until adulthood, demonstrating minimal skull defects with fenestration (cranium bifidum occultum). Posttraumatic encephaloceles have also been described. Mimics of encephalocele include dermoid/epidermoid cyst, nasal cerebral heterotopia (nasal glioma), sinus pericranii, and leptomeningeal cyst (growing fracture). To distinguish these various entities, US is used to evaluate superficial abnormalities, CT is used to evaluate bone, and MR is used to characterize brain and soft tissue abnormalities.

Reference:

Morón FE, Morriss MC, Jones JJ, et al. Lumps and bumps on the head in children: use of CT and MR imaging in solving the clinical diagnostic dilemma. *Radiographics*. 2004;24(6):1655-1674.

CUP, PING-PONG

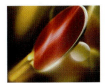

Modalities:
XR, CT, MR

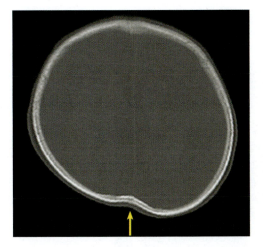 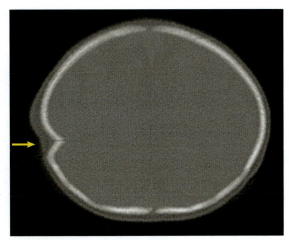

FINDINGS:

- Axial CT shows mild indentation of the posterior calvarium (arrow).
- Axial CT in a different patient shows inversion of the right coronal suture, with overlying scalp swelling (arrow).

DIAGNOSIS:

Pediatric skull fracture

DISCUSSION:

Compared to the adult skull, the pediatric skull is thin and incompletely ossified, causing it to be more fragile as well as more elastic. Mild focal trauma produces a smooth calvarial depression with intact periosteum, known as a "ping-pong" fracture (analogous to "greenstick" fractures of the long bones). This can also result from in utero pressure on the skull or vaginal/forceps delivery, and associated intracranial injury is rare. Surgical elevation of the fracture can be performed for cosmetic purposes, but is not necessary. As the brain grows, the overlying bone spontaneously re-expands and becomes level with the rest of the skull.

References:

Mogbo KI, Slovis TL, Canady AI, et al. Appropriate imaging in children with skull fractures and suspicion of abuse. *Radiology*. 1998;208(2):521-524.

Sorar M, Fesli R, Gürer B, et al. Spontaneous elevation of a ping-pong fracture: case report and review of the literature. *Pediatr Neurosurg*. 2012;48(5):324-326.

DISAPPEARING, PHANTOM, VANISHING

Modalities:
XR, CT

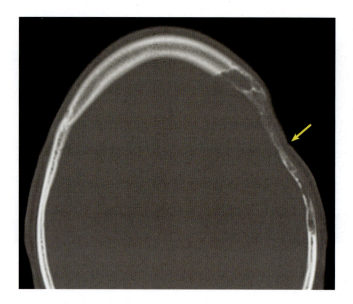

FINDINGS:

Axial CT shows a left frontal bone lytic lesion (arrow) with diploic thinning and septations.

DIFFERENTIAL DIAGNOSIS:

- Gorham disease
- Langerhans cell histiocytosis
- Fibrous dysplasia
- Paget disease
- Hemangioma
- Plasmacytoma
- Osteomyelitis

DISCUSSION:

Gorham disease, also known as phantom or vanishing bone disease, is an extremely rare skeletal condition involving proliferation of vascular and lymphatic channels within bone. This causes a derangement in osteoclastic activity, with replacement of normal bone by angiomatous/fibrous tissue and minimal osteoblastic response. The most commonly affected sites are the skull, jaw, shoulder, ribs, pelvis, and spine. The differential for lytic skull lesions includes Langerhans cell histiocytosis, fibrous dysplasia, hemangioma, early Paget disease, plasmacytoma, dermoid/epidermoid cyst, hyperparathyroidism, metastasis, and infection. Clinical history and time course are helpful, but biopsy is required for definitive diagnosis. Treatment is controversial, with options including medical therapy (bisphosphonates, interferon), percutaneous sclerotherapy or cementation, radiation, and surgery.

Reference:

Papadakis SA, Khaldi L, Babourda EC, et al. Vanishing bone disease: review and case reports. *Orthopedics*. 2008;31(3):278.

DISH, FLAT, FLOATING

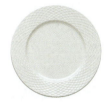

Modalities:
XR, CT

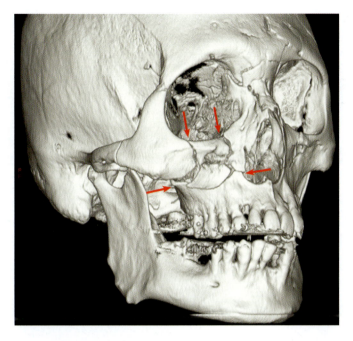

FINDINGS:

3D CT reconstruction shows multiple facial fractures (arrows) with midface flattening.

DIFFERENTIAL DIAGNOSIS:

- Le Fort fracture
- Facial smash fracture

DISCUSSION:

The facial skeleton is a complex structure that is stabilized by horizontal and vertical buttresses. Disruption of the facial buttresses following blunt or penetrating trauma produces various characteristic fracture patterns. Le Fort fractures are caused by high-impact trauma to the midface, resulting in fractures through the pterygoid plates and multiple facial buttresses. Type I Le Fort fracture, also known as Guérin fracture or "floating palate," involves the inferior portions of the medial and lateral maxillary buttresses, separating the maxillary arch from the face. Type II Le Fort fracture, also known as "pyramidal" fracture or "floating maxilla," courses through the inferior orbital rims, superior medial and inferior lateral maxillary buttresses to produce a pyramid-shaped maxillary fragment. Type III Le Fort fracture, also known as craniofacial dissociation or "floating face," involves the superior medial and superior lateral maxillary buttresses. Facial smash fractures are even more severe injuries with comminution of the facial bones and calvarium. An important subtype is the naso-orbitoethmoid (NOE) complex fracture, caused by high-impact force to the nose with disruption of the medial maxillary buttresses. There is involvement of the nasal bones, medial orbital walls, and ethmoid sinuses. The Markowitz and Manson classification includes type I (single bone fragment, intact medial canthal tendon attachment); II (comminuted fracture, intact medial canthal tendon attachment); and III (avulsed medial canthal tendon). Surgical repair involves extensive facial reconstruction with fixation of the fractured buttresses.

References:

Hopper RA, Salemy S, Sze RW. Diagnosis of midface fractures with CT: what the surgeon needs to know. *Radiographics*. 2006;26(3):783-793.

Winegar BA, Murillo H, Tantiwongkosi B. Spectrum of critical imaging findings in complex facial skeletal trauma. *Radiographics*. 2013;33(1):3-19.

DOT, HONEYCOMB, SPOKE/WAGON WHEEL, SUNBURST, WEB

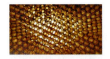

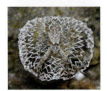

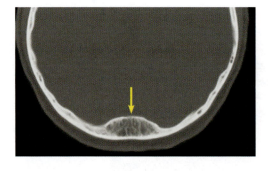

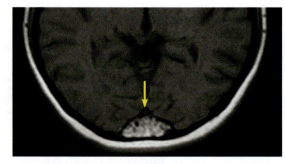

Modalities:
XR, CT, MR

FINDINGS:

Axial CT and T1-weighted MR show a lytic expansile occipital bone lesion (arrows) with thickened trabeculae.

DIAGNOSIS:

Calvarial hemangioma

DISCUSSION:

Intraosseous hemangiomas are benign vascular tumors that represent 0.2% of calvarial neoplasms, and are more common in middle-aged females. Histologically, they consist of endothelium-lined vascular spaces that may be venous, cavernous, and/or capillary. Two distinct morphologies have been described. The sessile type infiltrates the diploic space, while the globular type focally expands the diploë and can project out into the scalp or intracranially to produce a "dural tail." The frontal and parietal bones are most frequently involved. At imaging, the characteristic "honeycomb" or "sunburst" appearance is created by traversing vascular channels with compensatory thickening of residual bony trabeculae. If atypical or aggressive features are present, biopsy should be performed to exclude primary (plasmacytoma, sarcoma) and metastatic malignant tumors. Other benign lytic calvarial lesions include meningioma, fibrous dysplasia, epidermoid, eosinophilic granuloma, early Paget disease, giant cell tumor, and aneurysmal bone cyst. Clinical history and time course aid in diagnosis.

References:

Bastug D, Ortiz O, Schochet SS. Hemangiomas in the calvaria: imaging findings. *AJR Am J Roentgenol.* 1995;164(3):683-687.

Politi M, Romeike BF, Papanagiotou P, et al. Intraosseous hemangioma of the skull with dural tail sign: radiologic features with pathologic correlation. *AJNR Am J Neuroradiol.* 2005;26(8):2049-2052.

DOUBLE DISC

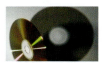

Modality:
MR

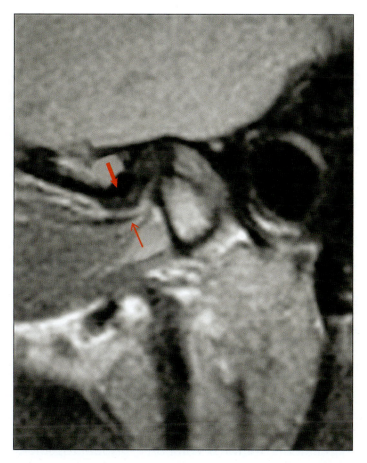

FINDINGS:

Sagittal T2-weighted MR in closed-mouth position shows a dysmorphic and anteriorly subluxed articular disc (thick arrow) and thickened inferior head of the lateral pterygoid muscle (thin arrow).

DIAGNOSIS:

Temporomandibular joint dysfunction

DISCUSSION:

The temporomandibular joint (TMJ) is a complex diarthrodial joint which coordinates rotatory and translational movements between the articular disc (meniscus), mandibular condyle, and glenoid fossa of the temporal bone. TMJ dysfunction is a common cause of myofascial pain and masticatory difficulty. Dynamic MR with closed and open-mouth views in sagittal and coronal planes is used to evaluate joint function. Normally, the TMJ disc has a biconcave appearance, with the thinnest portion (intermediate zone) centered over the condylar head in both closed- and open-mouth views. In closed-mouth position, the disc-condyle complex is located in the glenoid fossa. As the mouth begins to open, the digastric muscle forces the disc-condyle complex downward, causing it to rotate in the lower joint space. Subsequently, the inferior head of the lateral pterygoid muscle (LPM) pulls the disc-condyle complex anteriorly under the articular eminence. With full mouth opening, the condyle comes to rest beneath the anterior band of the meniscus. In cases of TMJ derangement, the inferior LPM may hypertrophy in an attempt to stabilize the disc and condyle. On sagittal images, the thickened inferior LPM is located caudal to the articular disc and produces the "double disc" sign.

Reference:

Tomas X, Pomes J, Berenguer J, et al. MR imaging of temporomandibular joint dysfunction: a pictorial review. *Radiographics*. 2006;26(3):765-781.

DRIVEN SNOW

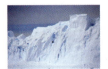

Modalities:
XR, CT

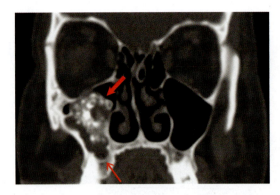
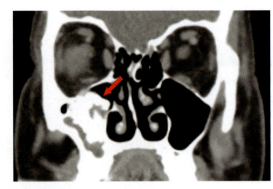

FINDINGS:

Coronal CT shows a soft tissue mass extending from the right maxilla (thin arrow) into the maxillary sinus, with dense spherical calcifications (thick arrows).

DIAGNOSIS:

Pindborg tumor

DISCUSSION:

Pindborg tumor, or calcifying epithelial odontogenic tumor (CEOT), is a benign and locally invasive primary jaw tumor, comprising less than 1% of all odontogenic lesions. Patients are typically in the third to fifth decades of life. Pathologically, Pindborg tumor is composed of odontogenic epithelial cells in a fibrous stroma. The stroma produces amyloid-like eosinophilic deposits, while epithelial cells calcify to yield a "driven snow" appearance at imaging. The central (intraosseous) type of CEOT is most common, and usually affects the posterior mandible. Lesions are focally expansile and can be associated with the crown of an impacted tooth. The peripheral (extraosseous) type is rare, and usually involves the anterior maxillary gingiva.

Reference:

Dunfee BL, Sakai O, Pistey R, et al. Radiologic and pathologic characteristics of benign and malignant lesions of the mandible. *Radiographics*. 2006;26(6):1751-1768.

EGGSHELL, STELLATE

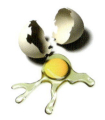

Modalities:
XR, CT

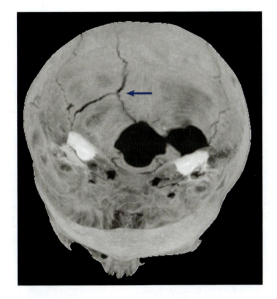
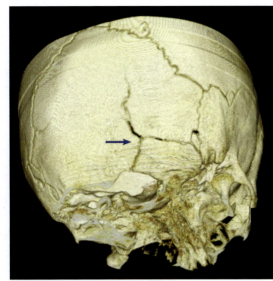

FINDINGS:

3D CT reconstructions show a comminuted right occipital bone fracture (arrows).

DIAGNOSIS:

Pediatric skull fracture

DISCUSSION:

Compared to the adult skull, the pediatric skull is thin and incompletely ossified, causing it to be more fragile as well as more elastic. Severe trauma crushes the skull at the point of impact, creating a comminuted "eggshell" fracture with multiple radiating fracture lines. Eggshell fractures raise concern for nonaccidental trauma (NAT), particularly when the clinical history is discordant with the severity of injury. Other suspicious findings include retinal hemorrhage, intracranial hemorrhage or ischemia, and injuries of different ages. A skeletal survey should be ordered to evaluate for extent of trauma. It is important to distinguish eggshell fractures from normal synchondroses, accessory fissures, and vascular grooves. Compared to true fractures, these entities are less linear and well defined, do not cross sutures or produce diastasis, and are not associated with skull deformities or soft tissue swelling.

References:

Ciurea AV, Gorgan MR, Tascu A, et al. Traumatic brain injury in infants and toddlers, 0-3 years old. *J Med Life*. 2011;4(3):234-243.

Mogbo KI, Slovis TL, Canady AI, et al. Appropriate imaging in children with skull fractures and suspicion of abuse. *Radiology*. 1998;208(2):521-524.

Sanchez T, Stewart D, Walvick M, et al. Skull fracture vs. accessory sutures: how can we tell the difference? *Emerg Radiol*. 2010;17(5):413-418.

ELEPHANT TRUNK, JUG HANDLE

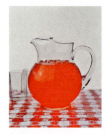

Modalities:
XR, CT

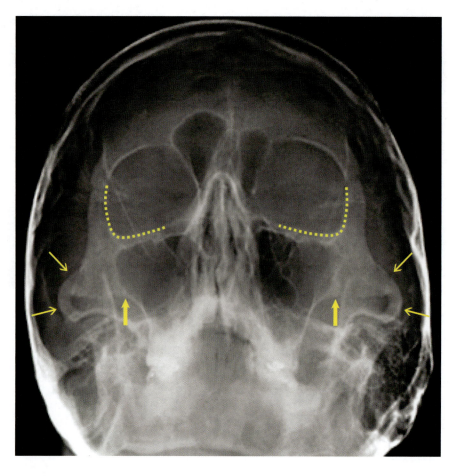

FINDINGS:

PA Waters radiograph shows normal contours of the orbital rims (dotted lines), zygomatic arches (thin arrows), and maxilla (thick arrows).

DIAGNOSIS:

Normal skull radiograph

DISCUSSION:

The Waters (occipitomental) view on skull radiography is used to screen for facial fractures and provide views of the orbital rims, nasal bones, zygoma, and maxilla. A useful search pattern involves the three lines of Dolan: orbital, zygomatic, and maxillary. These form the "elephant of Rogers," with the orbital line representing the elephant's ear, zygomatic line representing the elephant's forehead and trunk, and the maxillary line representing the elephant's chin and trunk. Disruption of these normal lines raises concern for orbital and/or zygomaticomaxillary complex fractures, which should be further evaluated by CT.

Reference:

Dolan KD, Jacoby CG. Facial fractures. *Semin Roentgenol.* 1978;13(1):37-51.

FLOATING DISC, PSEUDOMENISCUS

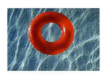

Modality:
MR

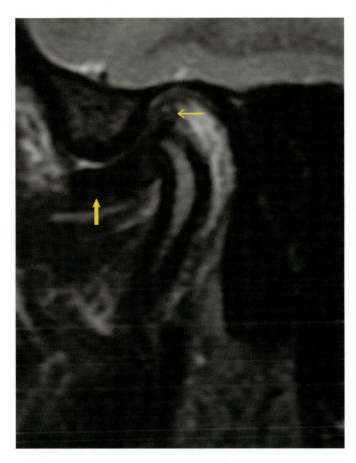

FINDINGS:

Sagittal T2-weighted MR in closed-mouth position shows anterior dislocation of the articular disc (thick arrow), with irregular morphology and hypointense signal. There is thickening of the posterior meniscal attachment (thin arrow) within the glenoid fossa.

DIAGNOSIS:

Temporomandibular disc displacement

DISCUSSION:

The temporomandibular joint (TMJ) is a complex diarthrodial joint which coordinates rotatory and translational movements between the articular disc (meniscus), mandibular condyle, and glenoid fossa of the temporal bone. TMJ dysfunction is a common cause of myofascial pain and masticatory difficulty. Dynamic MR with closed and open-mouth views in sagittal and coronal planes is used to evaluate joint function. Normally, the TMJ disc has a biconcave appearance, with the thinnest portion (intermediate zone) centered over the condylar head in both closed- and open-mouth views. In closed-mouth position, the disc-condyle complex is located in the glenoid fossa. As the mouth begins to open, the digastric muscle forces the disc-condyle complex downward, causing it to rotate in the lower joint space. Subsequently, the inferior head of the lateral pterygoid muscle (LPM) pulls the disc-condyle complex anteriorly under the articular eminence. With full mouth opening, the condyle comes to rest beneath the anterior band of the meniscus. The pathologic "floating" disc occurs when the disc becomes displaced away from its normal position over the mandibular condyle, either due to internal derangement or trauma. In patients with anterior disc displacement, disc stretching and reactive thickening of the posterior meniscal attachment creates a "pseudomeniscus" in the glenoid fossa. Uncovering of the mandibular condyle produces joint instability and degenerative changes.

Reference:

Tomas X, Pomes J, Berenguer J, et al. MR imaging of temporomandibular joint dysfunction: a pictorial review. *Radiographics*. 2006;26(3):765-781.

FLOATING/HANGING TEETH

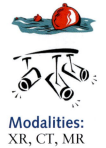

Modalities:
XR, CT, MR

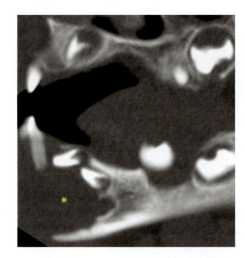
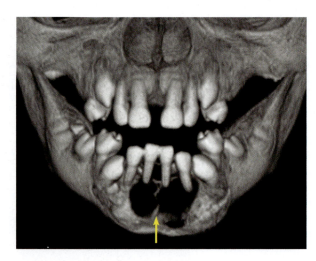

FINDINGS:

- Sagittal oblique CT MPR shows an expansile lytic mandibular lesion (asterisk), with severely disorganized teeth that are surrounded by soft tissue.
- 3D CT reconstruction shows the lytic lesion (arrow) surrounding and displacing the mandibular central and lateral incisors.

DIFFERENTIAL DIAGNOSIS:

- Langerhans cell histiocytosis
- Infection
- Malignancy

DISCUSSION:

Langerhans cell histiocytosis (LCH), previously known as histiocytosis X, is a proliferative disorder of Langerhans cells in the bone marrow, skin, and/or lymph nodes. Unifocal LCH (eosinophilic granuloma) affects the skeletal and/or pulmonary systems. Multifocal unisystem LCH (Hand-Schüller-Christian disease) is characterized by exophthalmos, diabetes insipidus, and lytic calvarial lesions. Multifocal multisystem LCH (Letterer-Siwe disease) is an acute disseminated disease affecting multiple organs. Lesions involving the maxilla and mandible can produce "floating teeth" with destruction of the alveolar ridge, lamina dura, and dental follicles. Erupted teeth are displaced away from the bone, appearing to "float" or "hang" in soft tissue without bony support. Unerupted teeth may also be displaced or resorbed. Rarely, infection or tumor can produce the "floating tooth" appearance. Contrast-enhanced CT or MR is warranted to evaluate for enhancing masses and fluid collections.

Reference:

Keusch KD, Poole CA, King DR. The significance of "floating teeth" in children. *Radiology.* 1966;86(2):215-219.

FLUFFY, SPECKLED

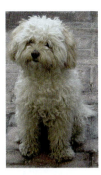

Modalities:
XR, CT

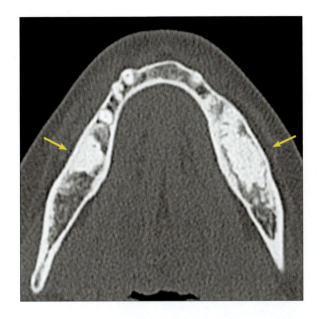

FINDINGS:

Axial CT shows amorphous calcifications within the medullary cavity of the anterior mandible (arrows), with surrounding lucent halos.

DIFFERENTIAL DIAGNOSIS:

- Cemento-osseous dysplasia
- Ossifying fibroma
- Odontoma
- Condensing osteitis

DISCUSSION:

Cemento-osseous (cemental) dysplasia is the most common fibro-osseous lesion of the mandible and maxilla, and represents a benign proliferation of fibroblasts within the periodontal ligaments. The condition is most common in African-American females in the fourth and fifth decades. Periapical cemento-osseous dysplasia mostly affects African-Americans and tends to involve the anterior mandible. Focal cemento-osseous dysplasia can also affect Caucasians and favors the posterior mandible. Both types can progress to the florid form, diffusely affecting the mandible and/or maxilla. Disease progresses from lytic to sclerotic, with the intermediate (cementoblastic) stage demonstrating "fluffy" sclerosis with lucent margins, and finally maturing into sclerotic lesions. Ossifying fibroma, also known as cemento-ossifying or cementifying fibroma, is a benign lesion containing fibrous tissue and bony trabeculae. Lesions typically occur in the posterior mandible, with an encapsulated and expansile appearance. There is a radiolucent rim and varying degrees of internal calcification, depending on the stage of maturation. The juvenile form, which is seen in young males, is rapidly growing and destructive. Odontoma is the most common odontogenic tumor of the mandible, and represents a hamartomatous malformation with production of mature enamel, dentin, cementum, and pulp. The compound type produces identifiable toothlike structures (denticles or abortive teeth), and is generally seen in the anterior maxilla. The complex type has amorphous calcifications, and favors the posterior mandible or anterior maxilla. There is a thin radiolucent rim, and adjacent teeth may be impacted or resorbed. Condensing osteitis, also known as sclerosing osteomyelitis or Garré disease, is periapical inflammation secondary to chronic periodontal infection. There is sclerotic bone formation adjacent to the affected teeth, with "onion-skin" periostitis.

Reference:

Dunfee BL, Sakai O, Pistey R, et al. Radiologic and pathologic characteristics of benign and malignant lesions of the mandible. *Radiographics*. 2006;26(6):1751-1768.

FRONTAL BOSSING

Modalities:
XR, CT, MR

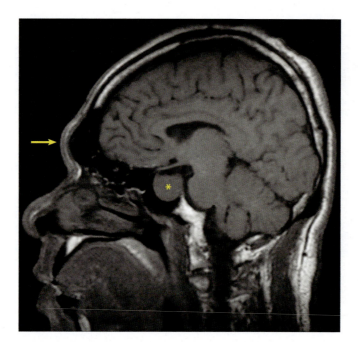

FINDINGS:

Sagittal T1-weighted MR shows enlarged pituitary gland (asterisk), facial soft tissue swelling, and enlarged frontal sinuses with prominent supraorbital ridge (arrow).

DIFFERENTIAL DIAGNOSIS:

- Acromegaly
- Skeletal dysplasias
- Other congenital disorders

DISCUSSION:

Acromegaly is an acquired disorder in which there is overproduction of growth hormone by the anterior pituitary gland, usually secondary to a pituitary adenoma. Because the epiphyseal plates close at puberty, bone expansion occurs in the transverse direction. There is also soft tissue swelling and visceromegaly. Patients display characteristic coarsened facies with prominent supraorbital ridge (frontal bossing), large nose, thickened lips/tongue, and square prognathic jaw. In young children, the differential for frontal bossing is wide. External hydrocephalus refers to benign enlargement of the bifrontal subarachnoid spaces, an asymptomatic condition of infancy that resolves with age. Rickets due to vitamin D deficiency results in softening of the skull (craniotabes) with prominence of the frontal bones and suture lines ("hot-cross-bun" skull). Sagittal synostosis (dolichocephaly) demonstrates frontal and occipital bossing, due to compensatory growth of the coronal and lambdoid sutures. Patients with mucopolysaccharidosis, achondroplasia, thanatophoric dysplasia, and other skeletal dysplasias can demonstrate coarse facies, frontal bossing, and J-shaped sella. Gorlin-Goltz (basal cell nevus) syndrome includes multiple basal cell carcinomas, palmar and plantar pits, keratocystic odontogenic tumors, intracranial calcifications, and skeletal anomalies. Congenital syphilis causes gummatous osteomyelitis, saddle-nose deformity, and narrow notched (Hutchinson) teeth. Trimethadione use during pregnancy has also been reported as a cause of frontal bossing. Clinical history, laboratory values, and associated systemic findings aid in diagnosis.

Reference:

Chanson P, Salenave S. Acromegaly. *Orphanet J Rare Dis.* 2008;3:17.

GEOGRAPHIC

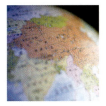

Modalities:
XR, CT

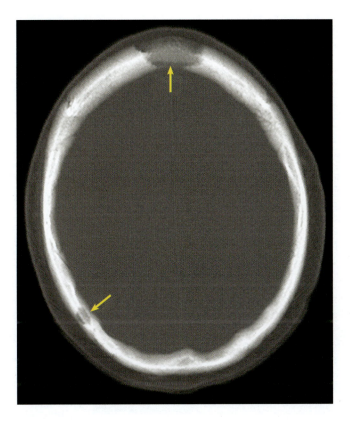

FINDINGS:

Axial CT shows asymmetric lytic lesions in the frontal and right parietal calvarium (arrows), surrounded by normal bone.

DIFFERENTIAL DIAGNOSIS:

- Langerhans cell histiocytosis
- Metastasis

DISCUSSION:

Langerhans cell histiocytosis (LCH), previously known as histiocytosis X, is a proliferative disorder of Langerhans cells in the bone marrow, skin, and/or lymph nodes. Unifocal LCH (eosinophilic granuloma) affects the skeletal and/or pulmonary systems. Multifocal unisystem LCH (Hand-Schüller-Christian disease) is characterized by exophthalmos, diabetes insipidus, and lytic skull lesions. Multifocal multisystem LCH (Letterer-Siwe disease) is an acute disseminated disease affecting multiple organs. Bone involvement is lytic with ill-defined margins and periosteal reaction in the acute phase, and well-defined with sclerotic margins in the chronic phase. Asymmetric erosion of the inner and outer tables of the skull produces a "beveled edge" sign in tangential views and a "bullseye" appearance en face. There may be a central fragment of devascularized bone, known as a "button sequestrum." Multiple confluent lesions may produce a "geographic" skull, with large lytic areas surrounded by normal bone. Lesions within the maxilla and mandible can result in "floating teeth." Lytic skull lesions that mimic LCH include dermoid/epidermoid cyst, hemangioma, fibrous dysplasia, early Paget disease, hyperparathyroidism, multiple myeloma, metastasis, and infection. Clinical history and time course aid in diagnosis.

References:

David R, Oria RA, Kumar R, et al. Radiologic features of eosinophilic granuloma of bone. *AJR Am J Roentgenol*. 1989;153(5):1021-1026.

Stull MA, Kransdorf MJ, Devaney KO. Langerhans cell histiocytosis of bone. *Radiographics*. 1992;12(4):801-823.

GEOGRAPHIC, JIGSAW, MOSAIC

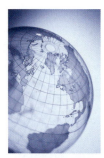

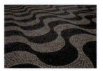

Modalities:
XR, CT, MR

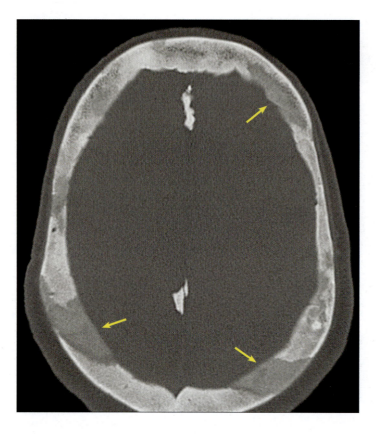

FINDINGS:

Axial CT shows an expanded calvarium with sharply marginated lytic lesions (arrows), separated by areas of sclerosis.

DIAGNOSIS:

Paget disease, intermediate phase

DISCUSSION:

Paget disease, also known as osteodystrophia deformans, is a chronic metabolic disorder characterized by increased bone turnover and remodeling. The cause is unknown, but has been linked to chronic paramyxovirus infection and mutations in bone remodeling proteins. Disease progresses in three stages: lytic (incipient active), in which osteoclasts predominate; mixed lytic/sclerotic (active), in which osteoblast repair and osteoclast resorption occur simultaneously; and sclerotic (late inactive), in which osteoblasts predominate. Paget disease involves the skull in 25%-65% of cases. The lytic phase is known as osteoporosis circumscripta and manifests as sharply marginated, lucent lesions favoring the frontal and occipital bones. This is the only form of Paget disease that demonstrates peripheral, rather than diffuse, tracer uptake on radionuclide bone scans. The intermediate phase yields a "jigsaw" or "mosaic" pattern with thickened cortex, trabecular disorganization, and alternating islands of lysis/sclerosis. On MR, this may produce a "speckled" appearance due to a combination of granulation tissue, hypervascularity, and edema. The sclerotic phase produces a "cotton-wool" appearance with fluffy areas of sclerosis that can cross sutures. Advanced disease produces the "Tam o' Shanter" (Scottish bonnet) appearance with a broad and flattened calvarium. Late complications of Paget disease include hydrocephalus, cranial neuropathies, syringohydromyelia, and sarcomatous transformation.

References:

Smith SE, Murphey MD, Motamedi K, et al. From the archives of the AFIP. Radiologic spectrum of Paget disease of bone and its complications with pathologic correlation. *Radiographics*. 2002;22(5):1191-1216.

Theodorou DJ, Theodorou SJ, Kakitsubata Y. Imaging of Paget disease of bone and its musculoskeletal complications: review. *AJR Am J Roentgenol*. 2011;196(6 Suppl):S64-S75.

GOURD, HOURGLASS, J-SHAPED SELLA, OMEGA, PEAR, SHOE

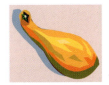

Modalities:
XR, CT, MR

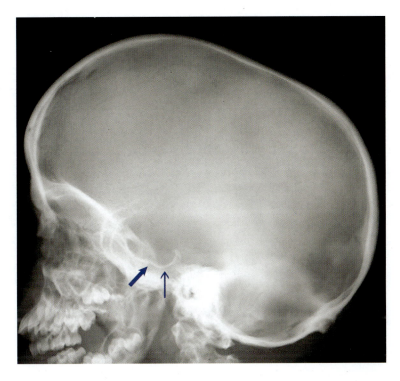

FINDINGS:

Lateral radiograph shows a dysmorphic skull with elongation and flattening of the sulcus chiasmaticus and tuberculum sellae (thick arrow), and normal rounding of the sellar floor (thin arrow).

DIFFERENTIAL DIAGNOSIS:

- Parasellar mass
- Chronic hydrocephalus
- Congenital syndromes
- Skeletal dysplasias
- Normal variant

DISCUSSION:

The "J-shaped" sella refers to an elongated sella with flattening of the tuberculum sellae, producing a shallow optic groove (sulcus chiasmaticus). The normal rounding of the sellar floor is preserved. Sellar/suprasellar lesions, such as optic glioma, aneurysm, and pituitary adenoma, can erode the anterior sella. Other conditions producing this appearance are chronic mild hydrocephalus, mucopolysaccharidoses, Down syndrome, neurofibromatosis, congenital hypothyroidism (cretinism), achondroplasia, chondrodysplasia, osteogenesis imperfecta, and other skeletal dysplasias. In addition, this finding can be seen in 5% of normal children and resolves with age.

Reference:

Burrows EH. The so-called J-sella. *Br J Radiol.* 1964;37:661-669.

GRANULAR, HAIR ON END

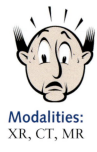

Modalities:
XR, CT, MR

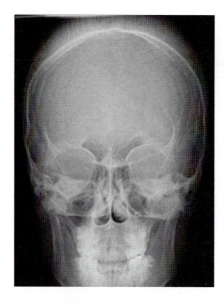

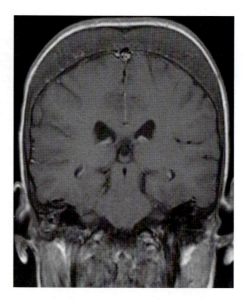

FINDINGS:

- PA radiograph shows multiple linear calvarial striations with indistinctness of the outer table.
- Coronal T1-weighted MR shows an expanded diploic space with alternating hyperintense marrow and hypointense trabeculations.

DIFFERENTIAL DIAGNOSIS:

- Thalassemia major
- Other causes of chronic anemia

DISCUSSION:

Chronic anemia induces compensatory red marrow hyperplasia and increases in circulating hematopoietic factors. Within the skull, there is resulting expansion of the diploic space. In the early stages, the skull appears porous and "granular" with indistinctness of the outer table. "Doughnut" lesions can be seen with sclerotic rims and lucent centers, which are thought to represent islands of active red marrow. Progressive trabecular destruction results in thickening of the residual trabeculae, which are interspersed with hyperplastic marrow. This produces a "hair on end" appearance with linear bone spicules extending through the entire width of the cranial vault. This finding is most commonly observed in thalassemia major, but can also occur in sickle cell disease, iron deficiency anemia, hemolytic anemia, spherocytosis, osteopetrosis, and following use of bone marrow-stimulating agents. Widely metastatic neuroblastoma can mimic the "hair on end" appearance due to aggressive periosteal reaction. This finding is caused by ossification of Sharpey fibers along the periosteum, rather than true diploic expansion.

Reference:

Hollar MA. The hair-on-end sign. *Radiology.* 2001;221(2):347-348.

GROUND GLASS, HAZY

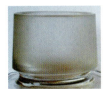

Modalities:
XR, CT

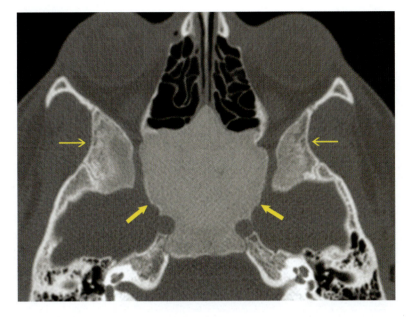

FINDINGS:

Axial CT shows smooth expansion and uniform sclerosis of the clivus (thick arrows) and sphenoid (thin arrows).

DIAGNOSIS:

Fibrous dysplasia

DISCUSSION:

Bone tumors may be composed of osseous, cartilaginous, and/or fibrous tissue. The pattern of calcification may provide clues to the underlying tumor matrix. Osseous tumors demonstrate dense "cloudlike" calcification, chondroid tumors show curvilinear "arc and ring" calcification, and fibrous tumors have a "ground glass" or "hazy" appearance without calcification. Benign fibrous neoplasms include fibrous dysplasia, fibroxanthoma (fibrous cortical defect, non-ossifying fibroma), ossifying fibroma (osteofibrous dysplasia), and desmoplastic fibroma. Fibrous dysplasia is a condition in which normal mature lamellar bone is replaced by immature woven bone. Smooth expansion of the medullary cavity occurs, with varying amounts of lysis and sclerosis. The "ground glass" imaging appearance is classic, and this is a "don't touch" lesion in which biopsy may confound the diagnosis and lead to unnecessary surgery. Malignant fibrous tumors include fibrosarcoma and pleomorphic undifferentiated sarcoma (previously known as malignant fibrous histiocytoma). At imaging, features concerning for an aggressive lesion include a wide zone of transition, deep endosteal scalloping or cortical breakthrough, irregular periosteal reaction, and soft-tissue extension.

Reference:

Fitzpatrick KA, Taljanovic MS, Speer DP, et al. Imaging findings of fibrous dysplasia with histopathologic and intraoperative correlation. *AJR Am J Roentgenol.* 2004;182(6):1389-1398.

GROUND GLASS, PEPPER POT, SALT AND PEPPER

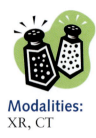

Modalities:
XR, CT

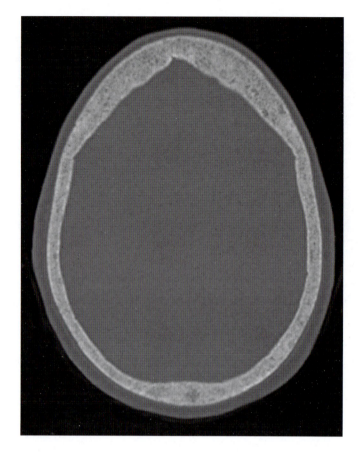

FINDINGS:

Axial CT shows numerous lytic and sclerotic foci throughout the calvarium.

DIAGNOSIS:

Hyperparathyroidism

DISCUSSION:

Parathyroid hormone (PTH), which is produced by the parathyroid glands, regulates serum calcium and phosphate levels by increasing bone osteoclastic activity, intestinal calcium absorption, and renal calcium resorption. Hyperparathyroidism (HPTH) refers to overactivity of the parathyroid glands that may be primary, secondary, or tertiary. Primary HPTH is caused by intrinsic parathyroid abnormalities (adenoma, hyperplasia, carcinoma) and results in elevated blood calcium levels. Secondary HPTH develops in response to low blood calcium levels, as seen in chronic renal failure and vitamin D deficiency. Tertiary HPTH represents autonomous parathyroid activity following longstanding secondary HPTH. In all cases, increased osteoclastic activity leads to diffuse osteomalacia with fibrous replacement of bone (osteitis fibrosa cystica). Diffuse resorption occurs in subperiosteal, intracortical, endosteal, trabecular, subchondral, subligamentous, and subtendinous locations. Brown tumors (osteoclastomas) are expansile collections of fibrous tissue, disorganized woven bone, and hemorrhage. Lesions appear lytic in the initial phase, but may become sclerotic as the process heals. The characteristic "salt and pepper" appearance of the skull reflects chronic HPTH with multifocal resorption and sclerosis.

References:

McDonald DK, Parman L, Speights VO Jr. Best cases from the AFIP: primary hyperparathyroidism due to parathyroid adenoma. *Radiographics*. 2005;25(3):829-834.

Murphey MD, Sartoris DJ, Quale JL, et al. Musculoskeletal manifestations of chronic renal insufficiency. *Radiographics*. 1993;13(2):357-379.

GROWING FRACTURE

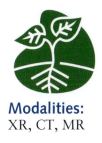

Modalities:
XR, CT, MR

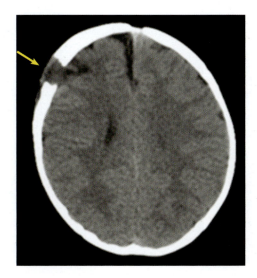

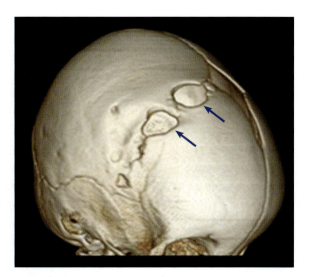

FINDINGS:

- Axial CT shows a distracted right frontal bone fracture with transcalvarial herniation of leptomeninges (arrow) and underlying encephalomalacia.
- 3D CT reconstruction shows scalloped erosions (arrows) along the fracture margins.

DIAGNOSIS:

Leptomeningeal cyst

DISCUSSION:

Compared to the adult skull, the pediatric skull is thin and incompletely ossified, causing it to be more fragile as well as more elastic. Since the dura mater is more adherent in children, skull fractures carry an increased risk of dural tear and underlying brain injury. In distracted fractures, the arachnoid and pia mater can herniate out through the defect to produce a leptomeningeal cyst. This interposed tissue inhibits bone healing, and CSF pulsations cause progressive bone erosion, colloquially known as a "growing fracture." At imaging, the margins of the fracture are angular and scalloped, with an intervening encephalocele. The underlying brain is encephalomalacic and may also herniate into the fracture (traumatic meningoencephalocele).

References:

Ciurea AV, Gorgan MR, Tascu A, et al. Traumatic brain injury in infants and toddlers, 0-3 years old. *J Med Life*. 2011;4(3):234-243.

Mogbo KI, Slovis TL, Canady AI, et al. Appropriate imaging in children with skull fractures and suspicion of abuse. *Radiology*. 1998;208(2):521-524.

HARLEQUIN EYE

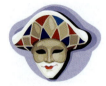

Modalities:
XR, CT, MR

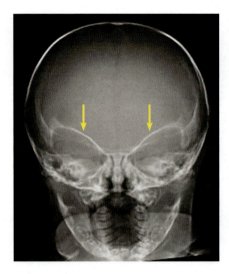
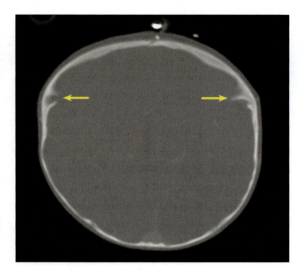

FINDINGS:

- PA radiograph shows bilaterally elevated lesser sphenoid wings (arrows). The greater sphenoid wings are intact, as evidenced by normal innominate lines.
- Axial CT shows premature fusion of both coronal sutures (arrows).

DIAGNOSIS:

Coronal synostosis

DISCUSSION:

The fibrous sutures of the infant skull serve to absorb mechanical forces and allow for cranial expansion during brain growth. Normally, the frontal suture closes between 3 and 9 months; the sagittal, coronal, and lambdoid sutures fuse between 20-40 years; and the squamosal suture closes after 60 years of age. Craniosynostosis refers to the premature fusion of one or more sutures due to genetic, metabolic, mechanical, and/or environmental factors. This prevents bone growth perpendicular to the fused suture, necessitating compensatory expansion parallel and distal to the involved suture. Coronal synostosis, or brachycephaly (Greek for "short head"), represents 30% of all craniosynostoses and has a female preponderance. Premature fusion of the coronal sutures yields a skull that is foreshortened in the anteroposterior direction with recessed frontal bones, flattened occiput, and deformation of the skull base. The "harlequin eye" deformity represents elevation of the lesser wing of the sphenoid. The greater wing of the sphenoid is preserved, yielding a normal innominate line on radiography. Unilateral coronal synostosis is usually sporadic, whereas bilateral coronal synostosis is seen as part of various syndromes (Apert, Beare-Stevenson, Crouzon, Jackson-Weiss, Muenke, Pfeiffer, Saethre-Chotzen). Associated craniofacial and extremity malformations can aid in the diagnosis.

References:

Nagaraja S, Anslow P, Winter B. Craniosynostosis. *Clin Radiol*. 2013;68(3):284-292.

Rice DP. *Craniofacial Sutures: Development, Disease, and Treatment*. Basel: Karger; 2008.

HIGH HEAD, STEEPLE, TOWER

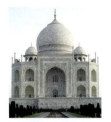

Modalities:
XR, CT, MR

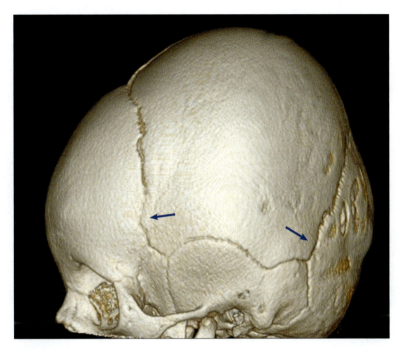

FINDINGS:

3D CT reconstruction shows partial fusion of the coronal and lambdoid sutures (arrows), with a tall and pointed skull.

DIAGNOSIS:

Compound coronal synostosis

DISCUSSION:

The fibrous sutures of the infant skull serve to absorb mechanical forces and allow for cranial expansion during brain growth. Normally, the frontal suture closes between 3 and 9 months; the sagittal, coronal, and lambdoid sutures fuse between 20-40 years; and the squamosal suture closes after 60 years of age. Craniosynostosis refers to the premature fusion of one or more sutures due to genetic, metabolic, mechanical, and/or environmental factors. This prevents bone growth perpendicular to the fused suture, necessitating compensatory expansion parallel and distal to the involved suture. Compound synostosis of the coronal sutures with the sagittal and/or lambdoid sutures is variably known as acrocephaly (Greek for "tall head"), hypsicephaly ("high head"), oxycephaly ("sharp head"), and turricephaly ("tower head"). This results in vertical growth of the skull with a pointed appearance. The skull base is not involved. Frequently associated conditions include central nervous system abnormalities, Chiari malformations, and various syndromes (Crouzon, Pfeiffer).

References:

Nagaraja S, Anslow P, Winter B. Craniosynostosis. *Clin Radiol*. 2013;68(3):284-292.

Rice DP. *Craniofacial Sutures: Development, Disease, and Treatment*. Basel: Karger; 2008.

HUTCHINSON/NOTCHED TEETH, MULBERRY MOLARS

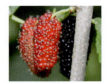

Modalities:
XR, CT

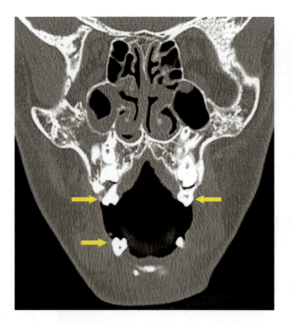 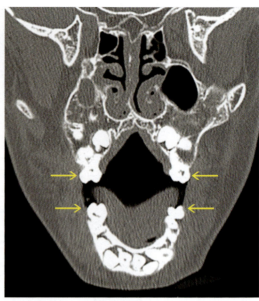

FINDINGS:

Coronal CT shows widely spaced and notched incisors (thick arrows) and molars (thin arrows). Several dysmorphic unerupted teeth are also present.

DIAGNOSIS:

Congenital syphilis

DISCUSSION:

Congenital syphilis is caused by the spirochete bacterium *Treponema pallidum*. This occurs due to maternal transmission of infection during pregnancy or at birth. Patients can present early (0-2 years) or late (after 2 years). Early symptoms and signs include fever, rash, syphilitic rhinitis ("snuffles"), anemia, jaundice, hepatosplenomegaly, and lymphadenopathy. Prompt antibiotic treatment with penicillin is essential to minimize morbidity and mortality, before late complications develop. Sir Jonathan Hutchinson described the classic triad of widely spaced and notched incisors (Hutchinson teeth), interstitial keratitis, and sensorineural hearing loss. "Mulberry" molars may also be seen, characterized by hypoplastic enamel with rounded rudimentary cusps. Other facial findings include recurrent periostitis with frontal bossing (Olympian brow), saddle nose deformity, palatal perforation, short maxilla, and protruding mandible. Involvement of the CNS (neurosyphilis) can be asymptomatic or present as acute syphilitic leptomeningitis, chronic meningovascular syphilis, general paresis, or tabes dorsalis (dorsal column myelopathy).

Reference:

Walker GJ, Walker DG. Congenital syphilis: a continuing but neglected problem. *Semin Fetal Neonatal Med.* 2007;12(3):198-206.

LACUNAR, LUCKENSCHÄDEL

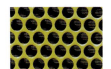

Modalities:
XR, US, CT, MR

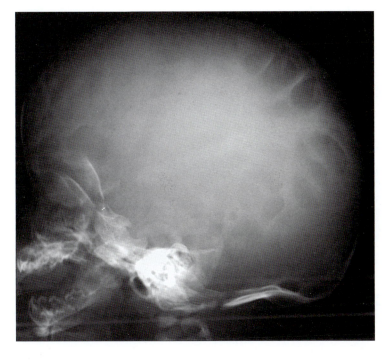

FINDINGS:

Lateral radiograph shows a dysmorphic skull with several ovoid lucencies, separated by thick branching ridges of bone.

DIAGNOSIS:

Luckenschädel skull

DISCUSSION:

Luckenschädel (German for "lacunar skull") is a membranous skull dysplasia usually associated with Chiari II malformation and less commonly with encephalocele, aqueductal stenosis, arthrogryposis multiplex congenita, and phenylketonuria. Abnormal collagen development results in delayed calvarial ossification, with several islands of non-ossified fibrous bone. At imaging, these lesions appear as well-circumscribed ovoid areas of calvarial thinning (craniolacunae). These are usually separated by dense branching strips of ossified bone ("honeycomb" appearance), though multiple craniolacunae can coalesce into larger defects (craniofenestra). The upper calvarium is most frequently affected. Luckenschädel skull may be present prenatally, and is typically evident at birth. It is a self-limiting condition that fades by 3-6 months and disappears by 1 year of age. In contrast, convolutional (digital) markings are mild gyral impressions on the posterior calvarium, normally seen during periods of rapid brain growth (3-7 years). "Beaten brass" skull is an acquired abnormality in patients with chronic increased intracranial pressure. Multifocal scalloping of the inner table is separated by thin nonbranching linear markings. The anterior and lower portions of the calvarium are preferentially affected. This finding is not present at birth, and only becomes prominent after several months of age.

References:

Glass RB, Fernbach SK, Norton KI, et al. The infant skull: a vault of information. *Radiographics*. 2004;24(2):507-522.

Naidich TP, Pudlowski RM, Naidich JB, et al. Computed tomographic signs of the Chiari II malformation, part I: skull and dural partitions. *Radiology*. 1980;134(1):65-71.

LEMON

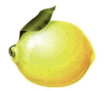

Modalities:
US, MR

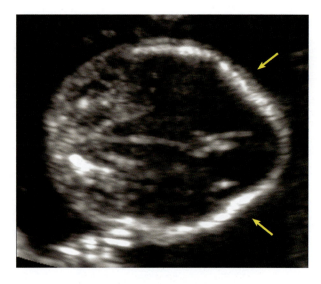

FINDINGS:

Fetal US, axial plane, shows concavity of the frontal bones (arrows).

DIFFERENTIAL DIAGNOSIS:

- Open neural tube defect
- Normal variant

DISCUSSION:

The fetal "lemon" sign refers to flattening or concavity of the frontal bones, rather than the typical convex appearance. It is crucial to obtain a true axial view at the level of the ventricles, as this sign can be mimicked by angling caudally and anteriorly to include the orbits. The "lemon" sign is thought to result from low CSF pressures with resulting deformation of the elastic calvarium. It is best seen in the second trimester of pregnancy and decreases in conspicuity with age, possibly due to progressive calvarial ossification and/or development of hydrocephalus. In high-risk pregnancies, the "lemon" sign is an important indicator for open neural tube defects such as spina bifida and encephalocele. There is an association with Chiari II malformation, Dandy-Walker, callosal agenesis, cystic hygroma, diaphragmatic hernia, hydronephrosis, umbilical vein varix, two-vessel cord, thanatophoric dysplasia, and fetal triploidy. A full fetal survey should be performed to evaluate for CNS anomalies such as ventriculomegaly, microcephaly, posterior fossa anomalies ("banana" sign), and spinal dysraphism. In low-risk pregnancies, a "mild lemon" sign can be present without posterior fossa anomalies, suggesting normal variation in fetal skeletal development.

References:

Ball RH, Filly RA, Goldstein RB, et al. The lemon sign: not a specific indicator of meningomyelocele. *J Ultrasound Med.* 1993;12(3):131-134.

Thomas M. The lemon sign. *Radiology.* 2003;228(1):206-207.

LONE RANGER

Modality:
NM

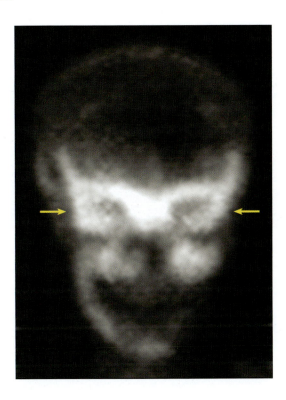

FINDINGS:

Anterior planar ⁹⁹ᵐTc-MDP scan shows avid periorbital uptake (arrows).

DIAGNOSIS:

Hyperparathyroidism

DISCUSSION:

Parathyroid hormone (PTH) is produced by the parathyroid glands, and regulates serum calcium levels by increasing bone osteoclastic activity, intestinal calcium absorption, and renal calcium resorption. HPTH refers to overactivity of the parathyroid glands and may be primary, secondary or tertiary. Primary HPTH is caused by intrinsic parathyroid abnormalities (adenoma, hyperplasia, carcinoma) and results in elevated blood calcium levels. Secondary HPTH occurs in response to low blood calcium levels, as seen in chronic renal failure and vitamin D deficiency. Tertiary HPTH represents autonomous parathyroid activity following longstanding secondary HPTH. In all cases, increased osteoclastic activity leads to diffuse osteomalacia with fibrous replacement of bone (osteitis fibrosa cystica). Diffuse resorption occurs in subperiosteal, intracortical, endosteal, trabecular, subchondral, subligamentous, and subtendinous locations. Brown tumors (osteoclastomas) are expansile collections of fibrous tissue, disorganized woven bone, and hemorrhage. Lesions appear lytic in the initial phase, and may become sclerotic in the healing phase. Radionuclide bone scanning using technetium-99m methylene diphosphonate (MDP) reveals a "superscan" appearance, with increased tracer uptake throughout the skeleton, and relatively decreased activity in the kidneys and soft tissues. Homogeneous "mask"-like periorbital uptake has been described and produces the characteristic "Lone Ranger" sign. Other causes of periorbital uptake (infection, hemorrhage, metastases) tend to be more discrete and asymmetric. In children, metastatic neuroblastoma ("raccoon eyes"), rhabdomyosarcoma, and nonaccidental trauma can also yield multifocal calvarial and facial uptake. I-123 metaiodobenzylguanidine (MIBG) scan is more sensitive and specific than conventional bone scan for evaluating neuroblastoma disease burden.

References:

Bohdiewicz PJ, Gallegos E, Fink-Bennett D. Raccoon eyes and the MIBG super scan: scintigraphic signs of neuroblastoma in a case of suspected child abuse. *Pediatr Radiol.* 1995;25(Suppl 1):S90-S92.

Pradeep DJ, Clunie GP, Watts RA, et al. Hyperparathyroid bone disease—an unusual and memorable condition. *Ann Rheum Dis.* 2006;65(9):1244.

PEPPER POT, PUNCHED OUT, RAINDROP

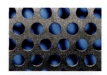

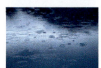

Modalities:
XR, CT

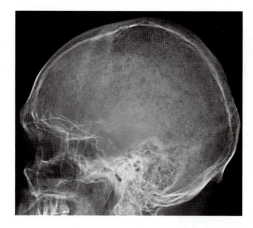

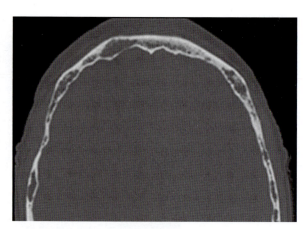

FINDINGS:

Lateral radiograph and axial CT show numerous permeative calvarial lytic lesions.

DIFFERENTIAL DIAGNOSIS:

- Multiple myeloma
- Metastases
- Langerhans cell histiocytosis

DISCUSSION:

Multiple myeloma (MM), a plasma cell dyscrasia, is the most common primary bone malignancy in adults and the second most common hematologic malignancy in Western countries. At imaging, disseminated multiple myeloma typically appears as numerous intramedullary lytic lesions with a well-defined or "punched-out" morphology. In adults, this appearance may also be seen with diffuse lytic metastases (such as renal cell or thyroid carcinoma), though margins tend to be less well-circumscribed. The permeative distribution of multiple myeloma and metastases should be distinguished from the "pseudopermeative" appearance of aggressive osteoporosis, radiation changes, and intraosseous hemangioma. These processes affect the cortex, rather than the medullary cavity, but can be difficult to localize when widespread. Careful inspection of tangential radiographs and/or cross-sectional imaging are required. In children, the differential includes Langerhans cell histiocytosis (LCH), which tends to produce fewer lesions with asymmetric involvement of the inner and outer tables ("beveled edge" and "bullseye" signs). Lytic metastases from Ewing sarcoma, neuroblastoma, and leukemia tend to be more aggressive with poorly defined borders.

References:

Delorme S, Baur-Melnyk A. Imaging in multiple myeloma. *Eur J Radiol.* 2009;70(3):401-408.

Helms CA, Munk PL. Pseudopermeative skeletal lesions. *Br J Radiol.* 1990;63(750):461-467.

POTT PUFFY TUMOR

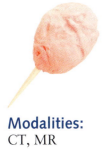

Modalities:
CT, MR

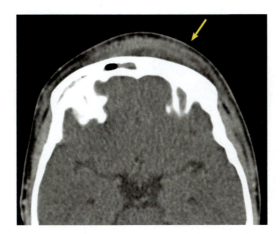 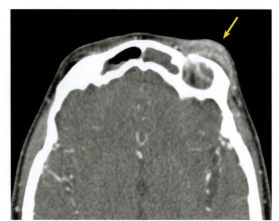

FINDINGS:

- Axial noncontrast CT shows subcutaneous edema and fat stranding in the left frontal scalp (arrow).
- Axial contrast-enhanced CT shows opacification of the left frontal sinus, defect in the left orbital roof, and subperiosteal abscess (arrow).

DIAGNOSIS:

Pott puffy tumor

DISCUSSION:

Pott puffy tumor, first described by Sir Percival Pott in 1760, refers to osteomyelitis with subperiosteal abscess complicating acute sinusitis, trauma, drug inhalation, or surgery. This usually involves the frontal sinuses of adolescent patients, who present with superficial forehead swelling. Intracranial extension can occur with epidural abscess, subdural empyema, cerebral abscess, and/or venous thrombosis. Prompt surgical intervention is indicated with abscess drainage, debridement of necrotic tissue, and long-term antibiotic therapy.

Reference:

Acke F, Lemmerling M, Heylbroeck P, et al. Pott's puffy tumor: CT and MRI findings. *JBR-BTR.* 2011;94(6):343-345.

QUADRIPOD, TRIMALAR, TETRAPOD, TRIPOD

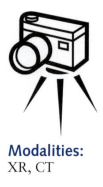

Modalities:
XR, CT

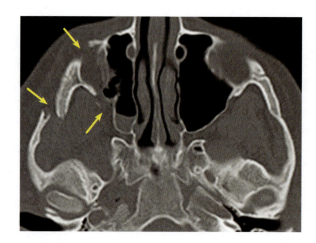

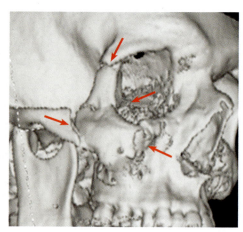

FINDINGS:

- Axial CT shows a distracted right zygomaticomaxillary complex fracture (arrows), with tripod-shaped bony fragment.
- 3D CT reconstruction shows disruption of all four sutures (arrows) of the right zygomaticomaxillary complex.

DIAGNOSIS:

Zygomaticomaxillary complex fracture, type B

DISCUSSION:

The facial skeleton is a complex structure that is stabilized by horizontal and vertical buttresses. Disruption of the facial buttresses following blunt and/or penetrating trauma produces various characteristic fracture patterns. Zygomaticomaxillary complex (ZMC) fractures are the second most common facial fractures and result from direct trauma to the malar eminence. The Zingg classification includes type A, B, and C fractures. Type A fractures are low-energy incomplete fractures that can involve the zygomatic arch (A1), lateral orbital wall (A2), or inferior orbital rim (A3). Type B are known as tetrapod fractures and involve all four sutures of the ZMC: zygomaticofrontal suture superiorly, zygomaticomaxillary suture medially, zygomaticotemporal suture posterolaterally, and zygomaticosphenoid suture posteromedially. Disruption of the first three sutures can be identified on radiography, while the fourth suture requires CT for evaluation. Type C fractures are complex multifragment fractures with additional comminution of the zygomatic bone. Complications include trismus; globe, optic nerve, and infraorbital nerve injury; and extraocular muscle entrapment. Minor fractures can be treated conservatively, but complex fractures require complete surgical exposure with open reduction and internal fixation.

Reference:

Bogusiak K, Arkuszewski P. Characteristics and epidemiology of zygomaticomaxillary complex fractures. *J Craniofac Surg.* 2010;21(4):1018-1023.

SALT AND PEPPER, SNOWFLAKE

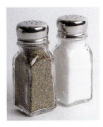

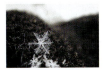

Modalities:
XR, CT

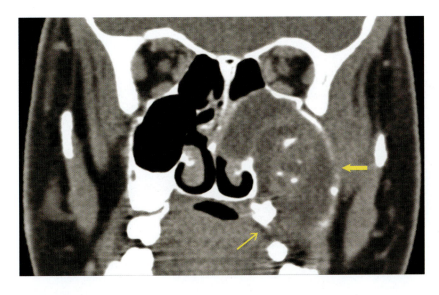

FINDINGS:

Coronal CT shows an expansile, partially calcified mass associated with a left maxillary tooth (thin arrow), with apical extension into the left maxillary sinus (thick arrow) and nasal cavity.

DIAGNOSIS:

Adenomatoid odontogenic tumor

DISCUSSION:

Adenomatoid odontogenic tumor (AOT) is a rare tumor that typically affects young female patients in the second decade of life. It arises from the enamel organ or dental lamina, usually in the anterior maxilla or mandible. The follicular type is associated with the crown and often root of an unerupted tooth, while the extrafollicular type is located adjacent to the roots of erupted permanent teeth. The peripheral (extraosseous) type of AOT is rare and occurs in the gingiva. At imaging, AOT appears as a well-circumscribed lytic lesion with flocculent internal calcifications, yielding a "salt and pepper" appearance. Apical extension past the cementoenamel junction is common. AOT is frequently misdiagnosed as a dentigerous (follicular) cyst. However, a dentigerous cyst should not extend beyond the cementoenamel junction, and lacks internal mineralization. Primary sinonasal masses, such as inverted papilloma and esthesioneuroblastoma, may demonstrate radiodensities representing calcification or residual bone. However, these lesions are not typically seen in association with teeth.

References:

Dunfee BL, Sakai O, Pistey R, et al. Radiologic and pathologic characteristics of benign and malignant lesions of the mandible. *Radiographics*. 2006;26(6):1751-1768.

Som PM, Lidov M. The significance of sinonasal radiodensities: ossification, calcification, or residual bone? *AJNR Am J Neuroradiol*. 1994;15(5):917-922.

SPALDING

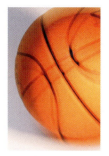

Modalities:
XR, US, MR

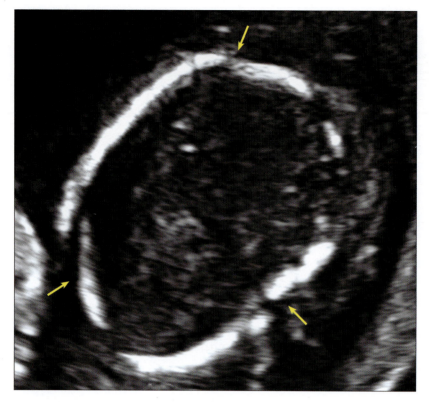

FINDINGS:

Fetal US, axial plane, shows a deformed skull with overlapping sutures (arrows) and separation from underlying brain.

DIAGNOSIS:

Fetal demise

DISCUSSION:

Spalding sign, described by Alfred Baker Spalding in 1922, refers to widely separated and overriding cranial sutures. This is a late finding of fetal demise, usually occurring 4-7 days after the initial event. Other signs of fetal demise include Deuel halo, a radiolucent band around the skull due to scalp edema and separation; and gas within the fetus and portal/umbilical veins. Occasionally, Spalding sign can be seen in live fetuses prior to 20 weeks of gestation, but remains a poor prognostic sign. Associations include extrinsic pressure or severe contractions during labor; oligohydramnios; microcephaly; and craniosynostosis. A biophysical profile should be performed to examine fetal heart rate, movement, tone, breathing, and amniotic fluid volume.

References:

Shaff MI. An evaluation of the radiological signs of fetal death. *S Afr Med J*. 1975;49(18):736-738.

Thomson JL. The differential diagnosis of Spalding's sign. *Br J Radiol*. 1950;23(266):122-124, illust.

STEPLADDER, TENNIS RACKET

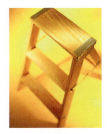

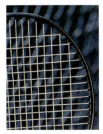

Modalities:
XR, CT, MR

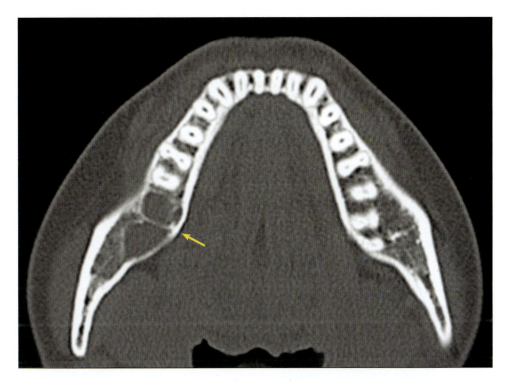

FINDINGS:

Axial CT shows a right mandibular lytic lesion with thin linear septation (arrow).

DIFFERENTIAL DIAGNOSIS:

- Odontogenic myxoma
- Ameloblastoma
- Nonodontogenic bone tumor

DISCUSSION:

Odontogenic myxoma is a rare benign, locally invasive tumor arising from odontogenic connective tissue, which usually affects patients in the second or third decades. The majority are multilocular and located in the mandibular ramus or posterior body. These demonstrate multiple internal septations that are classically thin and straight, with a "tennis racket" appearance. Septa can also be thick and curved, in which case they are indistinguishable from ameloblastoma. Other types of odontogenic myxoma include unilocular, osteolytic, and mixed lytic/sclerotic. Nonodontogenic bone tumors (aneurysmal bone cyst, fibrous dysplasia) can also demonstrate a lytic septated appearance.

References:

Dunfee BL, Sakai O, Pistey R, et al. Radiologic and pathologic characteristics of benign and malignant lesions of the mandible. *Radiographics*. 2006;26(6):1751-1768.

Zhang J, Wang H, He X, et al. Radiographic examination of 41 cases of odontogenic myxomas on the basis of conventional radiographs. *Dentomaxillofac Radiol*. 2007;36(3):160-167.

STRAWBERRY

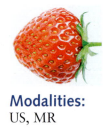

Modalities:
US, MR

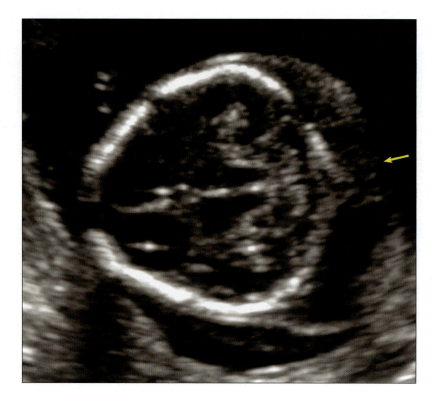

FINDINGS:

Fetal US, axial plane, shows a flattened occiput and pointed frontal bones. There is also a thick nuchal fold (arrow).

DIFFERENTIAL DIAGNOSIS:

- Trisomy 18 (Edwards syndrome)
- Other chromosomal abnormalities

DISCUSSION:

The fetal "strawberry" skull refers to flattening of the occiput with pointed frontal bones. This finding is thought to reflect hypoplasia of the face, frontal lobes, and hindbrain. It is seen with severe chromosomal anomalies, particularly trisomy 18 (Edwards syndrome). A full fetal survey should be performed to identify additional anomalies such as choroid plexus cysts, cystic hygroma, clenched hands, rocker-bottom feet, congenital heart disease, gastrointestinal malformations, and genitourinary anomalies. Due to the high incidence of chromosomal malformations, amniocentesis should be performed for fetal karyotyping.

References:

Nicolaides KH, Salvesen DR, Snijders RJ, Gosden CM. Strawberry-shaped skull in fetal trisomy 18. *Fetal Diagn Ther*. 1992;7(2):132-137.

Yeo L, Guzman ER, Day-Salvatore D, et al. Prenatal detection of fetal trisomy 18 through abnormal sonographic features. *J Ultrasound Med*. 2003;22(6):581-590; quiz 591-592.

STUCK DISC

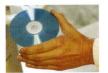

Modality:
MR

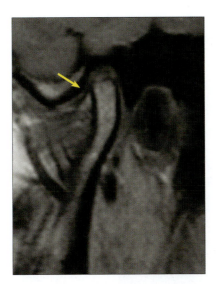
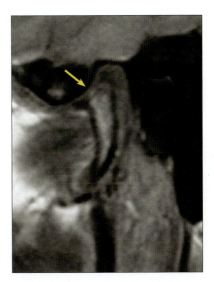

FINDINGS:

Sagittal T2-weighted MR in closed and open-mouth positions show fixation of the articular disc (arrows) within the glenoid fossa and restricted motion of the mandibular condyle.

DIAGNOSIS:

Temporomandibular disc adhesions

DISCUSSION:

The temporomandibular joint (TMJ) is a complex diarthrodial joint that coordinates rotatory and translational movements between the articular disc (meniscus), mandibular condyle, and glenoid fossa of the temporal bone. TMJ dysfunction is a common cause of myofascial pain and masticatory difficulty. Dynamic MR with closed and open-mouth views in sagittal and coronal planes is used to evaluate joint function. Normally, the TMJ disc has a biconcave appearance, with the thinnest portion (intermediate zone) centered over the condylar head in both closed- and open-mouth views. In closed-mouth position, the disc-condyle complex is located in the glenoid fossa. As the mouth begins to open, the digastric muscle forces the disc-condyle complex downward, causing it to rotate in the lower joint space. Subsequently, the inferior head of the lateral pterygoid muscle (LPM) pulls the disc-condyle complex anteriorly under the articular eminence. With full mouth opening, the condyle comes to rest beneath the anterior band of the meniscus. The pathologic "stuck disc" is seen in the setting of disc adhesions. The disc becomes fixed within the glenoid fossa in both closed- and open-mouth views, with resulting limitation of condylar translation.

Reference:

Tomas X, Pomes J, Berenguer J, et al. MR imaging of temporomandibular joint dysfunction: a pictorial review. *Radiographics*. 2006;26(3):765-781.

TAM O' SHANTER

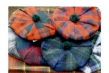

Modalities:
XR, CT, MR

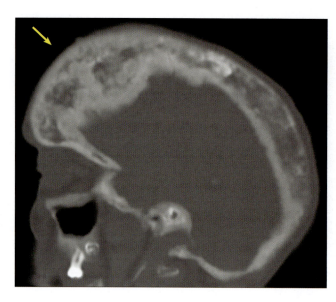

FINDINGS:

Sagittal CT shows severe calvarial expansion (arrow) with disorganized and sclerotic bone.

DIAGNOSIS:

Paget disease, advanced

DISCUSSION:

Paget disease, also known as osteodystrophia deformans, is a chronic metabolic disorder characterized by increased bone turnover and remodeling. The cause is unknown, but has been linked to chronic paramyxovirus infection and mutations in bone remodeling proteins. Disease progresses in three stages: lytic (incipient active), in which osteoclasts predominate; mixed lytic/sclerotic (active), in which osteoblast repair and osteoclast resorption occur simultaneously; and sclerotic (late inactive), in which osteoblasts predominate. Paget disease involves the skull in 25%-65% of cases. The lytic phase is known as osteoporosis circumscripta and manifests as sharply marginated, lucent lesions favoring the frontal and occipital bones. The intermediate phase yields a "jigsaw" or "mosaic" pattern with thickened cortex, trabecular disorganization, and alternating islands of lysis/sclerosis. The sclerotic phase produces a "cotton-wool" appearance with fluffy areas of sclerosis that can cross sutures. Advanced disease produces the "Tam o' Shanter" (Scottish bonnet) appearance with a broad and flattened calvarium. Late complications of Paget disease include hydrocephalus, cranial neuropathies, syringohydromyelia, and sarcomatous transformation.

References:

Smith SE, Murphey MD, Motamedi K, et al. From the archives of the AFIP. Radiologic spectrum of Paget disease of bone and its complications with pathologic correlation. *Radiographics.* 2002;22(5):1191-1216.

Theodorou DJ, Theodorou SJ, Kakitsubata Y. Imaging of Paget disease of bone and its musculoskeletal complications: review. *AJR Am J Roentgenol.* 2011;196(6 Suppl):S64-S75.

VOLCANO

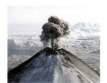

Modalities:
CT, MR

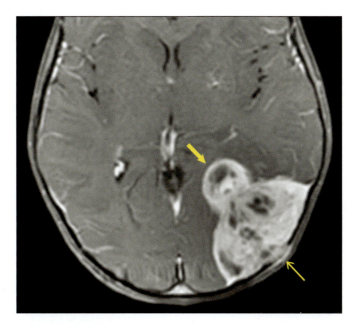

FINDINGS:

Axial contrast-enhanced T1-weighted MR shows an enhancing dural-based mass with dominant epidural component, endophytic subdural nodule (thick arrow), and transcalvarial invasion into the scalp (thin arrow).

DIFFERENTIAL DIAGNOSIS:

* Ewing sarcoma
* Neuroblastoma
* Aggressive metastases

DISCUSSION:

Rapidly growing dural-based masses erode superficially through the calvarium into the scalp, and deeply through the meninges into the brain parenchyma. In adults, such lesions usually represent metastases from breast, lung, melanoma, renal, prostate, or head and neck carcinoma. In the pediatric population, the differential includes Ewing sarcoma, neuroblastoma, lymphoma, and rhabdomyosarcoma. The "volcano" sign occurs when the intracranial portion of the mass consists solely of epidural and subdural components, without true intraaxial involvement. In such cases, the epidural component demonstrates a biconvex "lentiform" appearance, often with associated dural tails. The subdural component projects through a focal defect in the dura mater, producing a "waist" appearance with endophytic nodule indenting the brain. Without treatment, lesions will ultimately invade the leptomeninges and brain parenchyma.

References:

Maroldi R, Ambrosi C, Farina D. Metastatic disease of the brain: extra-axial metastases (skull, dura, leptomeningeal) and tumour spread. *Eur Radiol.* 2005;15(3):617-626.

Prabhu SP. "Volcano sign"—description of a sign of aggressive neoplastic epidural lesions with subdural extension. *Childs Nerv Syst.* 2009;25(4):399-402.

ABSENT PEDICLE, BLIND, MISSING OWL EYE, ONE EYED, WINKING OWL

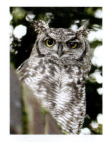

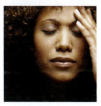

Modality:
XR

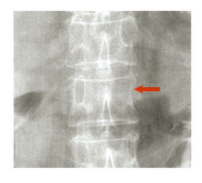

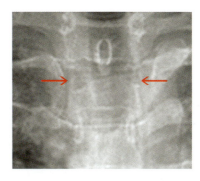

FINDINGS:

- AP radiograph shows absence of the left L1 pedicle (thick arrow).
- AP radiograph in a different patient shows absent bilateral T2 pedicles (thin arrows).

DIFFERENTIAL DIAGNOSIS:

- Metastasis
- Primary bone tumor
- Tuberculosis
- Congenitally absent pedicle

DISCUSSION:

On frontal radiography, the cortices of the vertebral pedicles appear as well-circumscribed ovoid radiodensities. Unilateral loss of the pedicle shadow produces the "winking owl" sign, while bilateral absence yields a "blind" vertebra. In adults, solitary pedicle lesions are usually metastases, but can also represent lymphoma and multiple myeloma. Other lytic lesions of the posterior elements include aneurysmal bone cyst, osteoblastoma/osteoid osteoma, and tuberculosis. Aneurysmal bone cysts are expansile "soap-bubble" lesions with internal fluid-blood levels. Osteoblastoma (>2 cm) and osteoid osteoma (<2 cm) are benign bone tumors with associated sclerotic periosteal reaction. Spinal tuberculosis (Pott disease) can cause vertebral destruction and paraspinal fluid collections. Another possibility is congenital absence of the pedicle, with ipsilateral pseudoenlargement of the neural foramen and a dysplastic "floating" transverse process.

Reference:

McLaughlin KJ, Kogon PL. The missing pedicle: a radiodiagnostic challenge. *J Can Chiropr Assoc.* 1989;33(4):187-190.

ACCORDION, CORDUROY (CLOTH), HONEYCOMB, JAIL BAR, POLKA DOT, SALT AND PEPPER, STRIATED

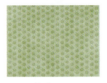

Modalities:
XR, CT, MR

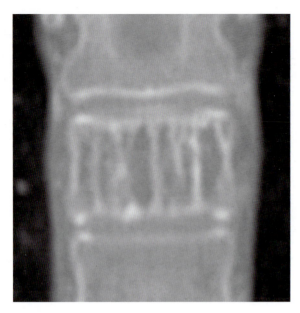

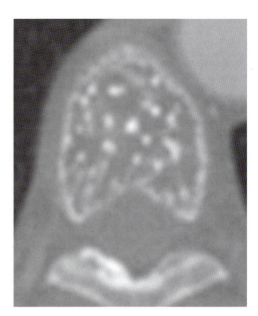

FINDINGS:

Coronal and axial CT show multiple prominent vertical trabeculations within a thoracic vertebra.

DIAGNOSIS:

Vertebral hemangioma

DISCUSSION:

Vertebral hemangioma is the most common benign tumor of the spine. Histologically, it consists of endothelium-lined vascular spaces, which may be cavernous (large vessels), capillary (small vessels), or mixed. Vascular proliferation results in osseous resorption and compensatory thickening of residual trabeculae. At imaging, the alternating lucent and sclerotic areas produce a "corduroy" appearance in long axis, "polka-dot" appearance en face, and "striated" pattern of enhancement.

References:

Murphey MD, Fairbairn KJ, Parman LM, et al. From the archives of the AFIP. Musculoskeletal angiomatous lesions: radiologic-pathologic correlation. *Radiographics*. 1995;15(4):893-917.

Yochum TR, Rowe LJ. *Essentials of Skeletal Radiology*. 3rd ed. Baltimore, MD: Lippincott Williams & Wilkins; 2004.

ANDERSSON

Modalities:
XR, CT, MR

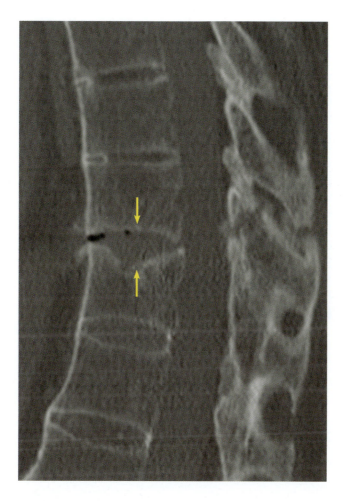

FINDINGS:

Sagittal CT shows concave erosions of thoracic vertebral endplates (arrows). There is multilevel paraspinous ossification.

DIFFERENTIAL DIAGNOSIS:

- Ankylosing spondylitis
- Infectious discitis

DISCUSSION:

At imaging, focal or asymmetric disc edema, enhancement, and endplate destruction are highly concerning for infectious discitis. This requires prompt antibiotic therapy and in some cases surgical intervention. However, in patients with ankylosing spondylitis (AS), inflammatory spondylodiscitis is a characteristic phenomenon that has been termed the Andersson lesion. The process begins in the central disc and produces symmetric concave erosions of the vertebral endplates. Other spinal manifestations of AS include peripheral spondylitis ("shiny corner"), vertebral squaring, ankylosis ("bamboo" spine), apophyseal joint fusion ("trolley track" sign), and spinous ligament enthesitis ("dagger" sign).

References:

Hermann KG, Althoff CE, Schneider U, et al. Spinal changes in patients with spondyloarthritis: comparison of MR imaging and radiographic appearances. *Radiographics*. 2005;25(3):559-569.

Lacout A, Rousselin B, Pelage JP. CT and MRI of spine and sacroiliac involvement in spondyloarthropathy. *AJR Am J Roentgenol*. 2008;191(4):1016-1023.

ANTERIOR VERTEBRAL SCALLOPING

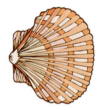

Modalities:
XR, CT, MR

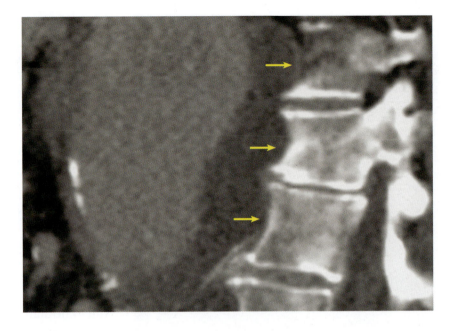

FINDINGS:

Sagittal contrast-enhanced CT shows a large abdominal aortic aneurysm with scalloping of the anterior lumbar vertebral bodies (arrows).

DIFFERENTIAL DIAGNOSIS:

- Abdominal aortic aneurysm
- Malignancy
- Chronic infection
- Tuberculosis
- Neurofibromatosis
- Down syndrome

DISCUSSION:

Anterior vertebral scalloping refers to abnormal concavity of the anterior vertebral cortex. This can be caused by pressure erosions from a large abdominal aortic aneurysm or bulky retroperitoneal lymphadenopathy, as seen in malignancy or chronic infection. Tuberculous spondylitis (Pott disease) with paraspinal abscesses tracking beneath the anterior longitudinal ligament can produce this appearance, but usually involves greater osseous destruction. Anterior vertebral scalloping can also reflect an underlying mesodermal dysplasia, which has been described in neurofibromatosis type I (NF1) and trisomy 21 (Down syndrome).

References:

Roche CJ, O'Keeffe DP, Lee WK, et al. Selections from the buffet of food signs in radiology. *Radiographics.* 2002;22(6):1369-1384.

Tsirikos AI, Ramachandran M, Lee J, et al. Assessment of vertebral scalloping in neurofibromatosis type 1 with plain radiography and MRI. *Clin Radiol.* 2004;59(11):1009-1017.

ARROW, BALLOON DISC, BIRD WING, CUPID BOW, DOUBLE HUMP, HATCHET, SEAGULL

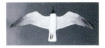

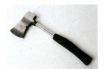

Modalities:
XR, CT, MR

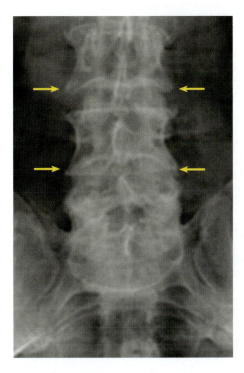

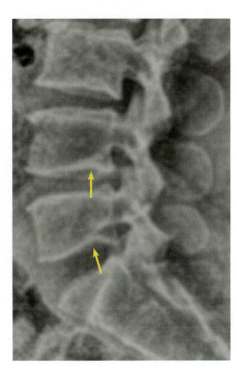

FINDINGS:

AP and lateral radiographs show paired paracentral concavities along the inferior and posterior endplates of lower lumbar vertebrae (arrows).

DIAGNOSIS:

Normal developmental variant

DISCUSSION:

The "Cupid bow" and "hatchet" contours describe parasagittal concavities along the inferior and posterior vertebral endplates, and are most commonly seen in the lower lumbar vertebrae. Histologically, there is focal absence of cartilage with direct insertion of annular fibers onto the vertebral body, resulting in endplate thickening and sclerosis. This represents a normal developmental variant with no known clinical significance. In contrast, the "codfish" vertebrae of osteopenia and the "Lincoln log" vertebrae of sickle cell anemia are broader in contour, affect the central instead of peripheral endplates, and are seen along the superior and inferior margins of multiple vertebrae.

References:

Chan KK, Sartoris DJ, Haghighi P, et al. Cupid's bow contour of the vertebral body: evaluation of pathogenesis with bone densitometry and imaging-histopathologic correlation. *Radiology.* 1997;202(1):253-256.

Dietz GW, Christensen EE. Normal "Cupid's bow" contour of the lower lumbar vertebrae. *Radiology.* 1976;121(3 pt 1):577-579.

ASSIMILATION, FAR OUT

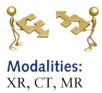

Modalities:
XR, CT, MR

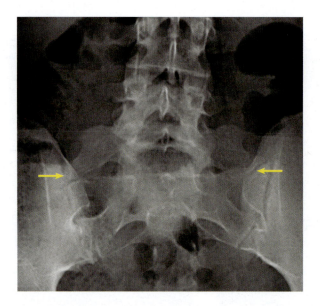

FINDINGS:

AP radiograph shows enlarged lumbar transverse processes that articulate with the sacrum (arrows).

DIAGNOSIS:

Lumbosacral transitional vertebra, type II

DISCUSSION:

Lumbosacral transitional vertebra (LSTV) is a congenital spinal anomaly in which there is sacralization of the lowest lumbar vertebra and/or lumbarization of the superior sacrum. Relative wedging of the lumbar vertebra and squaring of the sacral vertebra have been described. The Castellvi classification includes four different morphologies of LSTV. Type I demonstrates unilateral (Ia) or bilateral (Ib) dysplastic enlarged transverse processes. Type II exhibits unilateral (IIa) or bilateral (IIb) articulation between the transverse process and sacrum, forming a pseudoarthrosis or "assimilation" joint. Type III shows unilateral (IIIa) or bilateral (IIIb) osseous fusion of the transverse process and sacrum. Type IV consists of a unilateral type II and contralateral type III transition. The transverse processes have variable enlargement and degree of fusion to the sacrum. Bertolotti syndrome refers to lower back pain in the setting of LSTV, and is associated with Castellvi types II and IV. Theories for the etiology include extraforaminal nerve impingement between the enlarged lumbar transverse process and sacral ala ("far out" syndrome), degenerative changes at the anomalous facet, instability of the contralateral facet, and abnormal biomechanics at the level above the transitional articulation. Accurate enumeration of vertebrae is critical for surgical planning, and requires counting caudally from the cervical spine or identifying the iliolumbar ligaments, which typically arise from the L5 transverse processes.

References:

Konin GP, Walz DM. Lumbosacral transitional vertebrae: classification, imaging findings, and clinical relevance. *AJNR Am J Neuroradiol.* 2010;31(10):1778-1786.

Nardo L, Alizai H, Virayavanich W, et al. Lumbosacral transitional vertebrae: association with low back pain. *Radiology.* 2012;265(2):497-503.

Wiltse LL, Guyer RD, Spencer CW, et al. Alar transverse process impingement of the L5 spinal nerve: the far-out syndrome. *Spine (Phila Pa 1976).* 1984;9(1):31-41.

AXIS/C2/HARRIS RING, FAT C2

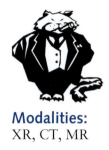

Modalities:
XR, CT, MR

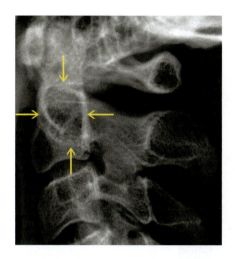

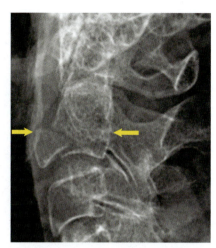

FINDINGS:

- Lateral radiograph in a normal patient shows an intact C2 ring (thin arrows) and normal C2-C3 alignment.
- Lateral radiograph in a patient with comminuted C2 fracture shows disruption of the Harris ring and widening of C2 (thick arrows).

DIAGNOSIS:

C2 body fracture

DISCUSSION:

The C2 vertebra (axis) consists of a body (centrum) and superior projection (dens, odontoid process, odontoid peg), which articulates with the anterior arch of C1 (atlas). Injuries to the atlantoaxial complex and upper cervical spine are common in elderly patients with osteopenia. These can be challenging to identify on frontal radiography, due to fracture obliquity and superimposed facial structures. AP open-mouth views are used to evaluate the dens and its relationship to the lateral masses of C1. This is useful for evaluating high (type I/II) dens fractures and atlantoaxial rotatory fixation. On lateral radiography, a normal elliptical shadow ("Harris ring") is formed by the anterior and posterior C2 body, superior articular facet, and inferior margin of the transverse foramen. Secondary signs of C2 fracture include prevertebral soft tissue swelling; disruption of the Harris ring; malalignment of C2 and C3; and the "fat C2" sign, in which the C2 vertebra appears widened relative to the superior endplate of C3. These findings indicate involvement of the C2 vertebral body, which can be seen in complex C2 fractures; low (type III) dens fractures; and traumatic spondylolisthesis ("hangman" fracture). CT and MR are used to characterize bone and soft tissue/ligamentous injury, respectively.

References:

Mirvis SE, Harris JH, Hopkins H. *The Radiology of Acute Cervical Spine Trauma*. 3rd ed. Lippincott Williams & Wilkins; 1996.

Pellei DD. The fat C2 sign. *Radiology*. 2000;217(2):359-360.

BAMBOO, POKER, RAT TAIL

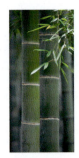

Modalities:
XR, CT, MR

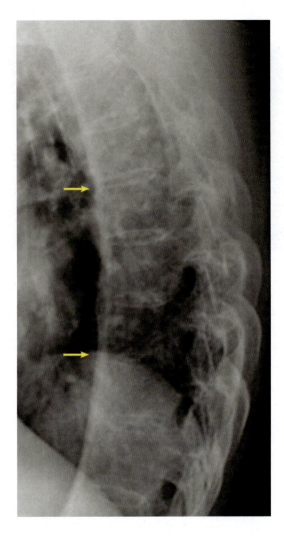

FINDINGS:

Lateral radiograph shows vertical bridging syndesmophytes (arrows) along multiple thoracic vertebrae.

DIAGNOSIS:

Seronegative spondyloarthropathy

DISCUSSION:

The "bamboo" spine refers to vertebral ankylosis caused by ossification of the intervertebral ligaments with formation of marginal syndesmophytes. This appearance is seen in inflammatory arthropathies, including ankylosing spondylitis (AS), enteropathic, psoriatic, reactive, and juvenile idiopathic arthritis. In AS and enteropathic arthritis, syndesmophyte formation is typically symmetric; in psoriatic and reactive arthritis, disease involvement is asymmetric. There is a predisposition for "chalk-stick" insufficiency fractures, which occur spontaneously or after minimal trauma. These can occur at the level of the disc (transdiscal) or through the vertebral body (transvertebral).

Reference:

Hermann KG, Althoff CE, Schneider U, et al. Spinal changes in patients with spondyloarthritis: comparison of MR imaging and radiographic appearances. *Radiographics.* 2005;25(3):559-569.

BAR, BLOCK, FUSED, (WASP) WAIST

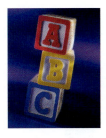

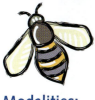

Modalities:
XR, CT, MR

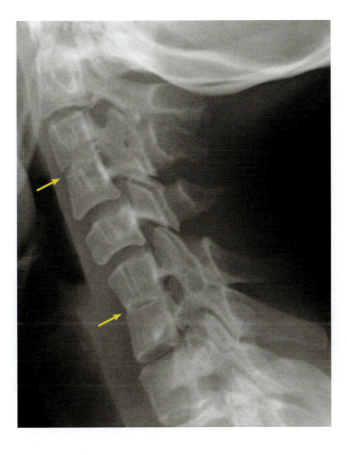

FINDINGS:

Lateral radiograph shows partial fusion of the C3-C4 and C6-C7 vertebrae, with hypoplastic intervertebral discs (arrows) and bridging of the posterior elements.

DIAGNOSIS:

Congenital vertebral fusion

DISCUSSION:

Vertebral fusion can be due to congenital or acquired causes. Congenital vertebral fusion results from errors in embryonic segmentation, and is most commonly seen in the cervical or lumbar spine. Adjacent vertebrae are partially or completely fused, with osseous "bars" joining the posterior elements. In addition, there is a hypoplastic intervertebral disc with decreased anteroposterior diameter, forming a characteristic "waist" with anterior vertebral concavity. Block vertebrae can occur sporadically or in association with various conditions including Klippel-Feil syndrome, VACTERL association, and various skeletal dysplasias. In contrast, acquired vertebral fusion is caused by inflammation, infection, surgery, or trauma. The intervertebral disc is obliterated without a focal "waist," and the spinous processes remain unfused.

References:

Castriota-Scanderbeg A, Dallapiccola B. *Abnormal Skeletal Phenotypes: From Simple Signs to Complex Diagnoses*. Berlin: Springer; 2005.

Kumar R, Guinto FC Jr, Madewell JE, et al. The vertebral body: radiographic configurations in various congenital and acquired disorders. *Radiographics*. 1988;8(3):455-485.

BAR, DOT AND DASH, TRAMLINE

Modalities:
NM, MR

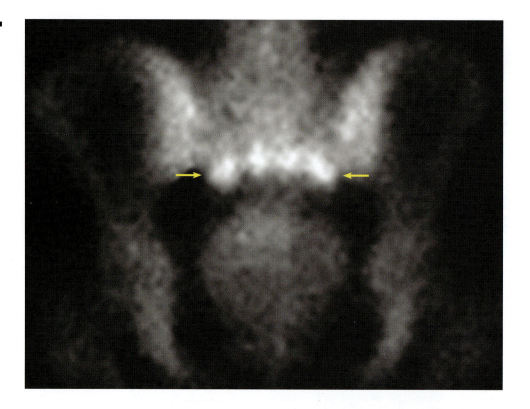

FINDINGS:

Anterior planar ^{99m}Tc-MDP bone scan shows horizontal foci of uptake across the sacral body (arrows), as well as vertical uptake in both sacral alae.

DIAGNOSIS:

Sacral insufficiency fracture

DISCUSSION:

Sacral insufficiency fracture is a common cause of lower back pain in patients with osteopenia or osteomalacia. Radionuclide bone scintigraphy with technetium-99m methylene disphosphonate (MDP) and MR are the most sensitive imaging examinations. On bone scan, incomplete sacral fractures demonstrate horizontal sacral uptake in a "bar" or "dot-dash" pattern. Complete fractures involve the sacral body and both sacral alae, creating an "H" appearance. On MR, bone marrow edema and enhancement follow a similar distribution. Treatment is conservative, with sacroplasty and/or surgery reserved for refractory cases. The differential includes metastases, which tend to be more discrete and asymmetric in distribution.

References:

Fujii M, Abe K, Hayashi K, et al. Honda sign and variants in patients suspected of having a sacral insufficiency fracture. *Clin Nucl Med.* 2005;30(3):165-169.

Lyders EM, Whitlow CT, Baker MD, et al. Imaging and treatment of sacral insufficiency fractures. *AJNR Am J Neuroradiol.* 2010;31(2):201-210.

BARREL, BOX, SQUARE

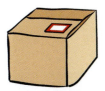

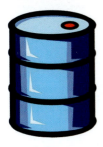

Modalities:
XR, CT, MR

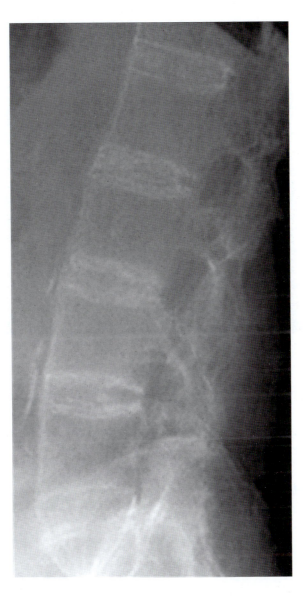

FINDINGS:

Lateral radiograph shows squared lumbar vertebrae with marginal syndesmophytes and disc calcifications.

DIFFERENTIAL DIAGNOSIS:

- Inflammatory arthritis
- Paget disease
- Down syndrome
- Turner syndrome

DISCUSSION:

Normal vertebrae demonstrate mild concavity along the anterior margins. Straightening or convex bulging ("box" or "barrel" vertebrae) is abnormal and can occur in inflammatory arthropathies including ankylosing spondylitis, rheumatoid arthritis, psoriatic arthritis, and reactive arthritis. In these conditions, enthesitis of the anterior longitudinal ligament results in bone remodeling. Paget disease can also produce "box"-shaped vertebrae, but these have an expanded appearance with cortical thickening ("picture frame" vertebra) and trabecular disorganization ("pumice" appearance). Occasionally, patients with Down or Turner syndromes can also demonstrate squaring of vertebrae.

References:

Kumar R, Guinto FC Jr, Madewell JE, et al. The vertebral body: radiographic configurations in various congenital and acquired disorders. *Radiographics*. 1988;8(3):455-485.

Yochum TR, Rowe LJ. *Essentials of Skeletal Radiology*. 3rd ed. Baltimore, MD: Lippincott Williams & Wilkins; 2004.

BASILAR IMPRESSION, BASILAR INVAGINATION

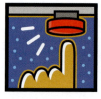

Modalities:
XR, CT, MR

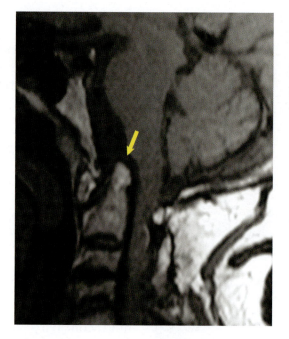
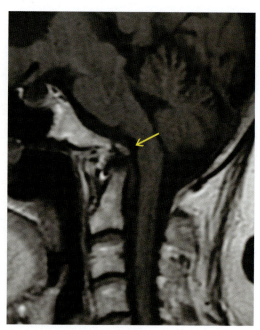

FINDINGS:

- Sagittal T1-weighted MR shows superior migration of the dens (thick arrow) beyond the clivus.
- Sagittal T1-weighted MR in a different patient shows platybasia and superior migration of both clivus and dens (thin arrow).

DIFFERENTIAL DIAGNOSIS:

- Basilar invagination
- Basilar impression

DISCUSSION:

Superior migration of the odontoid process above the level of the foramen magnum may be congenital or acquired. True basilar invagination refers to a primary developmental abnormality with prolapse of the odontoid into the skull base. This is seen with Down syndrome, Klippel-Feil syndrome, and Chiari malformation. Basilar impression, also known as acquired basilar invagination, refers to pathologic softening of the skull base with secondary upward migration of the dens and clivus. This occurs with rheumatoid arthritis, Paget disease, connective tissue disorders, hyperparathyroidism, osteomalacia, rickets, osteogenesis imperfecta, achondroplasia, mucopolysaccharidosis, and skeletal dysplasias. Platybasia, or flattening of the skull base, is commonly associated. If untreated, progressive odontoid migration can cause foramen magnum stenosis and brainstem impingement, requiring surgical decompression.

Reference:

Smoker WR, Khanna G. Imaging the craniocervical junction. *Childs Nerv Syst.* 2008;24(10): 1123-1145.

BATWING, BOWTIE, DOUBLE OUTLINE, FAN, HANGING, JUMPED, LOCKED, PERCHED

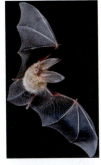

Modalities:
XR, CT, MR

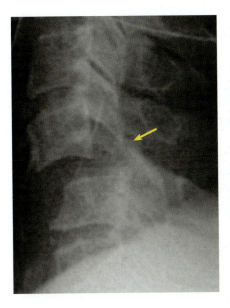

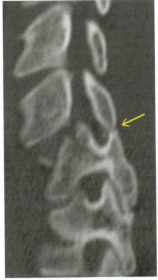

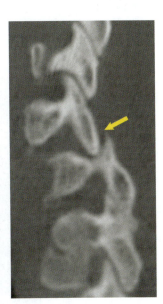

FINDINGS:

- Lateral radiograph shows anterior facet dislocation (arrow) in the lower cervical spine.
- Sagittal CT shows unilateral perched (thin arrow) and contralateral locked (thick arrow) facets.

DIAGNOSIS:

Facet dislocation

DISCUSSION:

The apophyseal (facet) joint is a synovial joint formed between the inferior articular process of a vertebra and the superior articular process of the vertebra below it. Facet joints stabilize the spine by limiting anterior translation, flexion, and excessive rotation. Unilateral facet dislocation is a mechanically stable injury, whereas bilateral facet dislocation is unstable. Mild injury leads to facet subluxation, which can be treated by closed reduction. Moderate displacement leads to "hanging" or "perched" facets, which articulate at a single point and can slip either anteriorly or posteriorly. Severe dislocation results in "locked" facets, with the inferior articular process of the cranial vertebra trapped between the caudal vertebral body and its superior articular process. Correction requires traction and occasionally open reduction. On lateral images, both perched and locked facets can demonstrate a "bowtie" appearance because of overriding of the inferior and superior articular processes. Oblique images demonstrate disruption of the normal "shingles on a roof" or imbricated appearance of normally aligned facets.

Reference:

Yetkin Z, Osborn AG, Giles DS, et al. Uncovertebral and facet joint dislocations in cervical articular pillar fractures: CT evaluation. *AJNR Am J Neuroradiol.* 1985;6(4):633-637.

BEAK, BOTTLE, BULLET, FLAME, HOOK, NOSE, NOTCH, SAIL, SPUR, STEPOFF, TONGUE, WEDGE

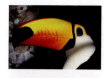

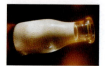

Modalities:
XR, CT, MR

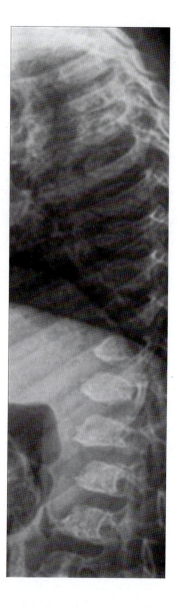

FINDINGS:

Lateral radiograph shows multiple anteriorly pointed vertebrae.

DIFFERENTIAL DIAGNOSIS:

- Mucopolysaccharidoses
- Lysosomal storage disorders
- Skeletal dysplasias
- Metabolic disorders

DISCUSSION:

"Beak" or "tongue" vertebrae demonstrate abnormally pointed or rounded anterior margins, which are thought to represent anterior herniation of the nucleus pulposus. This most commonly occurs at the thoracolumbar junction with associated focal kyphosis. The differential diagnosis is broad and includes mucopolysaccharidoses; lysosomal storage disorders; skeletal dysplasias (achondroplasia, thanatophoric dysplasia, spondyloepiphyseal dysplasia); metabolic disorders (hypothyroidism, phenylketonuria); trisomy 21 (Down syndrome); neuromuscular conditions (spinal muscular atrophy, myelomeningocele); and nonaccidental trauma. In hypothyroidism, posterior disc space widening and irregularity can create a "bottle" appearance. Skeletal changes of mucopolysaccharidosis (MPS) are known as dysostosis multiplex, and vary depending on the subtype of disease. MPS types I (Hurler-Scheie) and VI (Maroteaux-Lamy) usually show severe inferior beaking. MPS II (Hunter) demonstrates mild superior beaking. MPS IV (Morquio) typically has central beaked "flame" vertebrae. MPS III (Sanfilippo) vertebrae tend to be oval, rather than beaked.

References:

Castriota-Scanderbeg A, Dallapiccola B. *Abnormal Skeletal Phenotypes: From Simple Signs to Complex Diagnoses*. Berlin: Springer; 2005.

Swischuk LE. The beaked, notched, or hooked vertebra: its significance in infants and young children. *Radiology*. 1970;95(3):661-664.

BICONCAVE, COD(FISH), DISCAL BALLOONING, FISHBONE, FISH MOUTH, HOURGLASS, LENS, REYNOLD

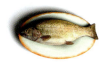

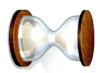

Modalities:
XR, CT, MR

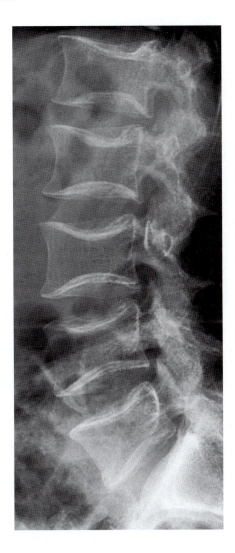

FINDINGS:

Lateral radiograph shows smooth central concavities along the superior and inferior vertebral endplates.

DIAGNOSIS:

Osteopenia

DISCUSSION:

"Codfish" vertebrae demonstrate smooth central concavities along the superior and inferior endplates, reflecting protrusion of the intervertebral discs into weakened bone. This appearance is seen in various conditions including osteopenia, rickets, hyperparathyroidism, sickle cell disease, eosinophilic granuloma, mucopolysaccharidoses, neurofibromatosis, and skeletal dysplasias.

References:

Kumar R, Guinto FC Jr, Madewell JE, et al. The vertebral body: radiographic configurations in various congenital and acquired disorders. *Radiographics.* 1988;8(3):455-485.

Yochum TR, Rowe LJ. *Essentials of Skeletal Radiology.* 3rd ed. Baltimore, MD: Lippincott Williams & Wilkins; 2004.

BLOWN OUT, FINGER IN BALLOON, HONEYCOMB, LATTICE, SOAP BUBBLE

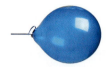

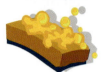

Modalities:
XR, CT, MR

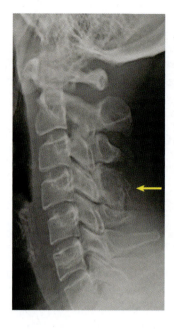 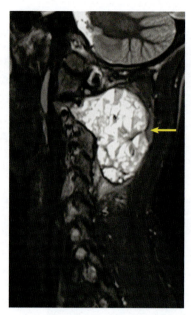

FINDINGS:

- Lateral radiograph shows an expansile lytic lesion of the C4 spinous process (arrow).
- Sagittal T2-weighted MR in a different patient shows an expansile lesion of the C3 posterior elements (arrow), with multiple septations and fluid-blood levels.

DIAGNOSIS:

Aneurysmal bone cyst

DISCUSSION:

Aneurysmal bone cyst (ABC) is a benign lytic tumor that consists histologically of multiple nonendothelialized blood and serum-filled spaces. The spine is involved in 3%-20% of cases, with a predilection for the posterior elements. Lesions can be intraosseous or extraosseous, developing on the surface of the bone with extension into the marrow ("finger in balloon" appearance). On radiography and CT, ABC has a lytic septated appearance resembling a "soap bubble." On MR, multiple fluid-blood levels can be identified, but are nonspecific. Solid components are rare and suggest either the solid variant of ABC or secondary ABC with a precursor lesion such as giant cell tumor. On radionuclide bone scintigraphy, tracer accumulates at the periphery with little activity in the center ("doughnut" sign). The differential for posterior element lesions includes metastases, which have a more aggressive imaging appearance; osteoid osteoma/osteoblastoma, which demonstrate sclerotic periosteal reaction; and tuberculosis, which causes frank osseous destruction with paraspinal fluid collections.

Reference:

Rodallec MH, Feydy A, Larousserie F, et al. Diagnostic imaging of solitary tumors of the spine: what to do and say. *Radiographics.* 2008;28(4):1019-1041.

BONE IN BONE, DOUBLE CONTOUR, ENDOBONE, GHOST

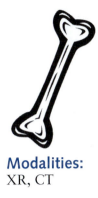

Modalities:
XR, CT

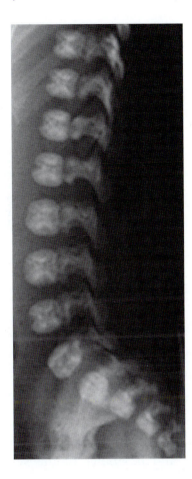

FINDINGS:

Lateral radiograph shows rectangular zones of sclerosis within the thoracolumbar vertebrae.

DIFFERENTIAL DIAGNOSIS:

- Mesenchymal dysplasia
- Metabolic bone disorders
- Systemic stress
- Normal infantile vertebrae

DISCUSSION:

"Bone in bone" vertebrae demonstrate internal sclerotic lines resembling a mini-vertebral body. In newborns, this finding can be a normal variant. Abnormal endosteal bone deposition is responsible for this appearance in mesenchymal dysplasias (type II osteopetrosis, infantile cortical hyperostosis, cleidocranial dysplasia, progressive diaphyseal dysplasia); metabolic bone disorders (Paget disease, idiopathic hypercalcemia, hypothyroidism, hypoparathyroidism, acromegaly, oxalosis); and nutritional deficiencies (rickets, scurvy). Systemic stress can also yield the "endobone" appearance, with growth arrest lines marking the position of the physis at the time of insult. This appearance may be seen with leukemia, hereditary anemias, lysosomal storage disorders, radiation, heavy metal poisoning, congenital syphilis, and Thorotrast exposure.

References:

Kumar R, Guinto FC Jr, Madewell JE, et al. The vertebral body: radiographic configurations in various congenital and acquired disorders. *Radiographics.* 1988;8(3):455-485.

Yochum TR, Rowe LJ. *Essentials of Skeletal Radiology.* 3rd ed. Baltimore, MD: Lippincott Williams & Wilkins; 2004.

BOWTIE, INVERTED T, SINGLE/SMOOTH LAYER

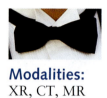

Modalities:
XR, CT, MR

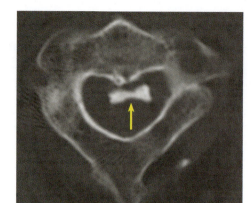 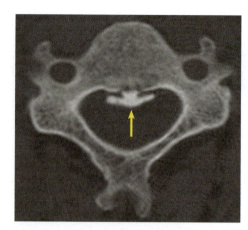

FINDINGS:

Axial CT in two different patients shows smooth unilayer ossification of the posterior longitudinal ligament (arrows).

DIAGNOSIS:

Ossification of the posterior longitudinal ligament

DISCUSSION:

The posterior longitudinal ligament (PLL) is located in the anterior spinal canal and contributes to stability, mobility, and flexibility of the vertebral column. It consists of three connective tissue layers: superficial, intermediate, and deep. The superficial layer is the most posterior, is intimately related to the dura mater, and spans several vertebral levels. The deep layer attaches directly to the intervertebral disc, and adheres to the other layers in the midline. Ossification of the PLL (OPLL) is common in elderly, male, and Asian patients. There is an association with diffuse idiopathic skeletal hyperostosis (DISH), ankylosing spondylitis (AS), and other spondyloarthropathies. The presence of OPLL predisposes to cord injury with minor trauma, especially in advanced cases with chronic spinal stenosis and cord compression. At imaging, the appearance of a single "smooth" layer of ossification suggests deep PLL involvement without dural invasion. In contrast, large irregular ossification ("modified single layer"), "double layered" ossification of the deep and superficial PLL, and/or extension into the lateral recesses ("C" sign) have been shown to correlate with dural invasion and risk of CSF leak at surgery.

References:

Epstein NE. Identification of ossification of the posterior longitudinal ligament extending through the dura on preoperative computed tomographic examinations of the cervical spine. *Spine (Phila Pa 1976)*. 2001;26(2):182-186.

Hida K, Iwasaki Y, Koyanagi I, et al. Bone window computed tomography for detection of dural defect associated with cervical ossified posterior longitudinal ligament. *Neurol Med Chir (Tokyo)* 1997;37:173-175.

Loughenbury PR, Wadhwani S, Soames RW. The posterior longitudinal ligament and peridural (epidural) membrane. *Clin Anat*. 2006;19(6):487-492.

BRAILSFORD BOW (LINE), DOUBLE VERTEBRA, GENDARME CAP, (INVERTED) NAPOLEON HAT

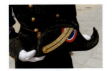

Modality:
XR

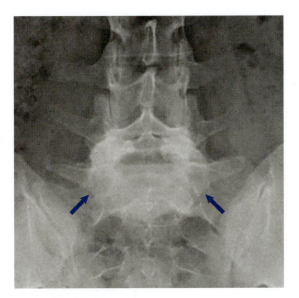
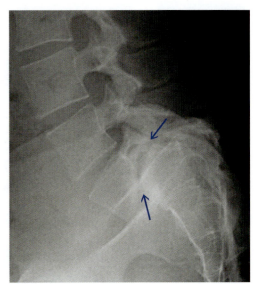

FINDINGS:

Frontal and lateral radiographs show grade V anterolisthesis of L5 on S1 (thin arrows) with superimposition on the frontal view (thick arrows).

DIAGNOSIS:

Severe L5-S1 spondylolysis

DISCUSSION:

Spondylolisthesis refers to abnormal displacement of a vertebral body relative to the vertebra below it. Etiologies are categorized using the Wiltse classification: type I (dysplastic), II (isthmic), III (degenerative), IV (traumatic), V (pathologic), and VI (postoperative). The Meyerding classification of anterolithesis, or anterior vertebral displacement, includes grade I (<25% displacement), II (25%-50%), III (50%-75%), IV (75%-100%), and V (>100%). Degenerative spondylolisthesis is caused by arthrosis at the facet joints without disruption of the pars interarticularis. There is concomitant anterior migration of the vertebra and posterior elements, resulting in grade I anterolisthesis and narrowing of the spinal canal. Isthmic spondylolisthesis, or spondylolysis, affects the pars interarticularis (isthmus) with separation of the vertebral body from the posterior elements. This results in grade II or higher anterolisthesis and widening of the spinal canal. Grade V anterolisthesis, or spondyloptosis, occurs when the vertebra is completely displaced and migrates inferiorly over the vertebra below it. Severe anterolisthesis is most common at L5-S1, where it creates a "double vertebra" or "inverted Napoleon hat" sign on frontal radiography due to superimposition of shadows.

Reference:

Talangbayan LE. The inverted Napoleon's hat sign. *Radiology*. 2007;243(2):603-604.

BURST

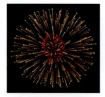

Modalities:
XR, CT, MR

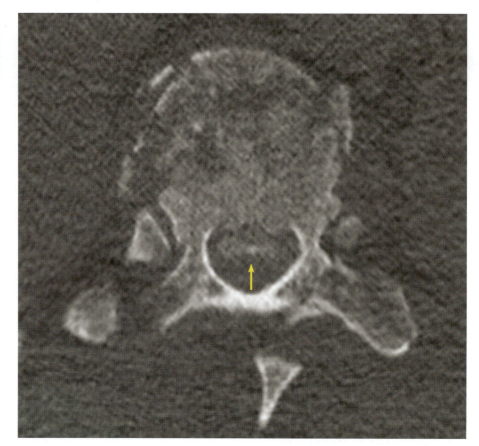

FINDINGS:

Axial CT shows an extensively comminuted fracture of the vertebral body and posterior elements. There is retropulsion of bone fragments into the spinal canal (arrow).

DIAGNOSIS:

Burst fracture

DISCUSSION:

A burst fracture is caused by high-energy axial loading as seen in motor vehicle accidents, seizures, or falls from great heights. Patients who jump and land on their feet may also have bilateral calcaneal fractures ("Don Juan" or "lover" fractures). Burst fractures most commonly occur at the thoracolumbar junction with three-column spinal injury. There is loss of vertebral height and extensive distraction of fracture fragments. Retropulsion of bone fragments into the spinal canal can cause cord compression, requiring emergent surgery.

Reference:

Bensch FV, Kiuru MJ, Koivikko MP, et al. Spine fractures in falling accidents: analysis of multidetector CT findings. *Eur Radiol.* 2004;14(4):618-624. Epub 2003 Oct 7.

BUTTERFLY, H, HONDA

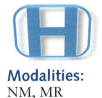

Modalities:
NM, MR

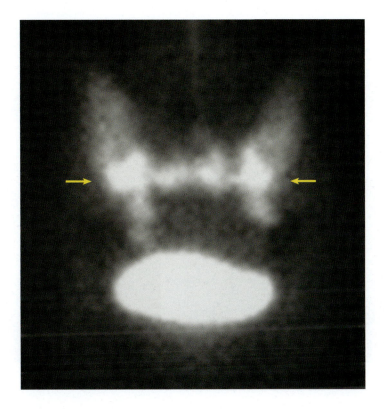

FINDINGS:

Anterior planar ^{99m}Tc-MDP bone scan shows horizontal uptake in the sacral body and vertical uptake (arrows) in both sacral alae.

DIAGNOSIS:

Sacral insufficiency fracture

DISCUSSION:

Sacral insufficiency fracture is a common cause of lower back pain in patients with osteopenia or osteomalacia. Radionuclide bone scintigraphy with technetium-99m methylene disphosphonate (MDP) and MR are the most sensitive imaging examinations. On bone scan, incomplete sacral fractures demonstrate horizontal sacral uptake in a "dot-dash" pattern. Complete fractures involve the sacral body and both sacral alae, creating an "H" appearance. On MR, bone marrow edema and enhancement follow a similar distribution. Treatment is conservative, with sacroplasty and/or surgery reserved for refractory cases. The differential includes metastases, which tend to be more discrete and asymmetric in distribution.

References:

Fujii M, Abe K, Hayashi K, et al. Honda sign and variants in patients suspected of having a sacral insufficiency fracture. *Clin Nucl Med.* 2005;30(3):165-169.

Lyders EM, Whitlow CT, Baker MD, et al. Imaging and treatment of sacral insufficiency fractures. *AJNR Am J Neuroradiol.* 2010;31(2):201-210.

BUTTERFLY, KISSING

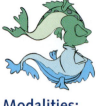

Modalities:
XR, CT, MR

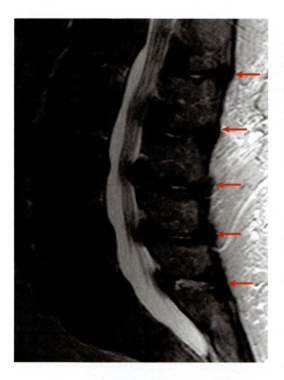 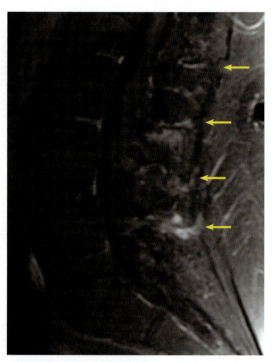

FINDINGS:

Sagittal T2-weighted and T1-weighted contrast-enhanced MR with fat saturation show hypertrophied spinous processes with edema and enhancement of the interspinous ligaments (arrows).

DIAGNOSIS:

Baastrup disease

DISCUSSION:

Baastrup disease, also known as spinous process impingement syndrome, commonly affects the elderly, athletes, and patients with lumbar hyperlordosis. In this condition, the lumbar spinous processes hypertrophy and closely appose each other in extension ("kissing" appearance). There is breakdown of the interspinous ligaments and formation of pseudoarthroses. Complications include adventitial bursitis, osteoarthritis, stress fractures, spondylolisthesis, and disc degeneration. Arthrography may demonstrate communications between the facet joints and interspinous spaces, forming a "butterfly" appearance. Therapeutic options include interspinous steroid injections and decompressive laminectomy.

Reference:

Kwong Y, Rao N, Latief K. MDCT findings in Baastrup disease: disease or normal feature of the aging spine? *AJR Am J Roentgenol.* 2011;196(5):1156-1159.

BUTTERFLY, SAGITTAL CLEFT

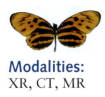

Modalities:
XR, CT, MR

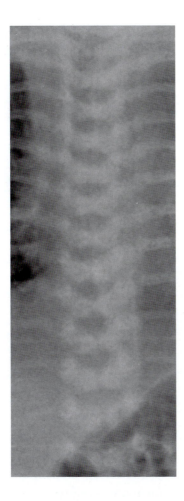

FINDINGS:

AP radiograph shows multiple thoracolumbar vertebrae with midline clefts.

DIAGNOSIS:

Butterfly vertebrae

DISCUSSION:

"Butterfly" vertebrae are composed of paramedian ossification centers that fail to fuse across the midline, due to persistent notochordal tissue. Type I ("double-D") vertebrae demonstrate a persistent sagittal cleft. On frontal radiography, the two halves of the vertebra have the shape of a capital "D." On lateral views, the vertebra retains its normal rectangular shape. Type II ("double-wedge") vertebrae have persistent sagittal and coronal clefts. On frontal radiography, the two halves of the vertebra have a triangular appearance with apices directed medially. On lateral views, there is also anterior wedging of the vertebra. Butterfly vertebrae can occur sporadically or in association with spinal dysraphism; Aicardi, Alagille, Crouzon, Jarcho-Levin, and Pfeiffer syndromes; and the VACTERL association.

References:

Cave P. Butterfly vertebra. *Br J Radiol.* 1958;31(369):503-506.

Rufener SL, Ibrahim M, Raybaud CA, et al. Congenital spine and spinal cord malformations—pictorial review. *AJR Am J Roentgenol.* 2010;194(3 Suppl):S26-S37.

C, DOUBLE LAYER, HOOK, MODIFIED SINGLE LAYER

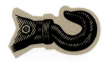

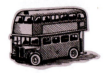

Modalities:
XR, CT, MR

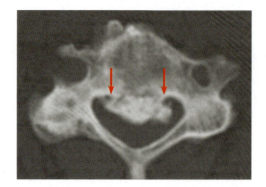

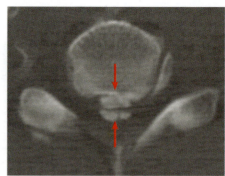

FINDINGS:

- Axial CT shows irregular ossification of the posterior longitudinal ligament extending into the lateral recesses (arrows).
- Axial CT in a different patient shows ossification of the superficial and deep layers of the posterior longitudinal ligament (arrows).

DIAGNOSIS:

Ossification of the posterior longitudinal ligament

DISCUSSION:

The posterior longitudinal ligament (PLL) is located in the anterior spinal canal and contributes to stability, mobility, and flexibility of the vertebral column. It consists of three connective tissue layers: superficial, intermediate, and deep. The superficial layer is the most posterior, is intimately related to the dura mater, and spans several vertebral levels. The deep layer attaches directly to the intervertebral disc, and adheres to the other layers in the midline. Ossification of the PLL (OPLL) is common in elderly, male, and Asian patients. There is an association with diffuse idiopathic skeletal hyperostosis (DISH), ankylosing spondylitis (AS), and other spondyloarthropathies. The presence of OPLL predisposes to cord injury with minor trauma, especially in advanced cases with chronic spinal stenosis and cord compression. At imaging, the appearance of a single "smooth" layer of ossification suggests deep PLL involvement without dural invasion. In contrast, large irregular ossification ("modified single layer"), "double layered" ossification of the deep and superficial PLL, and/or extension into the lateral recesses ("C" sign) have been shown to correlate with dural invasion and risk of CSF leak at surgery.

References:

Epstein NE. Identification of ossification of the posterior longitudinal ligament extending through the dura on preoperative computed tomographic examinations of the cervical spine. *Spine (Phila Pa 1976)*. 2001;26(2):182-186.

Hida K, Iwasaki Y, Koyanagi I, et al. Bone window computed tomography for detection of dural defect associated with cervical ossified posterior longitudinal ligament. *Neurol Med Chir (Tokyo)*. 1997;37:173-175.

Loughenbury PR, Wadhwani S, Soames RW. The posterior longitudinal ligament and peridural (epidural) membrane. *Clin Anat*. 2006;19(6):487-492.

CANDLE WAX

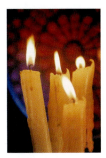

Modalities:
XR, CT, MR

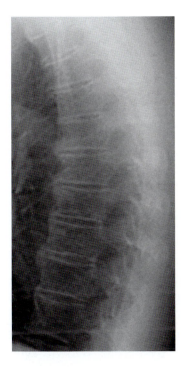

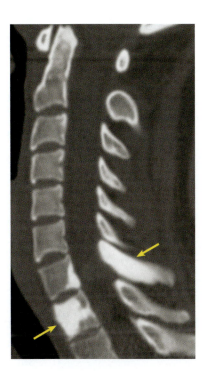

FINDINGS:

- Lateral radiograph in a patient with diffuse idiopathic skeletal hyperostosis shows paraspinal ossification with multilevel bridging osteophytes.
- Sagittal CT in a patient with melorheostosis shows segmental cortical and medullary hyperostosis (arrows) of the C7-T1 vertebrae.

DIFFERENTIAL DIAGNOSIS:

- Diffuse idiopathic skeletal hyperostosis
- Melorheostosis

DISCUSSION:

The dripping, flowing, or melted "candle wax" appearance has been used to describe both diffuse idiopathic skeletal hyperostosis (DISH) and melorheostosis. DISH is a chronic noninflammatory condition with ossification of paraspinal ligaments and entheses over at least four contiguous vertebral bodies. Associated conditions are ossification of the posterior longitudinal ligament (OPLL) and ossification of the vertebral arch ligaments (OVAL). Melorheostosis is a rare mesenchymal bone dysplasia that infrequently involves the spine, with cortical and medullary hyperostosis in a sclerotomal distribution.

References:

Belanger TA, Rowe DE. Diffuse idiopathic skeletal hyperostosis: musculoskeletal manifestations. *J Am Acad Orthop Surg.* 2001;9(4):258-267.

Ihde LL, Forrester DM, Gottsegen CJ, et al. Sclerosing bone dysplasias: review and differentiation from other causes of osteosclerosis. *Radiographics.* 2011;31(7):1865-1882.

CANINE, DOG, LONG, TALL, TOWER

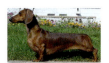

Modalities:
XR, CT, MR

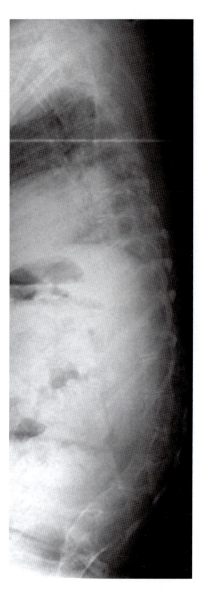

FINDINGS:

Lateral radiograph shows elongated vertebrae with increased craniocaudal and decreased anteroposterior dimension.

DIFFERENTIAL DIAGNOSIS:

- Mesenchymal dysplasia
- Neuromuscular disorder

DISCUSSION:

"Canine" vertebrae are elongated with increased craniocaudal and decreased anteroposterior dimension, analogous to the spine of a dog. This appearance can be seen in patients who are chronically supine with reduced axial loading and muscular stimulation. Other predisposing conditions include skeletal dysplasias, Down syndrome, congenital rubella, fibrodysplasia ossificans progressiva, and neuromuscular disorders (such as poliomyelitis). Focal vertebral caninization can be seen as a compensatory mechanism for adjacent vertebrae that have been shortened by infarction or infection.

References:

Kumar R, Guinto FC Jr, Madewell JE, et al. The vertebral body: radiographic configurations in various congenital and acquired disorders. *Radiographics*. 1988;8(3):455-485.

Yochum TR, Rowe LJ. *Essentials of Skeletal Radiology*. 3rd ed. Baltimore, MD: Lippincott Williams & Wilkins; 2004.

CARROT, CHALK STICK

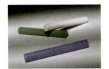

Modalities:
XR, CT, MR

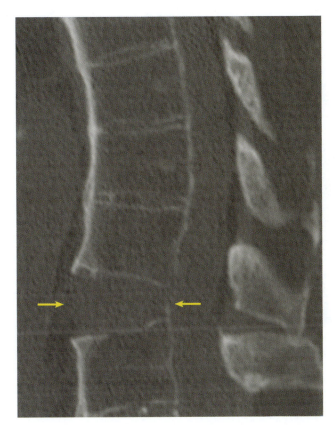

FINDINGS:

Sagittal CT shows multilevel bridging thoracic syndesmophytes, with a fracture through the intervertebral disc space (arrows).

DIFFERENTIAL DIAGNOSIS:

- Ankylosing spondylitis
- Diffuse idiopathic skeletal hyperostosis

DISCUSSION:

"Chalk stick" fracture is an insufficiency fracture that occurs spontaneously or after minimal trauma in patients with abnormal rigidity of the spine. This can occur at the level of the disc (transdiscal) or through the vertebral body (transvertebral), with failed healing leading to pseudoarthrosis and instability. Predisposing conditions include ankylosing spondylitis (AS) and diffuse idiopathic skeletal hyperostosis (DISH). AS is a chronic inflammatory seronegative spondyloarthropathy that affects the spine and sacroiliac joints. The disease is most common in young males, and there is a strong association with the HLA-B27 genotype. Other spinal manifestations of AS include peripheral spondylitis ("shiny corner"), marginal syndesmophytes ("trolley track" sign), spondylodiscitis (Andersson lesion), vertebral squaring, ankylosis ("bamboo" spine), apophyseal joint fusion ("trolley track" sign), and spinous ligament enthesitis ("dagger" sign). DISH is a chronic noninflammatory condition with ossification of paraspinal ligaments and entheses over at least four contiguous vertebral bodies. Associated conditions are ossification of the posterior longitudinal ligament (OPLL) and ossification of the vertebral arch ligaments (OVAL).

References:

Hermann KG, Althoff CE, Schneider U, et al. Spinal changes in patients with spondyloarthritis: comparison of MR imaging and radiographic appearances. *Radiographics.* 2005;25(3):559-569.

Taljanovic MS, Hunter TB, Wisneski RJ, et al. Imaging characteristics of diffuse idiopathic skeletal hyperostosis with an emphasis on acute spinal fractures: review. *AJR Am J Roentgenol.* 2009;193(3 suppl):S10-S19, quiz S20-S24.

CHAMPAGNE GLASS, MICKEY MOUSE, T, TRIANGLE

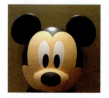

Modality:
NM

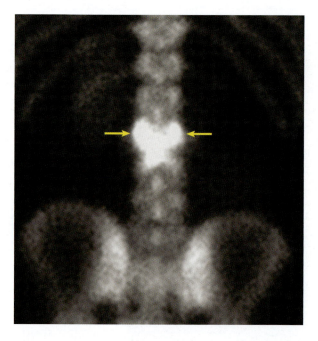

FINDINGS:

Anterior planar ^{99m}Tc-MDP bone scan shows increased uptake in the L2 vertebral body and pedicles (arrows).

DIAGNOSIS:

Paget disease

DISCUSSION:

Paget disease, also known as osteodystrophia deformans, is a chronic metabolic disorder characterized by increased bone turnover and remodeling. The cause is unknown, but has been linked to chronic paramyxovirus infection and mutations in bone remodeling proteins. Disease progresses in three stages: lytic (incipient active), in which osteoclasts predominate; mixed lytic/sclerotic (active), in which osteoblast repair and osteoclast resorption occur simultaneously; and sclerotic (late inactive), in which osteoblasts predominate. Paget disease involves the spine in 30%-75% of cases. Radionuclide bone scintigraphy shows increased tracer uptake, correlating with increased blood flow and osteoblastic activity. Symmetric uptake in the vertebral body and pedicles produces the "Mickey Mouse" sign. In contrast, metastases usually have a more discrete and asymmetric appearance. Radiographs can be ordered to confirm the characteristic trabecular coarsening and expansion of the pagetoid vertebra ("picture-frame" vertebra).

References:

Estrada WN, Kim CK. Paget's disease in a patient with breast cancer. *J Nucl Med*. 1993;34(7):1214-1216.

van Heerden BB, Prins MJ. The value of pinhole collimator imaging in the scintigraphic analysis of vertebral diseases. *S Afr Med J*. 1989;75(6):280-283.

CLASP KNIFE, HOOK, TONGUE

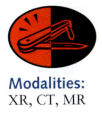

Modalities:
XR, CT, MR

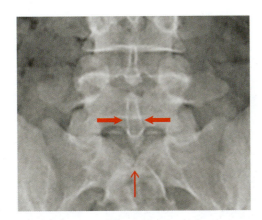
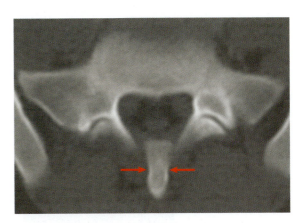

FINDINGS:

- AP radiograph shows spina bifida occulta at S1 (thin arrow) and an enlarged L5 spinous process (thick arrows).
- Axial CT shows the L5 spinous process (arrows) extending inferiorly and into the spinal canal at the site of the S1 posterior defect.

DIAGNOSIS:

Spina bifida engagement syndrome

DISCUSSION:

Spina bifida occulta is the mildest form of spina bifida, in which there is deficiency of the spinous process and/or laminae without herniation of intraspinal contents. This anomaly most commonly occurs at the lumbosacral junction, and is a common incidental finding that is estimated to affect 20% of the general population. However, in up to 2% of patients, spina bifida occulta of the upper sacrum can be associated with spinous process overgrowth at the level above the defect. This is variably known as spina bifida engagement syndrome, spina magna, or long spinous process syndrome. Anatomically, the L5 spinous process is contiguous with fibrocartilaginous tissue in the sacral defect and may adhere to the dura mater. Mechanical impingement can produce symptoms of low back pain and/or sacral radiculopathy. During lumbar extension, the L5 spinous process projects into the sacral arch defect, producing a "clasp-knife" imaging appearance with three distinct variations. Type I is the classic form, consisting of wide spina bifida occulta with an enlarged L5 spinous process ("hook" or "tongue" appearance). Type II is characterized by narrow spina bifida with an elongated L5 spinous process, forming pseudoarthroses with the S1 posterior elements. Type III is similar to type II, with the addition of a sacral ossicle.

References:

Goobar JE, Erickson F, Pate D, et al. Symptomatic clasp-knife deformity of the spinous processes. *Spine (Phila Pa 1976)*. 1988;13(8):953-956.

Yochum TR, Rowe LJ. *Essentials of Skeletal Radiology*. 3rd ed. Baltimore, MD: Lippincott Williams & Wilkins; 2004.

CLAW

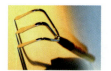

Modality:
MR

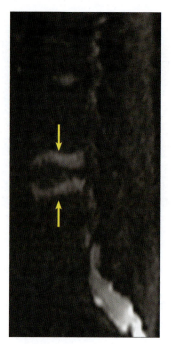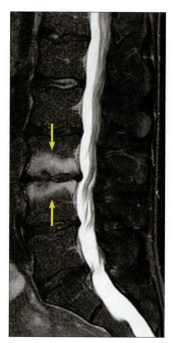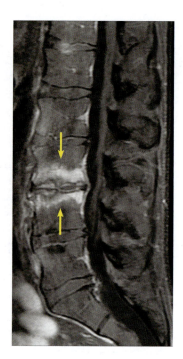

FINDINGS:

Sagittal DWI, T2-weighted, and contrast-enhanced T1-weighted MR with fat saturation show paired linear areas of reduced diffusion, edema, and enhancement surrounding the L3-L4 disc (arrows). Signal within the disc and vertebral endplates is relatively preserved.

DIAGNOSIS:

Degenerative disc disease

DISCUSSION:

Distinguishing between degenerative changes and infection in the spine can be challenging both clinically and radiologically. On MR, T2-weighted and contrast-enhanced T1-weighted images are used to identify disc edema and enhancement. These findings raise concern for infection, but can also be seen with severe inflammation secondary to degenerative disc disease. Recently, DWI has emerged as a highly sensitive and specific tool in distinguishing degenerative changes from infection. In particular, the "claw" sign refers to paired, well-defined linear areas of high signal surrounding a disc, with relatively normal signal within the disc and vertebral endplates. This finding has been shown to correlate with granulation tissue and edema along the advancing border of inflammation in patients with degenerative disc disease. The "claw" sign is readily distinguished from DWI findings of discitis, in which there is amorphous increased signal within and diffusely surrounding the disc.

Reference:

Tanenbaum LN. Clinical applications of diffusion imaging in the spine. *Magn Reson Imaging Clin N Am.* 2013;21(2):299-320.

COIN (ON END), FLAT, PANCAKE, SILVER DOLLAR, WAFER

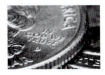

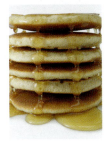

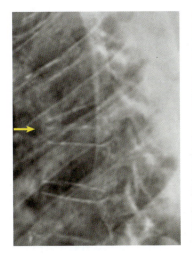

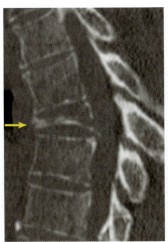

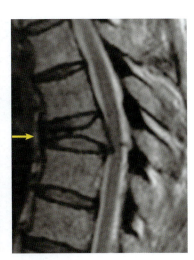

Modalities:
XR, CT, MR

FINDINGS:

Lateral radiograph, sagittal CT, and sagittal T2-weighted MR show a severe thoracic compression fracture (arrows), with near-complete loss of height and focal kyphosis. There is retropulsion into the spinal canal, contacting the ventral cord.

DIAGNOSIS:

Vertebra plana

DISCUSSION:

Complete vertebral collapse is known as vertebra plana when isolated, and platyspondyly when diffuse. This can develop following severe trauma or secondary to various conditions causing weakening of the bone. At imaging, there is a "coin on end" or "pancake" appearance with kyphotic angulation of the spine. In adults, the differential includes osteoporosis, metastasis, multiple myeloma, lymphoma/leukemia, avascular necrosis, and osteomyelitis. In children, considerations are eosinophilic granuloma, hemangioma, osteomyelitis, osteogenesis imperfecta, osteopetrosis, mucopolysaccharidoses, neurofibromatosis, lymphoma/leukemia, metastasis, and other skeletal dysplasias.

Reference:

Yochum TR, Rowe LJ. *Essentials of Skeletal Radiology*. 3rd ed. Baltimore, MD: Lippincott Williams & Wilkins; 2004.

COLLAR BUTTON, DUMBBELL, MUSHROOM

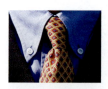

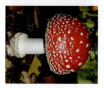

Modalities:
XR, CT, MR

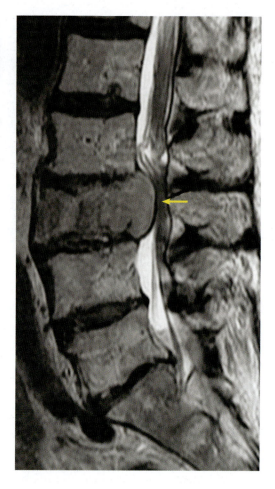

FINDINGS:

Sagittal T2-weighted MR shows an exophytic L3 mass projecting posteriorly into the spinal canal (arrow) and causing severe stenosis.

DIFFERENTIAL DIAGNOSIS:

- Chordoma
- Metastasis
- Osteomyelitis

DISCUSSION:

Notochordal remnants can be present along the midline spine from clivus to sacrum, and in the nucleus pulposus of intervertebral discs. Proliferation of notochordal tissue may produce a benign notochordal cell tumor (BNCT) or malignant chordoma. These involve the sacrococcygeal region in 50%, the spheno-occipital region in 35%, and the vertebral bodies in 15%. Vertebral chordomas are destructive, expansile lesions that extend posteriorly into the spinal canal, creating a "collar button" appearance. Lesions can span several vertebral levels and extend across intervertebral discs. Classically, there is heterogeneous "honeycomb" enhancement with bone destruction and soft-tissue components. Classic chordomas are iso- to hyperintense on T1-weighted MR, reflecting a combination of mucinous and hemorrhagic components. On T2-weighted MR, tumors are often hyperintense with scattered areas of hypointensity reflecting fibrosis, hemorrhage, and/or calcification. Because the imaging characteristics overlap with metastasis and infection, biopsy with demonstration of notochordal physaliferous cells is necessary for diagnosis.

References:

Nishiguchi T, Mochizuki K, Ohsawa M, et al. Differentiating benign notochordal cell tumors from chordomas: radiographic features on MRI, CT, and tomography. *AJR Am J Roentgenol.* 2011;196(3):644-650.

Rodallec MH, Feydy A, Larousserie F, et al. Diagnostic imaging of solitary tumors of the spine: what to do and say. *Radiographics.* 2008;28(4):1019-1041.

CORONAL CLEFT

Modalities:
XR, CT, MR

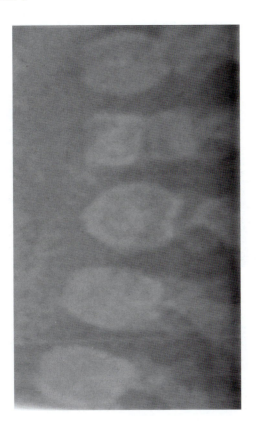

FINDINGS:

Lateral radiograph shows dysplastic lumbar vertebrae with vertically oriented clefts.

DIFFERENTIAL DIAGNOSIS:

- Prematurity
- Chondrodysplasia punctata
- Metatropic dysplasia
- Kniest dysplasia
- Trisomy 13 (Patau syndrome)

DISCUSSION:

"Coronal cleft" vertebrae consist of separate ventral and dorsal ossification centers that are separated by a cartilaginous plate. This appearance is most commonly seen in the lower thoracic or lumbar vertebrae, and reflects delayed skeletal maturation. Premature male infants are more likely to demonstrate this abnormality, which should resolve by 6 months of age. The differential also includes trisomy 13 (Patau syndrome) and complex mesenchymal dysplasias such as chondrodysplasia punctata, metatropic dysplasia, mesomelic dysplasia, and Kniest dysplasia.

Reference:

Kumar R, Guinto FC Jr, Madewell JE, et al. The vertebral body: radiographic configurations in various congenital and acquired disorders. *Radiographics.* 1988;8(3):455-485.

CRESCENT, SCIMITAR, SICKLE

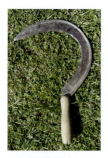

Modalities:
XR, CT, MR

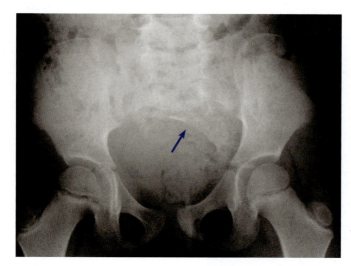

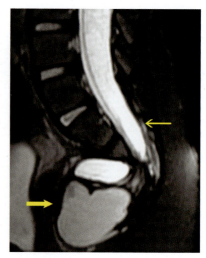

FINDINGS:

- AP radiograph shows a truncated sacrum (arrow).
- Sagittal T2-weighted MR shows sacral hypoplasia, complex presacral mass (thick arrow), and tethered cord with syringohydromyelia (thin arrow).

DIFFERENTIAL DIAGNOSIS:

- Sacral hypoplasia
- Sacral mass
- Spinal dysraphism

DISCUSSION:

The "scimitar" refers to a truncated curvilinear morphology of the sacrum that can reflect hypoplasia, tumor infiltration, or pressure erosions related to a spinal dysraphism. Currarino syndrome, formerly known as ASP association, is an autosomal dominant disorder caused by a mutation in the *MNX1* (*HLXB9*) homeobox gene. The classic triad of findings includes anorectal malformation, sacral hypoplasia or agenesis, and presacral mass. The presacral mass is most commonly an anterior meningocele or sacrococcygeal teratoma. Hereditary sacrococcygeal teratomas behave differently from their sporadic counterparts, with equal gender incidence, sacrococcygeal defects, more anterior location, less calcification, and lower malignant potential.

References:

Hunt PT, Davidson KC, Ashcraft KW, et al. Radiography of hereditary presacral teratoma. *Radiology*. 1977;122(1):187-191.

Pfluger T, Czekalla R, Koletzko S, et al. MRI and radiographic findings in Currarino's triad. *Pediatr Radiol*. 1996;26(8):524-527.

CUNEIFORM, WEDGE

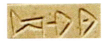

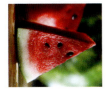

Modalities:
XR, CT, MR

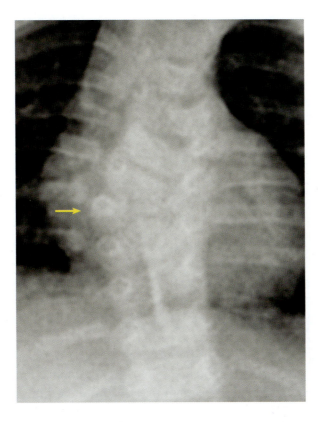

FINDINGS:

AP radiograph shows an isolated right thoracic hemivertebra (arrow) with associated dextroscoliosis. There are also multiple butterfly vertebrae.

DIAGNOSIS:

Hemivertebra

DISCUSSION:

A hemivertebra results from unilateral failure of ossification caused by agenesis, ischemia, or malalignment. Location may be lateral, dorsal, or ventral, with a "wedge" or "cuneiform" morphology. Isolated (unbalanced) hemivertebrae cause focal spinal curvature, while paired (balanced) hemivertebrae maintain spinal alignment. Depending on the presence of disc spaces and growth plates above and below the hemivertebra, it may be classified as fully segmented, semi-segmented, or nonsegmented. Incarcerated hemivertebrae lie within the spinal curve, while nonincarcerated (free) hemivertebrae are malaligned with the spinal column. There is an increased incidence of hemivertebrae in Aicardi syndrome, cleidocranial dysostosis, Gorlin syndrome, Jarcho-Levin syndrome, OEIS complex (omphalocele-exstrophy-imperforate anus-spinal defects), and VACTERL association (vertebral defects, anal atresia, cardiac defects, tracheo-esophageal fistula, renal anomalies, limb abnormalities).

References:

McMaster MJ, Singh H. Natural history of congenital kyphosis and kyphoscoliosis. A study of one hundred and twelve patients. *J Bone Joint Surg Am.* 1999;81(10):1367-1383.

Yochum TR, Rowe LJ. *Essentials of Skeletal Radiology.* 3rd ed. Baltimore, MD: Lippincott Williams & Wilkins; 2004.

CUP, H, LINCOLN LOG, STEP(OFF)

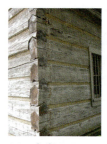

Modalities:
XR, CT, MR

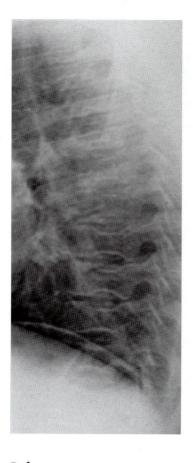

FINDINGS:

Lateral radiograph shows central rectangular depressions along the superior and inferior thoracic vertebral endplates.

DIFFERENTIAL DIAGNOSIS:

- Hemoglobinopathy
- Lysosomal storage disorder

DISCUSSION:

"Lincoln log" vertebrae have characteristic steplike depressions of the central endplates. This is thought to represent regional circulatory stasis and ischemia, with resulting growth arrest and subchondral bone infarcts. The peripheral endplates are preserved because of collateral blood supply. This finding has classically been described in sickle cell disease, but can be seen in other hemoglobinopathies including thalassemia major and hereditary spherocytosis, as well as Gaucher disease. Massive vertebral infarction can cause complete vertebral collapse (vertebra plana).

Reference:

Yochum TR, Rowe LJ. *Essentials of Skeletal Radiology*. 3rd ed. Baltimore, MD: Lippincott Williams & Wilkins; 2004.

DAGGER, RAILROAD/TROLLEY TRACK

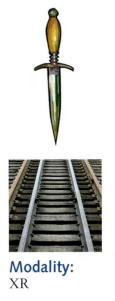

Modality:
XR

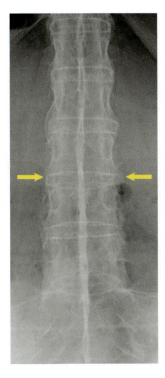

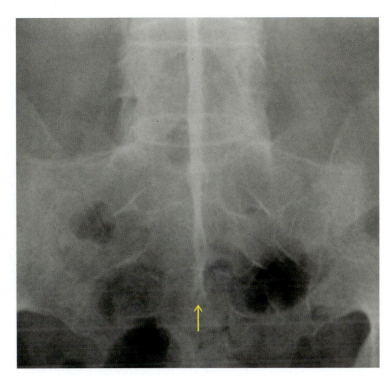

FINDINGS:

AP radiographs show multilevel ossification of the lumbar apophyseal joints (thick arrows) and spinous ligaments (thin arrow).

DIAGNOSIS:

Ankylosing spondylitis

DISCUSSION:

Ankylosing spondylitis (AS) is a chronic inflammatory seronegative spondylo-arthropathy that affects the spine and sacroiliac joints. The disease is most common in young males, and there is a strong association with the HLA-B27 genotype. The "dagger" sign refers to contiguous midline ossification of the interspinous and supraspinous ligaments. When combined with apophyseal (facet) joint ossification along the lateral paraspinal lines, this produces the "railroad track" sign. Other spinal manifestations of AS include peripheral spondylitis ("shiny corner"), spondylodiscitis (Andersson lesion), vertebral squaring, and ankylosis ("bamboo" spine).

Reference:

Hermann KG, Althoff CE, Schneider U, et al. Spinal changes in patients with spondyloarthritis: comparison of MR imaging and radiographic appearances. *Radiographics*. 2005;25(3):559-569.

DISSOLVING/OPEN PEDICLE, EMPTY (HOLE), SANDWICH

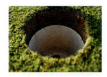

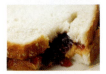

Modalities:
XR, CT, MR

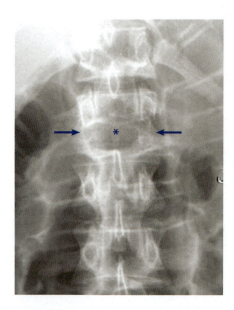

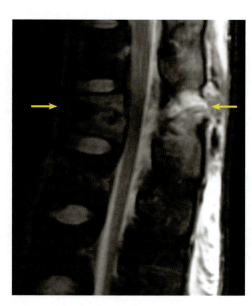

FINDINGS:

- AP radiograph shows a transverse fracture through the L1 vertebra and pedicles (arrows), with nonvisualization of the spinous process (asterisk).
- Sagittal T2-weighted MR shows three-column spinal injury with fracture hemorrhage (arrows) and surrounding edema. An epidural hematoma is also present.

DIAGNOSIS:

Chance fracture

DISCUSSION:

A Chance fracture is a flexion-distraction injury seen with lap seatbelt restraint during motor vehicle accidents, as well as falls from heights. The mechanism involves anterior compression and posterior distraction about a central fulcrum, usually at the thoracolumbar junction. At imaging, there is a horizontal fracture through the vertebral body, pedicles, laminae, and spinous process, with focal kyphosis. The anterior column is impacted, and the posterior elements are separated. On frontal radiography, disruption of the pedicles produces the "dissolving pedicle" sign, and splaying of the spinous processes forms an "empty hole." MR should be performed to evaluate for ligamentous and cord injury. The "sandwich" sign is seen on T2-weighted MR and consists of hypointense hemorrhage within fracture lines, surrounded by hyperintense marrow edema. Associated pancreatic, bowel, and mesenteric injuries are common.

References:

Bernstein MP, Mirvis SE, Shanmuganathan K. Chance-type fractures of the thoracolumbar spine: imaging analysis in 53 patients. *AJR Am J Roentgenol.* 2006;187(4):859-868.

Groves CJ, Cassar-Pullicino VN, Tins BJ, et al. Chance-type flexion-distraction injuries in the thoracolumbar spine: MR imaging characteristics. *Radiology.* 2005;236(2):601-608.

DOUBLE CANAL/FACET, INCOMPLETE RING

Modalities:
CT, MR

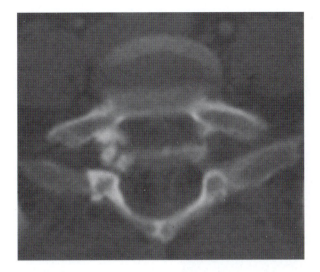

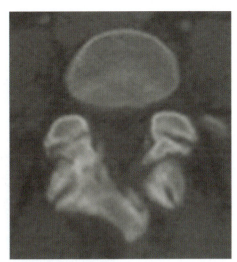

FINDINGS:

Axial CT shows L4-L5 spondylolysis with visualization of both spinal canals and facet joints at the same axial level.

DIAGNOSIS:

Spondylolysis

DISCUSSION:

Spondylolisthesis refers to abnormal displacement of a vertebral body relative to the vertebra below it. Etiologies are categorized using the Wiltse classification: type I (dysplastic), II (isthmic), III (degenerative), IV (traumatic), V (pathologic), and VI (postoperative). The Meyerding classification of anterolithesis, or anterior vertebral displacement, includes grade I (<25% displacement), II (25%-50%), III (50%-75%), IV (75%-100%), and V (>100%). Isthmic spondylolisthesis, or spondylolysis, affects the pars interarticularis (isthmus) with separation of the vertebral body from the posterior elements. On axial imaging, there is interruption of the normal vertebral ring with a "double" appearance of the spinal canal and facet joints.

Reference:

Helms CA, Vogler JB 3rd, Hardy DC. CT of the lumbar spine: normal variants and pitfalls. *Radiographics*. 1987;7(3):447-463.

DOUBLE CONTOUR, (PICTURE) FRAME, PUMICE, WINDOW

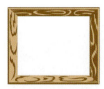

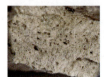

Modalities:
XR, CT, MR

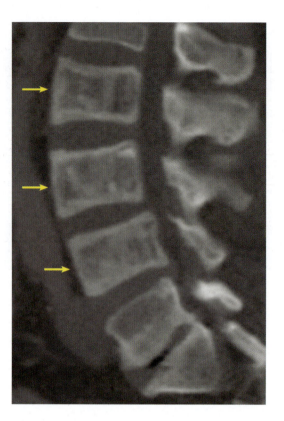

FINDINGS:

Sagittal CT shows expanded lumbar vertebrae with cortical thickening (arrows) and disorganized trabeculae.

DIAGNOSIS:

Paget disease

DISCUSSION:

Paget disease, also known as osteodystrophia deformans, is a chronic metabolic disorder characterized by increased bone turnover and remodeling. The cause is unknown, but has been linked to chronic paramyxovirus infection and mutations in bone remodeling proteins. Disease progresses in three stages: lytic (incipient active), in which osteoclasts predominate; mixed lytic/sclerotic (active), in which osteoblast repair and osteoclast resorption occur simultaneously; and sclerotic (late inactive), in which osteoblasts predominate. Paget disease involves the spine in 30%-75% of cases. In the intermediate phase, involved vertebrae appear expanded with cortical thickening and a relatively radiolucent center, known as the "square" or "picture frame" appearance. Bizarre disorganized trabeculae have been likened to a "pumice" stone. Late complications of spinal Paget disease include vertebral fracture/collapse, spinal stenosis, syringohydromyelia, neurovascular compromise, and sarcomatous transformation.

References:

Smith SE, Murphey MD, Motamedi K, et al. From the archives of the AFIP. Radiologic spectrum of Paget disease of bone and its complications with pathologic correlation. *Radiographics.* 2002;22(5):1191-1216.

Theodorou DJ, Theodorou SJ, Kakitsubata Y. Imaging of Paget disease of bone and its musculoskeletal complications: review. *AJR Am J Roentgenol.* 2011;196(6 suppl):S64-S75.

DOUBLE LINE

Modality:
MR

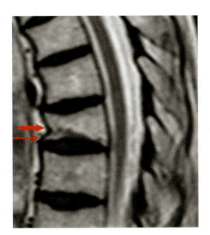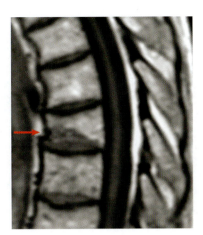

FINDINGS:

- Sagittal T2-weighted MR shows a thoracic vertebral compression fracture with parallel hyperintense (thin arrow) and hypointense (thick arrow) bands along the inferior endplate.
- Sagittal T1-weighted MR shows hypointense signal in both regions (arrow).

DIAGNOSIS:

Vertebral avascular necrosis

DISCUSSION:

Vertebral avascular necrosis (AVN) is a rare condition that typically results from a compression fracture with ischemic nonunion (Kümmel disease). Other predisposing conditions include osteoporosis, vascular disease, pregnancy, alcoholism, steroid excess, pancreatitis, renal disease, hemoglobinopathies, multiple myeloma, AIDS, chemotherapy, radiation, Gaucher disease, autoimmune disorders, bisphosphonate use, and dysbaric (Caisson) disease. Pathologically, disease progresses in four separate phases. The avascular phase involves interruption of blood supply with resulting infarction, usually of the anterior metaphyseal and/or peripheral arteries. The revascularization phase is marked by hyperemia with deposition of new bone and resorption of necrotic bone, leading to cortical fragmentation/collapse. The repair phase involves continued new bone deposition with variable healing. The deformity phase refers to end-stage AVN with secondary osteoarthritic changes. On MR, the "double line" sign is pathognomonic for AVN. T2-weighted sequences show parallel subchondral bands of high signal intensity, representing ischemic granulation tissue; and low signal intensity, representing necrotic bone. On T1-weighted sequences, both of these regions appear hypointense. Over time, progressive vertebral collapse occurs with accumulation of fluid ("fluid" sign) and/or air ("intravertebral vacuum cleft") within fracture lines.

References:

Yu CW, Hsu CY, Shih TT, et al. Vertebral osteonecrosis: MR imaging findings and related changes on adjacent levels. *AJNR Am J Neuroradiol.* 2007;28(1):42-47.

Zurlo JV. The double-line sign. *Radiology.* 1999;212(2):541-542.

DOUBLE SPINOUS PROCESS, GHOST

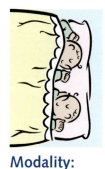

Modality:
XR

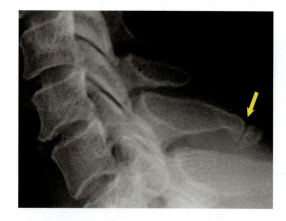

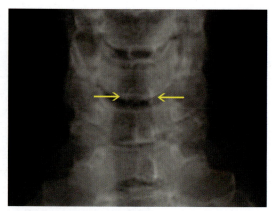

FINDINGS:

Lateral and AP radiographs show a lower cervical spinous process fracture (thick arrow) with fragmentation of the normal cortical shadow (thin arrows).

DIAGNOSIS:

Clay-shoveler fracture

DISCUSSION:

Clay-shoveler fracture is a stable spinous process avulsion fracture affecting the cervicothoracic junction, usually C6 or C7. On frontal radiography, downward displacement of the fracture fragment produces a "double spinous process" or "ghost" appearance. This injury was first described in Australian ditch diggers in 1933. When they tossed clay above their heads with long-handled shovels, the clay sometimes stuck to the shovel, producing a sudden and opposing force on the neck and back muscles. Transmission of force to the interspinous, supraspinous, and nuchal ligaments resulted in avulsion of a lower cervical spinous process. Today, these fractures are usually seen after motor vehicle accidents, sudden muscle contractions, or direct trauma.

Reference:

Lee P, Hunter TB, Taljanovic M. Musculoskeletal colloquialisms: how did we come up with these names? *Radiographics.* 2004;24(4):1009-1027.

DOUBLE VERTEBRA, EMPTY/NAKED FACET

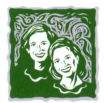

Modalities:
CT, MR

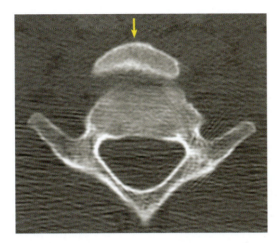

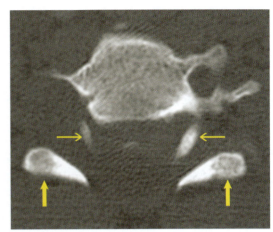

FINDINGS:

Axial CT shows C6-C7 facet dislocation with both vertebral bodies visualized at the same level (arrow). The superior articular processes of C7 (thick arrows) do not articulate with the inferior articular processes of C6. Bilateral uncovertebral joint dislocation is also noted (thin arrows).

DIAGNOSIS:

Facet dislocation

DISCUSSION:

The apophyseal (facet) joint is a synovial joint formed between the inferior articular process of a vertebra and the superior articular process of the vertebra below it. Facet joints stabilize the spine by limiting anterior translation, flexion, and excessive rotation. Unilateral facet dislocation is a mechanically stable injury, whereas bilateral facet dislocation is unstable. Mild injury leads to facet subluxation, which can be treated by closed reduction. Moderate displacement leads to "hanging" or "perched" facets, which articulate at a single point and can slip either anteriorly or posteriorly. Severe dislocation results in "locked" facets, with the inferior articular process of the cranial vertebra trapped between the caudal vertebral body and its superior articular process. On axial images, there is a "double vertebra" appearance with distracted or "naked" superior and inferior articular processes. Correction requires traction and occasionally open reduction.

References:

Lingawi SS. The naked facet sign. *Radiology.* 2001;219(2):366-367.

O'Callaghan JP, Ullrich CG, Yuan HA, et al. CT of facet distraction in flexion injuries of the thoracolumbar spine: the "naked" facet. *AJR Am J Roentgenol.* 1980;134(3):563-568.

DOWAGER HUMP, HUNCHBACK, ROUNDBACK

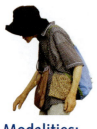

Modalities:
XR, CT, MR

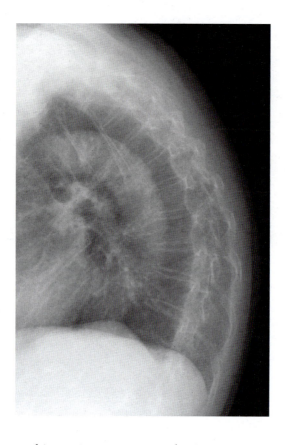

FINDINGS:

Lateral radiograph shows multilevel vertebral compression deformities with thoracic hyperkyphosis.

DIAGNOSIS:

Thoracic hyperkyphosis

DISCUSSION:

Exaggeration of thoracic kyphosis is common in elderly patients with multilevel compression fractures due to osteopenia, trauma, infection, inflammation, or neoplasia. Scheuermann disease (juvenile kyphosis) affects 4%-8% of adolescents. In this condition, disturbed growth of the vertebral endplates results in anterior vertebral wedging, multiple Schmorl nodes, and limbus vertebrae. This produces spinal deformity, back pain, and in severe cases neurologic compromise. Most cases are idiopathic, though there is an association with axial loading sports such as weightlifting and gymnastics. Surgical correction can be performed for symptomatic and cosmetic relief.

References:

Jung HS, Jee WH, McCauley TR, et al. Discrimination of metastatic from acute osteoporotic compression spinal fractures with MR imaging. *Radiographics*. 2003;23(1):179-187.

Swischuk LE, John SD, Allbery S. Disc degenerative disease in childhood: Scheuermann's disease, Schmorl's nodes, and the limbus vertebra: MRI findings in 12 patients. *Pediatr Radiol*. 1998;28(5):334-338.

(DRAPED) CURTAIN

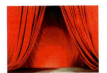

Modalities:
CT, MR

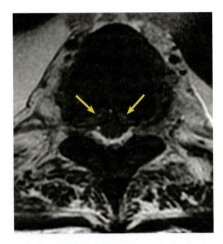
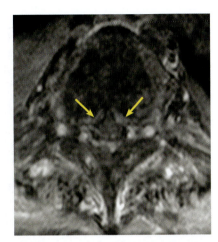

FINDINGS:

Axial T2-weighted and contrast-enhanced T1-weighted MR with fat saturation show enhancing soft tissue in the ventral epidural space (arrows), with midline sparing.

DIAGNOSIS:

Epidural metastasis

DISCUSSION:

Epidural metastasis is a serious complication of systemic cancer, with a high risk of spinal cord and nerve root compression. Early diagnosis and treatment are crucial to minimize neurologic damage from relentless tumor progression. In adults, the most common primary tumors are breast, lung, prostate, renal, melanoma, lymphoma, multiple myeloma, and sarcoma. In children, etiologies include Ewing sarcoma, neuroblastoma, germ cell tumors, and lymphoma. The majority of epidural metastases represent direct extension from a vertebral or paraspinal metastasis, with few lesions truly isolated to the epidural space. Gradually enlarging metastases can form the "draped curtain" sign, in which a bilobed mass occupies the ventral epidural space with midline sparing along the posterior longitudinal ligament. This appearance reflects tethering by the meningovertebral (Hoffmann) ligaments, which connect the dura mater to the osteofibrous walls of the spinal canal. Additional ligaments in the lateral and dorsal spinal canal can produce a "polygonal" appearance. Ligamentous sparing is not generally seen with epidural abscess or hematoma, given that these are rapidly enlarging fluid collections under high pressure.

References:

Mavrogenis AF, Pneumaticos S, Sapkas GS, et al. Metastatic epidural spinal cord compression. *Orthopedics*. 2009;32(6):431-439.

Shah LM, Salzman KL. Imaging of spinal metastatic disease. *Int J Surg Oncol*. 2011; Article ID 769753.

Shi B, Li X, Li H, et al. The morphology and clinical significance of the dorsal meningovertebral ligaments in the lumbosacral epidural space. *Spine (Phila Pa 1976)*. 2012;37(18):E1093-E1098.

DUMBBELL

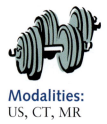

Modalities:
US, CT, MR

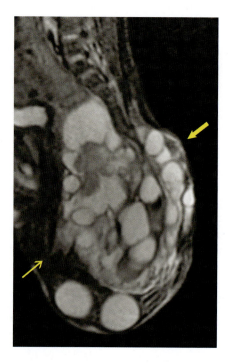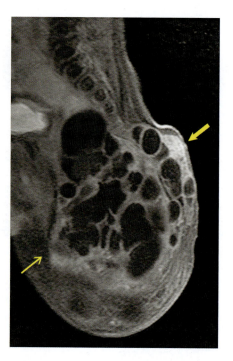

FINDINGS:

Sagittal T2-weighted and contrast-enhanced T1-weighted MR with fat saturation show a mixed solid and cystic mass with extrapelvic (thick arrows) and intrapelvic (thin arrows) components.

DIAGNOSIS:

Sacrococcygeal teratoma

DISCUSSION:

Sacrococcygeal teratoma is the most common solid tumor in neonates, and the most common sacrococcygeal germ cell tumor in children. It is a congenital tumor that arises from embryonic neural cell rests along the caudal spine and contains elements of all three germ cell layers (ectoderm, mesoderm, endoderm). At imaging, sacrococcygeal teratoma appears as a complex solid and cystic mass with variable amounts of soft tissue, fluid, fat, and calcification. The Altman classification includes type I (completely extrapelvic), II (primarily extrapelvic with small presacral component), III (primarily abdominopelvic with small external component), or IV (completely intrapelvic). Types II and III can demonstrate a "dumbbell" appearance spanning the sacrum. Complete surgical resection is advised, because of the potential for malignant transformation. There is also an association with spinal dysraphism: the Currarino triad consists of anorectal malformation, sacral hypoplasia or agenesis, and presacral mass.

Reference:

Kocaoglu M, Frush DP. Pediatric presacral masses. *Radiographics*. 2006;26(3):833-857.

EXTENSION TEARDROP

Modalities:
XR, CT, MR

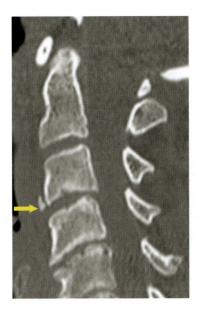 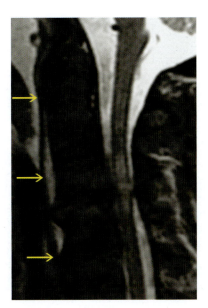

FINDINGS:

- Sagittal CT shows a fracture of the C3 anteroinferior endplate (thick arrow).
- Sagittal T2-weighted MR with fat saturation shows anterior longitudinal ligament injury (thin arrows) and cord edema at C3-C4.

DIFFERENTIAL DIAGNOSIS:

- Hyperextension teardrop fracture
- Hyperextension dislocation injury

DISCUSSION:

Hyperextension teardrop fracture is caused by cervical hyperextension injury with primary failure of the anterior spinal column. Stretching of the anterior longitudinal ligament (ALL) can avulse the anteroinferior endplates of cervical vertebrae. This produces a triangular or "teardrop" fragment with vertical dimension equal to or greater than transverse dimension. In elderly patients with osteopenia, low-force trauma can result in extension teardrop fractures of upper cervical vertebrae (particularly C2). In younger patients with normal bone density, extension teardrop fractures indicate high-force trauma and are typically seen in the lower cervical spine. There is a high incidence of prevertebral swelling and neurologic compromise, particularly central cord syndrome. Hyperextension dislocation injury involves all three columns of the spine and occurs with severe transient hyperextension. Avulsion of the annulus fibrosus can produce a bone fragment with transverse dimension exceeding vertical dimension. Neurologic compromise and central cord syndrome are almost always present.

Reference:

Rao SK, Wasyliw C, Nunez DB Jr. Spectrum of imaging findings in hyperextension injuries of the neck. *Radiographics*. 2005;25(5):1239-1254.

FAN, FLEXION TEARDROP, FLOATING

Modalities:
XR, CT, MR

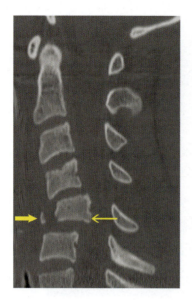
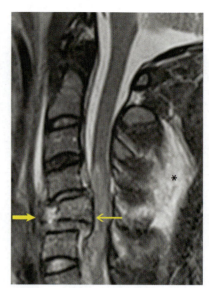

FINDINGS:

Sagittal CT and T2-weighted MR with fat saturation show three-column spinal injury with focal kyphosis and avulsion of the C5 anteroinferior endplate (thick arrows), retropulsion of the C5 vertebra (thin arrows), and edema of the posterior ligamentous complex (asterisk). Severe canal stenosis is present with T2-hyperintense edema and T2-hypointense hemorrhage in the anterior cord.

DIAGNOSIS:

Hyperflexion teardrop fracture

DISCUSSION:

Hyperflexion teardrop fracture is caused by extreme cervical flexion with axial loading. This is a three-column spinal injury involving the anterior longitudinal ligament (ALL), posterior longitudinal ligament (PLL), and posterior ligamentous complex. Lower cervical vertebrae are most frequently affected, particularly C5 and C6. Shearing through the anteroinferior vertebral endplate and intervertebral disc creates a triangular "teardrop" fragment. This typically measures at least half the height of the vertebral body, and remains aligned with the anterior spine. The remainder of the vertebra is fragmented and posteriorly separated from the spine, creating a "floating" appearance. Retropulsion of the vertebral body causes severe canal stenosis and neurologic symptoms in almost all cases. The classic manifestation is anterior cord syndrome with paraplegia or quadriplegia. Facet dislocation and kyphosis produce widening or "fanning" of the spinous processes. In contrast, hyperextension teardrop fractures affect the anterior spinal column, without vertebral displacement or distraction of the posterior elements.

Reference:

Kim KS, Chen HH, Russell EJ, et al. Flexion teardrop fracture of the cervical spine: radiographic characteristics. *AJR Am J Roentgenol.* 1989;152(2):319-326.

FLAT/STRAIGHT BACK

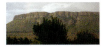

Modalities:
XR, CT, MR

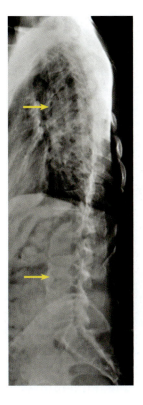

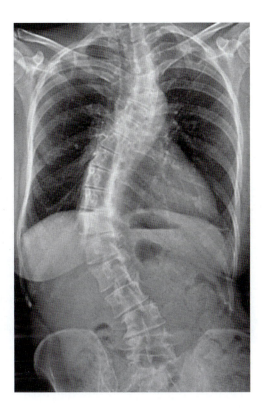

FINDINGS:

- Lateral radiograph shows loss of normal thoracic kyphosis and lumbar lordosis (arrows).
- AP radiograph shows severe rotatory scoliosis.

DIFFERENTIAL DIAGNOSIS:

- Scoliosis
- Arthritis
- Multilevel spinal fusion

DISCUSSION:

The normal spine demonstrates physiologic cervical lordosis, thoracic kyphosis, and lumbar lordosis. Scoliosis refers to abnormal curvature in the coronal plane. This may be corresponding decreased curvature in the sagittal plane, producing a "straight back" appearance with restriction of motion. Scoliosis can be primary (idiopathic) or secondary (neuromuscular, congenital, developmental, tumor-associated). Other causes of spinal straightening include arthritis and multilevel spinal fusion.

References:

Kim H, Kim HS, Moon ES, et al. Scoliosis imaging: what radiologists should know. *Radiographics*. 2010;30(7):1823-1842.

Malfair D, Flemming AK, Dvorak MF, et al. Radiographic evaluation of scoliosis: review. *AJR Am J Roentgenol*. 2010;194(3 suppl):S8-S22.

FLUID

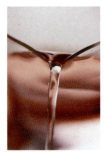

Modality:
MR

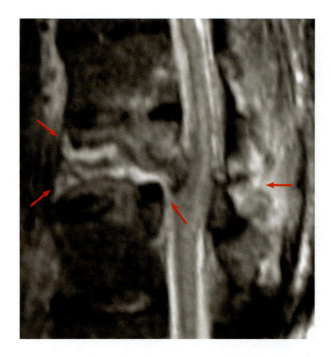

FINDINGS:

Sagittal T2-weighted MR shows a three-column spinal injury with fluid dissecting between fracture fragments (arrows). There is retropulsion of fracture fragments with epidural hematoma and cord compression.

DIAGNOSIS:

Benign compression fracture

DISCUSSION:

Vertebral compression fractures can occur secondary to benign (trauma, osteopenia, ischemia, inflammation, infection) or malignant (primary or metastatic tumor) causes. Imaging findings suggesting a benign fracture include flat or concave vertebral borders, normal marrow signal, multiple fractures, retropulsed fragments, fragments approximating the morphology of the original vertebra ("puzzle" sign), fluid ("fluid" sign) or air ("intravertebral vacuum" sign) within fracture lines, and bandlike subchondral fractures ("double line" sign). In the correct clinical setting, infection should also be considered. Discitis/osteomyelitis manifests with variable intradiscal and vertebral edema and enhancement, osseous destruction, and paraspinal fluid collections. Imaging features suggestive of malignancy include convex vertebral borders, abnormal marrow signal, marrow enhancement, reduced diffusion, involvement of the posterior elements, epidural/paraspinal masses, and other spinal metastases.

References:

Baur A, Stäbler A, Arbogast S, et al. Acute osteoporotic and neoplastic vertebral compression fractures: fluid sign at MR imaging. *Radiology.* 2002;225(3):730-735.

Jung HS, Jee WH, McCauley TR, et al. Discrimination of metastatic from acute osteoporotic compression spinal fractures with MR imaging. *Radiographics.* 2003;23(1):179-187.

FROG HEAD, WEDGE

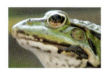

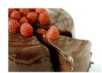

Modalities:
XR, CT, MR

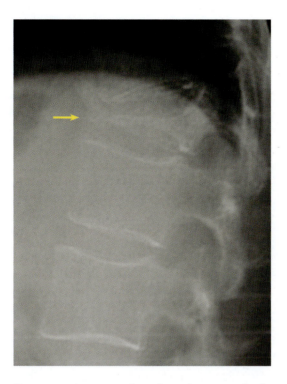

FINDINGS:

Lateral radiograph shows a vertebral compression fracture (arrow) with near-complete loss of height.

DIAGNOSIS:

Vertebral compression fracture

DISCUSSION:

Vertebral compression or "wedge" fractures can occur secondary to benign (trauma, osteopenia, ischemia, inflammation, infection) or malignant (primary or metastatic tumor) causes. Imaging findings suggesting a benign fracture include flat or concave vertebral borders, normal marrow signal, multiple fractures, retropulsed fragments, fragments approximating the morphology of the original vertebra ("puzzle" sign), fluid ("fluid" sign) or air ("intravertebral vacuum" sign) within fracture lines, and bandlike subchondral fractures ("double line" sign). In the correct clinical setting, infection should also be considered. Discitis/osteomyelitis manifests with variable intradiscal and vertebral edema and enhancement, osseous destruction, and paraspinal fluid collections. Imaging features suggestive of malignancy include convex vertebral borders, abnormal marrow signal, marrow enhancement, reduced diffusion, involvement of the posterior elements, epidural/paraspinal masses, and other spinal metastases.

References:

Jung HS, Jee WH, McCauley TR, et al. Discrimination of metastatic from acute osteoporotic compression spinal fractures with MR imaging. *Radiographics.* 2003;23(1):179-187.

Yochum TR, Rowe LJ. *Essentials of Skeletal Radiology.* 3rd ed. Baltimore, MD: Lippincott Williams & Wilkins; 2004.

GIBBUS

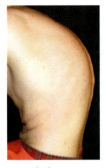

Modalities:
XR, CT, MR

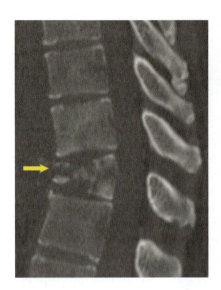

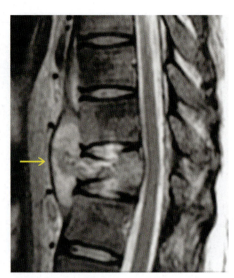

FINDINGS:

- Sagittal CT shows thoracic vertebral fragmentation and collapse (thick arrow), with associated kyphosis.
- Sagittal T2-weighted MR shows marrow/disc edema with destruction of the vertebral endplates and anterior cortex, as well as prevertebral abscess (thin arrow).

DIAGNOSIS:

Tuberculous spondylitis

DISCUSSION:

Vertebral compression fractures can occur secondary to trauma, osteopenia, infection, inflammation, ischemia, and neoplasia. This produces a "gibbus" deformity with abrupt kyphotic angulation. Classically, this has been described in end-stage tuberculous spondylitis (Pott disease) with vertebral fragmentation and collapse. Tuberculosis affects the musculoskeletal system in 1%-3% of cases. Of these, 50% involve the spine, favoring the lower thoracic and upper lumbar vertebrae. It is theorized that hematogenous spread via the Batson venous plexus seeds the anterior vertebral body adjacent to the endplate. Subsequent dissemination through intervertebral discs or paraspinal soft tissues can yield multilevel vertebral disease. Extravertebral extension results in formation of paraspinal abscesses (Pott abscesses) with subligamentous and/or retroperitoneal involvement. Abscess calcification, if present, is a specific imaging feature for TB. Remodeling of adjacent bone can produce anterior vertebral scalloping and/or contour irregularity ("gouge" defect). Mild sclerosis and periosteal reaction are present, as compared to bacterial osteomyelitis.

Reference:

Burrill J, Williams CJ, Bain G, et al. Tuberculosis: a radiologic review. *Radiographics*. 2007;27(5): 1255-1273.

GOOSE/SWAN NECK

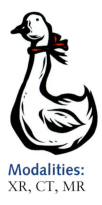

Modalities:
XR, CT, MR

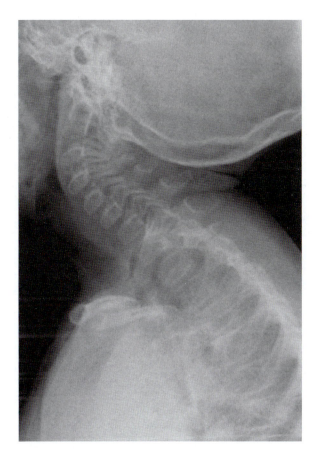

FINDINGS:

Lateral radiograph shows exaggerated cervical lordosis and thoracic kyphosis.

DIFFERENTIAL DIAGNOSIS:

- Mesenchymal dysplasias
- Neuromuscular disorders
- Degenerative spine disease
- Postlaminectomy

DISCUSSION:

The normal spine demonstrates physiologic cervical lordosis, thoracic kyphosis, and lumbar lordosis. Exaggerated curvature ("swan neck" deformity) can develop in mesenchymal dysplasias, neuromuscular disorders, and degenerative spine disease. This appearance is also seen following multilevel laminectomy without spinal fusion, which destabilizes the spine and predisposes to progressive vertebral subluxations/dislocations.

References:

Anderson SM. Spinal curves and scoliosis. *Radiol Technol.* 2007;79(1):44-65.

Yochum TR, Rowe LJ. *Essentials of Skeletal Radiology.* 3rd ed. Baltimore, MD: Lippincott Williams & Wilkins; 2004.

GOUGE, POTT

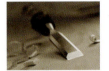

Modalities:
CT, MR

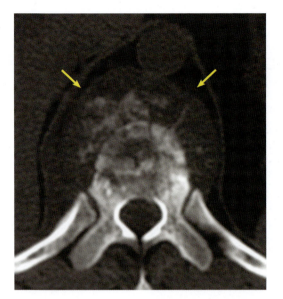 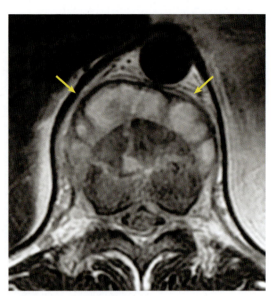

FINDINGS:

Axial CT and T2-weighted MR show vertebral fragmentation with partially calcified paravertebral abscess (arrows) bulging the anterior longitudinal ligament.

DIAGNOSIS:

Tuberculous spondylitis

DISCUSSION:

Tuberculosis affects the musculoskeletal system in 1%-3% of cases, of which 50% involve the spine (tuberculous spondylitis or Pott disease). The lower thoracic and upper lumbar vertebrae are most commonly affected. It is theorized that hematogenous spread via the Batson venous plexus seeds the anterior vertebral body adjacent to the endplate. Subsequent dissemination through intervertebral discs or paraspinal soft tissues can yield multilevel vertebral disease. Extravertebral extension results in formation of paraspinal abscesses (Pott abscesses) with subligamentous and/or retroperitoneal involvement. These appear as rim-enhancing, sometimes calcified fluid collections. Remodeling of adjacent bone can produce anterior vertebral scalloping and/or contour irregularity ("gouge" defect). Mild sclerosis and periosteal reaction are present, as compared to bacterial osteomyelitis. The "gouge" defect should be distinguished from the "wraparound" sign of spinal lymphoma, which involves the paravertebral and epidural spaces without bone disruption. In addition, lymphoma enhances homogeneously and rarely calcifies if untreated.

Reference:

Burrill J, Williams CJ, Bain G, et al. Tuberculosis: a radiologic review. *Radiographics*. 2007;27(5): 1255-1273.

H, U

H
U

Modalities:
XR, CT, MR

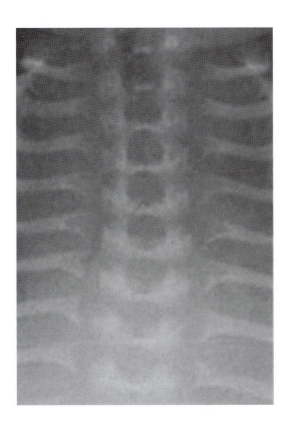

FINDINGS:

AP radiograph shows diffusely hypoplastic vertebrae with central flattening.

DIAGNOSIS:

Thanatophoric dysplasia, type II

DISCUSSION:

Thanatophoric (Greek for "death bringing") dysplasia is the most common lethal neonatal skeletal dysplasia. It is an autosomal dominant condition caused by mutations in the fibroblast growth factor receptor (FGFR3) on chromosome 4p. This is a rhizomelic dwarfism characterized by narrow chest and short ribs. Death occurs in utero or shortly after birth, due to respiratory insufficiency from pulmonary hypoplasia. Type I demonstrates frontal bossing, saddle nose, hypoplastic skull base, platyspondyly, and bowed long bones with "telephone receiver" femora. Type II is associated with pansynostosis (Kleeblattschädel skull), centrally flattened vertebrae ("H" or "U" morphology), and straight long bones. Narrowing of interpedicular distance in the lumbar spine is a specific finding for thanatophoric dysplasia or achondroplasia.

References:

Dighe M, Fligner C, Cheng E, et al. Fetal skeletal dysplasia: an approach to diagnosis with illustrative cases. *Radiographics*. 2008;28(4):1061-1077.

Hinck VC, Clark WM, Hopkins CE. Normal interpediculate distances (minimum and maximum) in children and adults. *Am J Roentgenol Radium Ther Nucl Med*. 1966;97(1):141-153.

HAMBURGER (BUN)

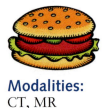

Modalities:
CT, MR

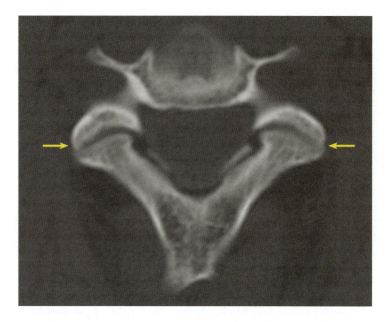

FINDINGS:

Axial CT shows normal cervical facet joints (arrows).

DIAGNOSIS:

Normal cervical facet joints

DISCUSSION:

The apophyseal (facet) joint is a synovial joint formed between the inferior articular process of a vertebra and the superior articular process of the vertebra below it. Facet joints stabilize the spine by limiting anterior translation, flexion, and excessive rotation. On axial images, these normally have a rounded "hamburger" appearance with symmetric articulation between the inferior articular process of the cranial vertebra, located posteriorly; and the superior articular process of the caudal vertebra, located anteriorly. Unilateral facet dislocation is a mechanically stable injury, whereas bilateral facet dislocation is unstable. Mild injury leads to facet subluxation, which can be treated by closed reduction. Moderate displacement leads to "hanging" or "perched" facets, which articulate at a single point and can slip either anteriorly or posteriorly. Severe dislocation results in "locked" facets, with the inferior articular process of the cranial vertebra trapped between the caudal vertebral body and its superior articular process. On axial images, this results in a "reverse hamburger" appearance with the inferior articular process of the cranial vertebra located anterior to the superior articular process of the caudal vertebra, and the joint surfaces facing in opposite directions. Correction requires traction and occasionally open reduction.

Reference:

Daffner SD, Daffner RH. Computed tomography diagnosis of facet dislocations: the "hamburger bun" and "reverse hamburger bun" signs. *J Emerg Med.* 2002;23(4):387-394.

HAMBURGER/SANDWICH VERTEBRA

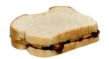

Modalities:
XR, CT

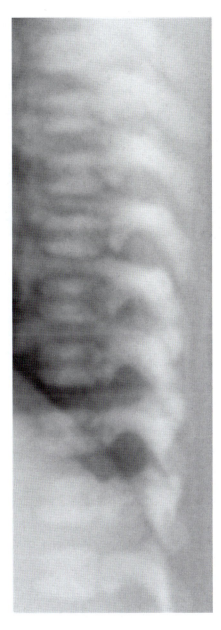

FINDINGS:

Lateral radiograph shows increased density of the thoracolumbar endplates.

DIFFERENTIAL DIAGNOSIS:

- Type II osteopetrosis
- Myelofibrosis
- Fluorosis
- Systemic stress

DISCUSSION:

"Sandwich" vertebrae demonstrate dense sclerosis of the superior and inferior vertebral endplates. The central vertebral bodies may be normal or mildly sclerotic, with well-defined contours. This finding can be seen in type II (autosomal dominant) osteopetrosis, also known as Albers-Schönberg disease; myelofibrosis; fluorosis; and after systemic stress. Type II osteopetrosis can also exhibit "bone in bone" vertebrae and sclerosis of the skull base. Myelofibrosis is a myeloproliferative disorder that is associated with cortical thinning of long bones and splenomegaly. Fluorosis is caused by exposure to high levels of fluoride and can produce endosteal sclerosis, periostitis, enthesophytes, and osteophytes. "Sandwich" vertebrae should be distinguished from the "rugger-jersey" spine of hyperparathyroidism (HPTH), in which sclerosis occurs subjacent to the vertebral endplates with associated subperiosteal resorption. The central vertebral bodies may be normal or lucent, with poorly defined borders. Another mimic is vertebral demineralization, in which the vertebral body appears hyperlucent, but the endplates are relatively preserved due to cortical buttressing. Over time, the entire vertebra becomes osteopenic. The intervertebral discs herniate into the weakened endplates and produce a "codfish" deformity.

References:

Kumar R, Guinto FC Jr, Madewell JE, et al. The vertebral body: radiographic configurations in various congenital and acquired disorders. *Radiographics*. 1988;8(3):455-485.

Yochum TR, Rowe LJ. *Essentials of Skeletal Radiology*. 3rd ed. Baltimore, MD: Lippincott Williams & Wilkins; 2004.

HEADPHONES

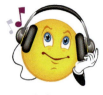

Modalities:
CT, MR

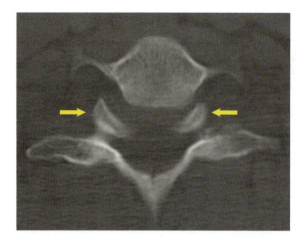
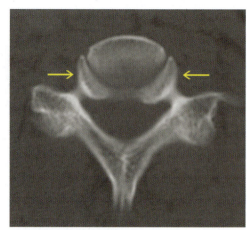

FINDINGS:

Axial CT shows C6-C7 facet dislocation with uncovertebral joint separation (thick arrows). At a higher level, the uncovertebral joints are intact (thin arrows).

DIAGNOSIS:

Cervical facet dislocation

DISCUSSION:

In the cervical spine, the articular pillars are stabilized by apophyseal (facet) and uncovertebral (Luschka) joints. Facet joints are synovial joints formed between the inferior and superior articular processes of adjacent vertebrae. They stabilize the spine by limiting anterior translation, flexion, and excessive rotation. Uncovertebral joints involve the lower five cervical vertebrae, and demonstrate features of both cartilaginous and synovial joints. They are not present at birth, but develop in the first decade of life and progressively enlarge. Uncovertebral joints are formed by hooklike uncinate processes at the superolateral borders of the C3 through T1 vertebrae, which articulate with the vertebral body one level above. These prevent posterior translation and limit lateral flexion. On axial images, the normal "headphones" appearance is created by the uncinate processes of the caudal vertebra concentrically surrounding the cranial vertebral body. Uncovertebral joint distraction is a secondary sign of facet dislocation, with unilateral or bilateral disruption of the "headphones" appearance. The cranial vertebra is anteriorly displaced from one or both uncinate processes. Unilateral facet dislocation is a mechanically stable injury, whereas bilateral facet dislocation is unstable.

References:

Palmieri F, Cassar-Pullicino VN, Dell'Atti C, et al. Uncovertebral joint injury in cervical facet dislocation: the headphones sign. *Eur Radiol.* 2006;16(6):1312-1315.

Yetkin Z, Osborn AG, Giles DS, et al. Uncovertebral and facet joint dislocations in cervical articular pillar fractures: CT evaluation. *AJNR Am J Neuroradiol.* 1985;6(4):633-637.

HEAP, HUMP, PEAR

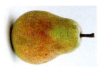

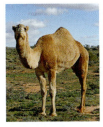

Modalities:
XR, CT, MR

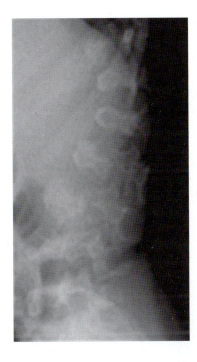
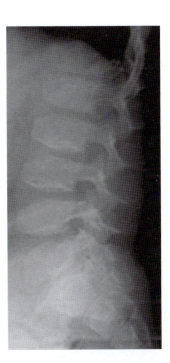

FINDINGS:

- Lateral radiograph in a patient with spondyloepiphyseal dysplasia congenita shows flattened and lobulated vertebrae.
- Lateral radiograph in a patient with spondyloepiphyseal dysplasia tarda shows deposition of bone along the posterior vertebral endplates.

DIAGNOSIS:

Spondyloepiphyseal dysplasia

DISCUSSION:

Spondyloepiphyseal dysplasia (SED) is a heterogeneous group of disorders characterized by undergrowth of the vertebrae and proximal epiphyseal centers, resulting in short-trunk dwarfism. The disease is classified into SED congenita and SED tarda, based on the age of onset. SED congenita is caused by an autosomal dominant mutation in the *COL2A1* gene for type II collagen on chromosome 12q13. It presents at birth with platyspondyly or "pear"-shaped vertebrae. Other manifestations include myopia, retinal detachment, sensorineural hearing loss, and cleft palate. SED tarda is an X-linked recessive disease that maps to the *TRAPPC2* (*SEDL*) gene. This affects the trafficking protein particle (TRAPP) complex, a crucial vesicular transport protein. It presents in adolescence or adulthood, with "heaped-up" bone along the posterior vertebral endplates.

References:

Poker N, Finby N, Archibald RM. Spondyloepiphysial dysplasia tarda. Four cases in childhood and adolescence, and some considerations regarding platyspondyly. *Radiology.* 1965;85(3):474-480.

Vanhoenacker FM, De Schepper AM, Parizel PM. Congenital abnormalities of the osseous spine: a radiological approach. *JBR-BTR.* 2005;88(1):37-41.

INTERVERTEBRAL VACUUM (PHENOMENON), PHANTOM NUCLEUS PULPOSUS

Modalities:
XR, CT, MR

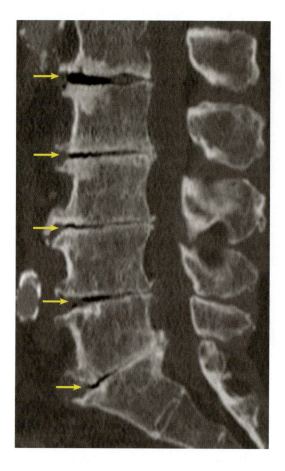

FINDINGS:

Sagittal CT shows lumbar spine degeneration with multilevel loss of disc space, intervertebral vacuum gas (arrows), endplate sclerosis, and marginal osteophytes.

DIFFERENTIAL DIAGNOSIS:

- Degenerative disc disease
- Vertebral collapse

DISCUSSION:

The "intervertebral vacuum" phenomenon refers to gas within the intervertebral disc. Air appears radiolucent on radiography and CT, and creates signal void with susceptibility on MR. The most common etiology is degenerative disc disease. It is theorized that degradation of the nucleus pulposus creates a potential space with low intradiscal pressure. This draws fluid and/or air out from the blood and surrounding tissues, consisting primarily of nitrogen with small amounts of oxygen and carbon dioxide. Schmorl nodes that herniate through the vertebral endplates can produce intravertebral foci of gas, which are distinct from the "intravertebral vacuum cleft" of avascular necrosis. Another common etiology is vertebral collapse with involvement of the disc space. Causes include osteoporosis, multiple myeloma, trauma, metastasis, and infection. In the absence of vertebral fracture, infection and malignancy are unlikely causes of the intervertebral vacuum phenomenon. These conditions cause increased intradiscal pressure that usually force gas out of the joint. If present, air collections tend to appear more focal and can extend into the soft tissues.

References:

D'Anastasi M, Birkenmaier C, Schmidt GP, et al. Correlation between vacuum phenomenon on CT and fluid on MRI in degenerative disks. *AJR Am J Roentgenol.* 2011;197(5):1182-1189.

Lafforgue PF, Chagnaud CJ, Daver LM, et al. Intervertebral disc vacuum phenomenon secondary to vertebral collapse: prevalence and significance. *Radiology.* 1994;193(3):853-858.

INTRAVERTEBRAL VACUUM (CLEFT)

Modalities:
XR, CT, MR

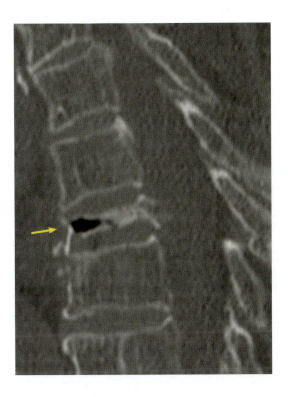

FINDINGS:

Sagittal CT shows a collapsed thoracic vertebra with internal gas (arrow).

DIFFERENTIAL DIAGNOSIS:

- Vertebral avascular necrosis
- Nonunited compression fracture

DISCUSSION:

The "intravertebral vacuum cleft" sign refers to gas located within a fractured vertebral body. Air appears radiolucent on radiography and CT, and creates signal void with susceptibility on MR. This finding has been described in nonunited vertebral compression fractures, and may be due to excessive motion and/or ischemia at the fracture site. Post-traumatic AVN is known as Kümmel disease and is associated with osteoporosis, vascular disease, pregnancy, alcoholism, steroid excess, pancreatitis, renal disease, hemoglobinopathies, multiple myeloma, AIDS, chemotherapy, radiation, Gaucher disease, autoimmune disorders, bisphosphonate use, and dysbaric (Caisson) disease. Pathologically, the disease progresses in four separate phases. The avascular phase involves interruption of blood supply with resulting infarction, usually of the anterior metaphyseal and/or peripheral arteries. The revascularization phase is marked by hyperemia with deposition of new bone and resorption of necrotic bone, leading to cortical fragmentation/collapse. The repair phase involves continued new bone deposition with variable healing. The deformity phase refers to end-stage AVN with secondary osteoarthritic changes. On MR, the "double line" sign corresponds to parallel subchondral layers of ischemic granulation tissue and necrotic bone. Over time, there is progressive vertebral collapse with formation of intravertebral clefts. Because of low pressure within the clefts, fluid ("fluid" sign) and/or air ("intravertebral vacuum cleft") may be drawn out from the blood and surrounding tissues, consisting primarily of nitrogen with small amounts of oxygen and carbon dioxide. If the fracture extends to the intervertebral disc space, an "intervertebral vacuum" sign can also be produced. Rarely, infection or malignancy may demonstrate intravertebral gas, but this is unlikely due to associated high pressures. If present, air collections tend to appear more focal and can extend into the soft tissues.

References:

Mirovsky Y, Anekstein Y, Shalmon E, et al. Vacuum clefts of the vertebral bodies. *AJNR Am J Neuroradiol.* 2005 Aug;26(7):1634-1640.

Theodorou DJ. The intravertebral vacuum cleft sign. *Radiology.* 2001;221(3):787-788.

Yu CW, Hsu CY, Shih TT, et al. Vertebral osteonecrosis: MR imaging findings and related changes on adjacent levels. *AJNR Am J Neuroradiol.* 2007;28(1):42-47.

INVERTED/REVERSE HAMBURGER (BUN)

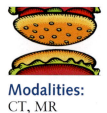

Modalities:
CT, MR

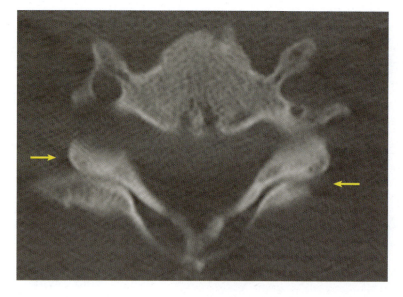

FINDINGS:

Axial CT shows C6-C7 facet dislocation with inversion of the normal facet joint orientation (arrows).

DIAGNOSIS:

Cervical facet dislocation

DISCUSSION:

The apophyseal (facet) joint is a synovial joint formed between the inferior articular process of a vertebra and the superior articular process of the vertebra below it. Facet joints stabilize the spine by limiting anterior translation, flexion, and excessive rotation. On axial images, these normally have a rounded "hamburger" appearance with symmetric articulation between the inferior articular process of the cranial vertebra, located posteriorly; and the superior articular process of the caudal vertebra, located anteriorly. Unilateral facet dislocation is a mechanically stable injury, whereas bilateral facet dislocation is unstable. Mild injury leads to facet subluxation, which can be treated by closed reduction. Moderate displacement leads to "hanging" or "perched" facets, which articulate at a single point and can slip either anteriorly or posteriorly. Severe dislocation results in "locked" facets, with the inferior articular process of the cranial vertebra trapped between the caudal vertebral body and its superior articular process. On axial images, this results in a "reverse hamburger" appearance with the inferior articular process of the cranial vertebra located anterior to the superior articular process of the caudal vertebra, and the joint surfaces facing in opposite directions. Correction requires traction and occasionally open reduction.

Reference:

Daffner SD, Daffner RH. Computed tomography diagnosis of facet dislocations: the "hamburger bun" and "reverse hamburger bun" signs. *J Emerg Med.* 2002;23(4):387-394.

IVORY, WHITE

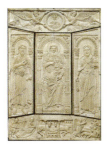

Modalities:
XR, CT

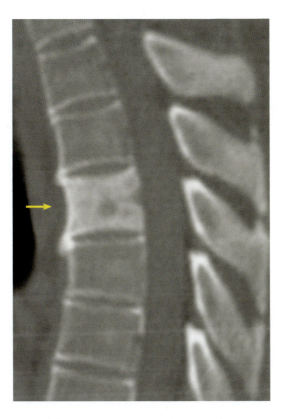

FINDINGS:

Sagittal CT shows isolated sclerosis of a thoracic vertebra (arrow).

DIFFERENTIAL DIAGNOSIS:

- Metastasis
- Lymphoma
- Paget disease
- Primary bone tumor
- Infection/inflammation

DISCUSSION:

The "ivory" vertebra is characterized by diffuse and uniform sclerosis when compared to adjacent vertebrae of normal density. In adults, this may represent confluent blastic metastases (such as prostate, breast, and lung carcinoma), lymphoma, or Paget disease. Lymphoma can induce an osteoblastic response, often with associated lymphadenopathy and paraspinal soft tissue ("wraparound" sign). Pagetoid vertebrae are expanded with cortical and trabecular disorganization, as well as diffuse sclerosis in the late phases. In children, ivory vertebrae are rare and may represent Hodgkin lymphoma or metastases from osteosarcoma, neuroblastoma, medulloblastoma, and Ewing sarcoma. Primary bone tumors, such as osteoblastoma, chordoma, plasmacytoma, and various sarcomas, can produce marked sclerotic periosteal reaction. Spinal tuberculosis (Pott disease), chronic bacterial osteomyelitis, postradiation necrosis, and stress reaction manifest with variable sclerosis and bone destruction. When no etiology is identified, the condition is known as idiopathic segmental sclerosis. When multiple "ivory" vertebrae are present, sclerosing bone dysplasias should be considered in the differential. These are a diverse group of disorders with hereditary, nonhereditary, and acquired causes. Hereditary sclerosing bone dysplasias affect endochondral and/or intramembranous ossification. These include osteopetrosis, pyknodysostosis, osteopoikilosis, osteopathia striata, progressive diaphyseal dysplasia, hereditary multiple diaphyseal sclerosis, and hyperostosis corticalis generalisata. Nonhereditary causes of bone sclerosis include intramedullary osteosclerosis, melorheostosis, and SAPHO syndrome (synovitis, acne, pustulosis, hyperostosis, and osteitis). Acquired conditions include renal osteodystrophy, sickle cell anemia, Erdheim-Chester disease, myelofibrosis, mastocytosis, and fluorosis.

References:

Graham TS. The ivory vertebra sign. *Radiology*. 2005;235(2):614-615.

Ihde LL, Forrester DM, Gottsegen CJ, et al. Sclerosing bone dysplasias: review and differentiation from other causes of osteosclerosis. *Radiographics*. 2011;31(7):1865-1882.

JIGSAW

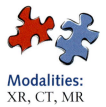

Modalities:
XR, CT, MR

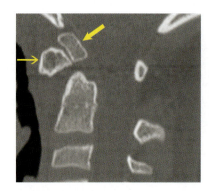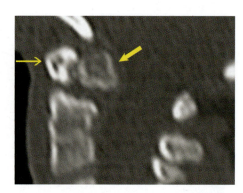

FINDINGS:

Sagittal CT in two different patients shows large ossicles (thick arrows) separate from the odontoid base and C2 body, and articulating with hyperplastic anterior C1 arches (thin arrows).

DIAGNOSIS:

Os odontoideum

DISCUSSION:

Os odontoideum is a developmental anomaly in which the odontoid process (dens) is hypoplastic and associated with a large ossicle in the expected region of the odontoid tip. There is an association with Down, Klippel-Feil, and Morquio syndromes, as well as multiple epiphyseal dysplasia. The etiology is unknown, but is thought to represent either congenital nonfusion or injury to the odontoid synchondrosis before 5-7 years of age. The craniocervical ligaments attach to the ossicle and do not restrict motion of the odontoid process/C2 body, resulting in atlantoaxial instability and variable degrees of cervicomedullary stenosis. At imaging, the odontoid is foreshortened and widely separated from the os odontoideum. The latter appears as a rounded and well-corticated ossicle in the expected location of the odontoid tip (orthotopic) or superiorly displaced toward the skull base (dystopic). Remodeling of the clivus and hyperplasia of the anterior arch of C1, which interdigitates with the os ("jigsaw" sign) are specific signs. Surgical correction is indicated for significant pain, instability, and/or neurologic deficits. Os odontoideum must be distinguished from persistent ossiculum terminale and acquired dens fracture. In persistent ossiculum terminale, also known as Bergman ossicle, the terminal ossification center fails to fuse with the odontoid by 12 years of age. At imaging, a tiny ossicle is present above the normal C1 arch and transverse ligament, and is not associated with instability. Dens fractures after 7 years of age appear as thin irregular lucencies, with preservation of the odontoid contour. Nonunion is common with type II fractures and in elderly osteopenic patients. However, fracture fragments have an angular morphology, and the C1 arch is not dysplastic.

Reference:

Fagan AB, Askin GN, Earwaker JW. The jigsaw sign. A reliable indicator of congenital aetiology in os odontoideum. *Eur Spine J*. 2004;13(4):295-300.

KEEL, PAPER THIN

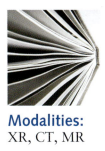

Modalities:
XR, CT, MR

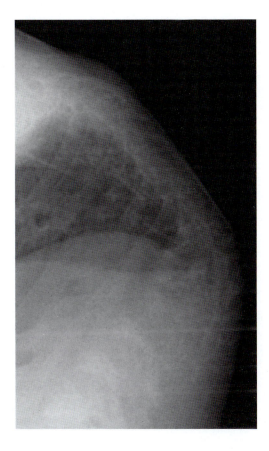

FINDINGS:

Lateral radiograph shows severe osteopenia with multilevel vertebral collapse and thoracic hyperkyphosis.

DIAGNOSIS:

Platyspondyly

DISCUSSION:

Platyspondyly refers to diffuse flattening of vertebrae, resembling the "keel" of a boat or "paper on edge." In adults, this appearance is commonly seen secondary to osteopenia and various systemic processes that weaken bone (infection, inflammation, ischemia, neoplasia). In children, the differential includes but is not limited to osteogenesis imperfecta, thanatophoric dysplasia, achondroplasia, achondrogenesis, mucopolysaccharidoses, lysosomal storage disorders, hypothyroidism, hypophosphatasia, congenital Cushing disease, metatropic dysplasia, spondyloepiphyseal dyplasia, and spondyloepimetaphyseal dysplasia.

References:

Klaus-Dietrich E, Blickman JG, Willich E, et al. *Differential Diagnosis in Pediatric Radiology*. Thieme; 1999.

Vanhoenacker FM, De Schepper AM, Parizel PM. Congenital abnormalities of the osseous spine: a radiological approach. *JBR-BTR*. 2005;88(1):37-41.

LIMBUS, RIM

Modalities:
XR, CT, MR

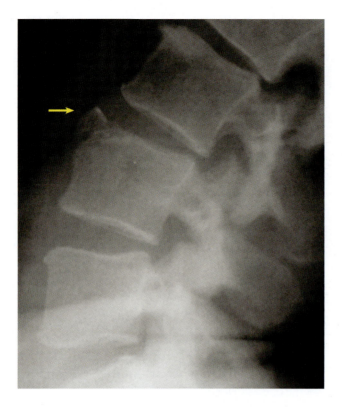

FINDINGS:

Lateral radiograph shows a triangular ossicle (arrow) offset from the main vertebral body.

DIAGNOSIS:

Limbus vertebra

DISCUSSION:

A limbus (Latin for "edge" or "border") vertebra is a developmental anomaly caused by intraosseous herniation of the nucleus pulposus through the peripheral vertebral endplate, separating the ring apophysis from the main vertebral body. This most commonly occurs at the anterosuperior corner of a mid-lumbar vertebra, but can occasionally involve the anteroinferior or posterior corners. Over time, the apophysis ossifies and appears as a triangular corticated bone fragment ("rim" lesion) that is offset from the vertebral body. The vast majority of limbus vertebrae are asymptomatic, though the posterior variant can occasionally cause neurologic symptoms. When the nucleus pulposus herniates more centrally, a Schmorl node is formed. Both limbus vertebrae and Schmorl nodes are seen in Scheuermann disease (juvenile kyphosis), a condition affecting 4%-8% of adolescents in which there is disturbed growth of the vertebral endplates.

Reference:

Ghelman B, Freiberger RH. The limbus vertebra: an anterior disc herniation demonstrated by discography. *AJR Am J Roentgenol.* 1976;127(5):854-855.

MARBLE, STONE

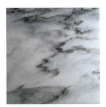

Modalities:
XR, CT

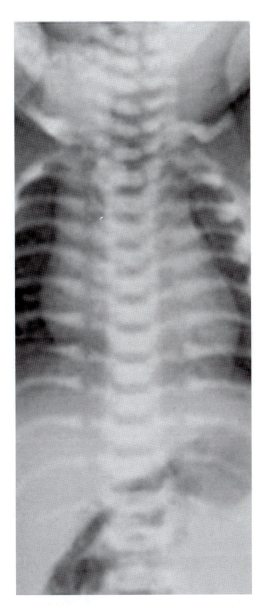

FINDINGS:

AP radiograph shows diffusely increased bone density.

DIAGNOSIS:

Sclerosing bone dysplasia

DISCUSSION:

Sclerosing bone dysplasias are a diverse group of disorders that can be hereditary, nonhereditary, or acquired. Hereditary sclerosing bone dysplasias affect endochondral and/or intramembranous ossification. These include osteopetrosis, pyknodysostosis, osteopoikilosis, osteopathia striata, progressive diaphyseal dysplasia, hereditary multiple diaphyseal sclerosis, and hyperostosis corticalis generalisata. Osteopetrosis is caused by endochondral defects of the primary spongiosa. Type I osteopetrosis, also known as congenital or malignant subtype, demonstrates autosomal recessive inheritance. There is uniform diffuse sclerosis throughout the skull, spine, and long bones creating a "marble" or "stone" appearance. Patients die in utero or shortly after birth. Type II osteopetrosis, also known as Albers-Schönberg disease, has autosomal dominant inheritance. Osseous sclerosis is less severe, with "bone-in-bone" or "sandwich" vertebrae. Pathologic fractures are common, due to decreased bone elasticity and impaired remodeling. Nonhereditary causes of bone sclerosis include intramedullary osteosclerosis, melorheostosis, and SAPHO syndrome (synovitis, acne, pustulosis, hyperostosis, and osteitis). Acquired conditions include blastic metastases, renal osteodystrophy, sickle cell anemia, Paget disease, Erdheim-Chester disease, myelofibrosis, mastocytosis, and fluorosis.

Reference:

Ihde LL, Forrester DM, Gottsegen CJ, et al. Sclerosing bone dysplasias: review and differentiation from other causes of osteosclerosis. *Radiographics.* 2011;31(7):1865-1882.

MINI BRAIN, SOAP BUBBLE, SPOKE WHEEL, WRINKLED

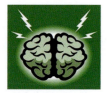

Modalities:
CT, MR

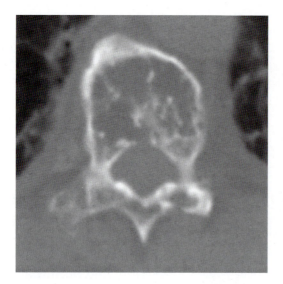
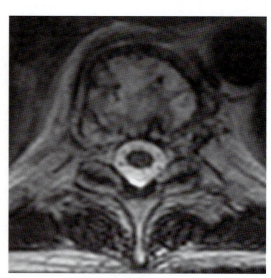

FINDINGS:

Axial CT and T2-weighted MR show an expansile vertebral lytic lesion with radiating bone struts.

DIAGNOSIS:

Vertebral plasmacytoma

DISCUSSION:

Plasmacytoma is a malignant plasma cell tumor that represents the unifocal form of multiple myeloma. Disease can affect bone (solitary bone plasmacytoma) or soft tissue (extramedullary plasmacytoma). The spine is affected in 25%-60% of cases. On CT, vertebral plasmacytoma appears as an expansile lytic lesion with radiating internal bone struts and lobulated cortical thickening ("mini brain") appearance. This is thought to represent indolent tumor proliferation within bone marrow, with compensatory hypertrophy of remaining trabeculae and mild surrounding periostitis. On MR, the involved marrow appears abnormally T1-hypointense, T2-hyperintense, and enhancing. To date, the "mini brain" appearance has not been reported with any other bone tumor. Patients eventually progress to multiple myeloma, usually within 2-4 years.

Reference:

Major NM, Helms CA, Richardson WJ. The "mini brain": plasmacytoma in a vertebral body on MR imaging. *AJR Am J Roentgenol.* 2000;175(1):261-263.

MOUSTACHE

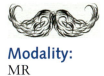

Modality:
MR

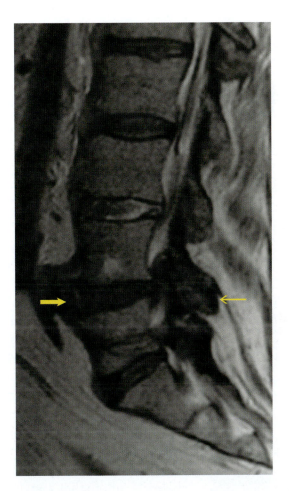

FINDINGS:

Sagittal T2-weighted MR shows contiguous low signal in the L4-L5 disc (thick arrow) and facet joint (thin arrow).

DIAGNOSIS:

Ankylosing spondylitis

DISCUSSION:

Ankylosing spondylitis (AS) is a chronic inflammatory seronegative spondyloarthropathy that affects the spine and sacroiliac joints. The disease is most common in young males, and there is a strong association with the HLA-B27 genotype. On paramedian sagittal T2-weighted MR, the combination of intervertebral disc fibrosis/ calcification and apophyseal (facet) joint arthrosis produces a hypointense "moustache." This finding has been identified at the level of greatest biomechanical stress in the spine, which is most likely to lead to neurological compromise requiring intervention. Other spinal manifestations of AS include peripheral spondylitis ("shiny corner"), spondylodiscitis (Andersson lesion), vertebral squaring, ankylosis ("bamboo" spine), apophyseal joint fusion ("trolley track" sign), and spinous ligament enthesitis ("dagger" sign).

Reference:

Behari S, Tungeria A, Jaiswal AK, et al. The "moustache" sign: localized intervertebral disc fibrosis and panligamentous ossification in ankylosing spondylitis with kyphosis. *Neurol India.* 2010;58(5):764-767.

NARROWING OF INTERPEDICULAR DISTANCE

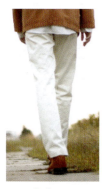

Modalities:
XR, CT, MR

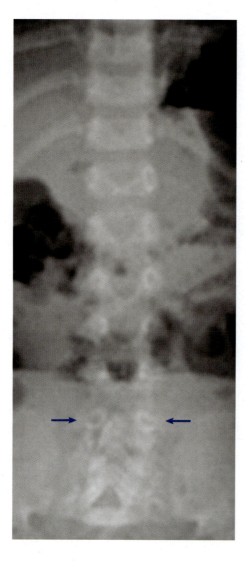

FINDINGS:

AP radiograph shows abnormally decreased interpedicular distance in the lower lumbar spine (arrows).

DIFFERENTIAL DIAGNOSIS:

- Achondroplasia
- Thanatophoric dysplasia

DISCUSSION:

On frontal radiography, the distance between pedicles gradually increases from the midthoracic to lumbar spine. Abnormal narrowing of interpedicular distance can occur in achondroplasia and thanatophoric dysplasia, both of which are caused by mutations in the fibroblast growth factor receptor (FGFR3) on chromosome 4p. Achondroplasia is the most common heritable nonlethal skeletal dysplasia, and follows an autosomal dominant inheritance pattern. The homozygous form is lethal, whereas heterozygous individuals demonstrate multiple skeletal anomalies including rhizomelic dwarfism, macrocephaly, frontal bossing, foramen magnum stenosis, bullet- or wedge-shaped ("cuneiform") vertebrae, posterior vertebral scalloping, kyphoscoliosis, and small squared "tombstone" iliac wings with narrow sciatic notches and horizontal acetabular roofs. Thanatophoric dysplasia is the most common lethal neonatal skeletal dysplasia. Patients demonstrate severe rhizomelic dwarfism with narrow chest and short ribs. Death occurs in utero or shortly after birth, due to respiratory insufficiency from pulmonary hypoplasia. Type I demonstrates frontal bossing, saddle nose, hypoplastic skull base, platyspondyly, and bowed long bones with "telephone receiver" femora. Type II is associated with pansynostosis (Kleeblattschädel skull), centrally flattened vertebrae ("H" or "U" morphology), and straight long bones.

References:

Dighe M, Fligner C, Cheng E, et al. Fetal skeletal dysplasia: an approach to diagnosis with illustrative cases. *Radiographics*. 2008;28(4):1061-1077.

Hinck VC, Clark WM, Hopkins CE. Normal interpediculate distances (minimum and maximum) in children and adults. *Am J Roentgenol Radium Ther Nucl Med*. 1966;97(1):141-153.

PARROT BEAK

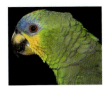

Modalities:
XR, CT, MR

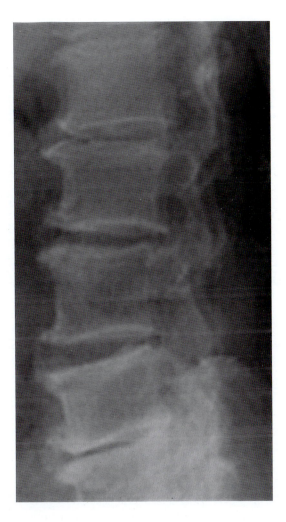

FINDINGS:

Lateral radiograph shows lumbar spine degeneration with multilevel anterior osteophytes.

DIAGNOSIS:

Osteophytosis

DISCUSSION:

Osteophytes are small, hook-shaped bony projections that develop at joint margins because of degeneration, instability, and/or abnormal stresses. There is an association with advanced age, degenerative disc disease, diffuse idiopathic skeletal hyperostosis (DISH), various arthritides, and other diseases causing mechanical instability. Certain conditions, such as acromegaly and fluorosis, can also cause increased bone deposition with osteophyte formation.

Reference:

Kumar R, Guinto FC Jr, Madewell JE, et al. The vertebral body: radiographic configurations in various congenital and acquired disorders. *Radiographics.* 1988;8(3):455-485.

POLKA DOT, SPOTTED

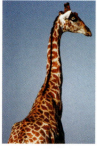

Modalities:
XR, CT, MR

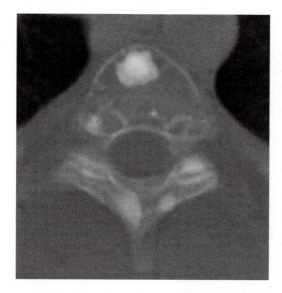

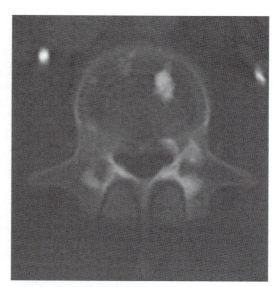

FINDINGS:

Axial CT shows multiple rounded sclerotic foci throughout the spine.

DIFFERENTIAL DIAGNOSIS:

- Osteopoikilosis
- Blastic metastases

DISCUSSION:

Osteopoikilosis is a rare sclerosing bone dysplasia with hereditary (autosomal dominant) and sporadic forms. Multiple islands of compact (cortical) bone (enostoses) are present within the medullary cavity (cancellous bone or spongiosa). These usually have a round or oval morphology, creating a "polka dot" or "spotted" appearance. Peripheral margins blend into the surrounding trabeculae, producing mild contour irregularity ("brush," "cumulus cloud," "feather," "spiculated," "thorny" appearance). Predominant locations are near joints and in the appendicular skeleton. Lesion size is usually 1-2 mm, but can measure up to 10 mm. In older patients, the differential includes multiple blastic metastases, such as from prostate or breast carcinoma. Metastases are large, inhomogeneous, and predominate in the axial skeleton. Prostate cancer metastasis is very rare when serum prostate specific antigen (PSA) is less than 10 nanograms per milliliter (ng/mL), and more likely when PSA exceeds 20 ng/mL. Radionuclide bone scintigraphy may aid in diagnosis: metastases demonstrate avid tracer uptake, while osteopoikilosis usually shows absent or mild tracer uptake.

Reference:

Ihde LL, Forrester DM, Gottsegen CJ, et al. Sclerosing bone dysplasias: review and differentiation from other causes of osteosclerosis. *Radiographics.* 2011;31(7):1865-1882.

PORTOBELLO MUSHROOM

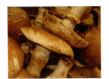

Modalities:
CT, MR

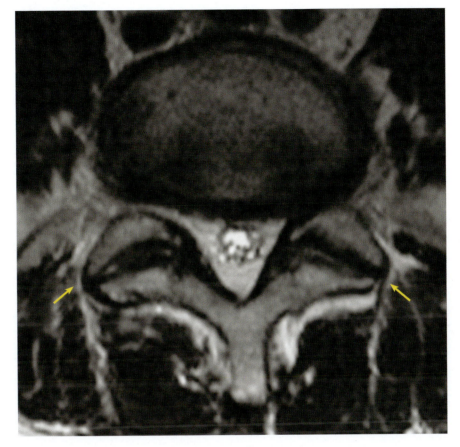

FINDINGS:

Axial T2-weighted MR shows facet arthropathy (arrows) with joint space narrowing and bone overgrowth. There is also a diffuse disc bulge and epidural lipomatosis.

DIAGNOSIS:

Facet arthropathy

DISCUSSION:

The apophyseal (facet) joint is a synovial joint formed between the inferior articular process of a vertebra and the superior articular process of the vertebra below it. Facet joints stabilize the spine by limiting anterior translation, flexion, and excessive rotation. On axial images, these normally have a rounded "hamburger" appearance with symmetric articulation between the inferior articular process of the cranial vertebra, located posteriorly; and the superior articular process of the caudal vertebra, located anteriorly. With facet arthropathy, joint space narrowing and bone overgrowth can produce a "Portobello mushroom" appearance.

Reference:

Helms CA, Major NM, Anderson MW, et al. *Musculoskeletal MRI*. 2nd ed. Philadelphia: Saunders; 2008.

POSTERIOR VERTEBRAL SCALLOPING

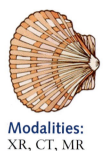

Modalities:
XR, CT, MR

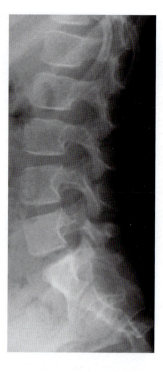 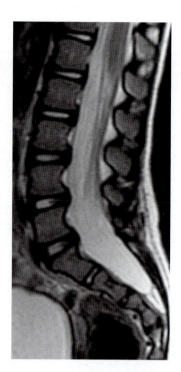

FINDINGS:

Lateral radiograph and sagittal T2-weighted MR show abnormal posterior concavity of lumbar vertebral bodies.

DIFFERENTIAL DIAGNOSIS:

- Increased intraspinal pressure
- Dural ectasia
- Small spinal canal
- Skeletal disorders
- Normal variant

DISCUSSION:

Posterior vertebral scalloping refers to abnormal concavity of the posterior vertebral cortex. Mild physiologic scalloping can be seen in healthy adults. More severe focal scalloping can be caused by disc herniation or expansile spinal tumors. Diffuse vertebral scalloping can be seen in chronic communicating hydrocephalus, with increased CSF pressures; dural ectasia (Marfan, Ehlers-Danlos, neurofibromatosis, ankylosing spondylitis), due to weakening of the dura mater; congenital skeletal disorders (achondroplasia, mucopolysaccharidoses, osteogenesis imperfecta, metatropic dysplasia), with restricted spinal growth; and acromegaly, with vertebral resorption and soft tissue hypertrophy.

Reference:

Wakely SL. The posterior vertebral scalloping sign. *Radiology.* 2006;239(2):607-609.

PSEUDODYSRAPHISM

Modality:
US

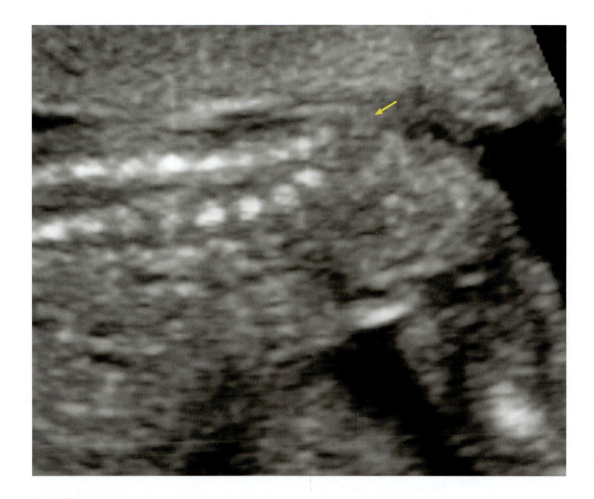

FINDINGS:

Fetal US, sagittal oblique plane, shows a pseudodefect of the sacrum (arrow). True sagittal and axial views failed to demonstrate a neural tube defect.

DIAGNOSIS:

Normal fetal spine

DISCUSSION:

Evaluation of the spine for neural tube defects is a crucial part of the ultrasonographic fetal survey. However, true sagittal and axial views must be obtained, as angled views may produce artifacts that mimic a spinal defect.

Reference:

Dennis MA, Drose JA, Pretorius DH, et al. Normal fetal sacrum simulating spina bifida: "pseudodysraphism." *Radiology.* 1985;155(3):751-754.

PUZZLE

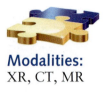

Modalities:
XR, CT, MR

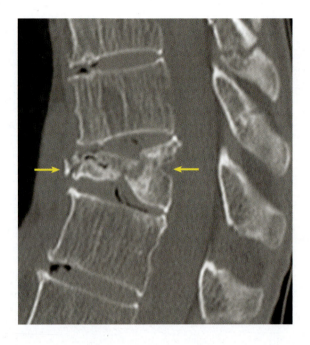

FINDINGS:

Sagittal CT shows a comminuted thoracic vertebral fracture (arrows), with fragments approximating the original vertebral contour. There is diffuse osseous demineralization.

DIAGNOSIS:

Benign compression fracture

DISCUSSION:

Vertebral compression fractures can occur secondary to benign (trauma, osteopenia, ischemia, inflammation, infection) or malignant (primary or metastatic tumor) causes. Imaging findings suggesting a benign fracture include flat or concave vertebral borders, normal marrow signal, multiple fractures, retropulsed fragments, fragments approximating the morphology of the original vertebra ("puzzle" sign), fluid ("fluid" sign) or air ("intravertebral vacuum" sign) within fracture lines, and bandlike subchondral fractures ("double line" sign). In the correct clinical setting, infection should also be considered. Discitis/osteomyelitis manifests with variable intradiscal and vertebral edema and enhancement, osseous destruction, and paraspinal fluid collections. Imaging features suggestive of malignancy include convex vertebral borders, abnormal marrow signal, marrow enhancement, reduced diffusion, involvement of the posterior elements, epidural/paraspinal masses, and other spinal metastases.

References:

Jung HS, Jee WH, McCauley TR, et al. Discrimination of metastatic from acute osteoporotic compression spinal fractures with MR imaging. *Radiographics*. 2003;23(1):179-187.

Yousem DI, Zimmerman RD, Grossman RI. *Neuroradiology: The Requisites*. 3rd ed. St Louis, MO: Mosby; 2010.

ROMANUS, SHINY CORNER, SHINY ODONTOID

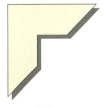

Modalities:
XR, CT, MR

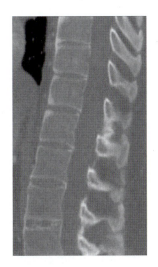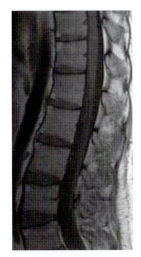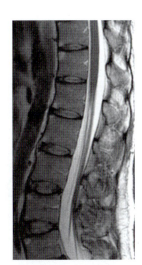

FINDINGS:

- Sagittal CT shows sclerosis along multiple anterior vertebral corners. Also noted are box-shaped vertebrae and calcifications of the interspinous ligaments and intervertebral discs.
- Sagittal T1-weighted and T2-weighted MR show hyperintensities along antero-superior and anteroinferior vertebral corners.

DIAGNOSIS:

Ankylosing spondylitis

DISCUSSION:

Ankylosing spondylitis (AS) is a chronic inflammatory seronegative spondyloar-thropathy that affects the spine and sacroiliac joints. The disease is most common in young males, and there is a strong association with the HLA-B27 genotype. The earliest imaging manifestation is peripheral spondylitis, affecting the vertebral corners along the attachments of the annulus fibrosus ("shiny corner"). This is frequently observed in the odontoid process and thoracolumbar spine in an anterior, posterior, or combined (marginal) location. On MR, active lesions demonstrate edema and enhancement, while inactive lesions undergo postinflammatory fatty degeneration. In the late stages, sclerosis can be appreciated on radiography or CT. Other spinal manifestations of AS include spondylodiscitis (Andersson lesion), vertebral squaring, ankylosis ("bamboo" spine), apophyseal joint fusion ("trolley track" sign), and spinous ligament enthesitis ("dagger" sign).

References:

Hermann KG, Althoff CE, Schneider U, et al. Spinal changes in patients with spondyloarthritis: comparison of MR imaging and radiographic appearances. *Radiographics*. 2005;25(3):559-569.

Kim NR, Choi JY, Hong SH, et al. "MR corner sign": value for predicting presence of ankylosing spondylitis. *AJR Am J Roentgenol*. 2008;191(1):124-128.

Lacout A, Rousselin B, Pelage JP. CT and MRI of spine and sacroiliac involvement in spondyloarthropathy. *AJR Am J Roentgenol*. 2008;191(4):1016-1023.

RUGGER JERSEY

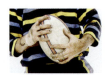

Modalities:
XR, CT

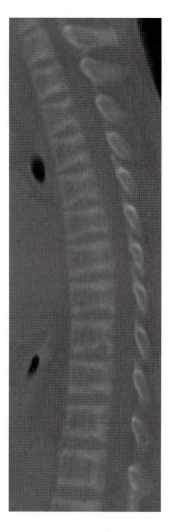

FINDINGS:

Sagittal CT shows sclerosis subjacent to thoracolumbar vertebral endplates, with associated subperiosteal resorption.

DIAGNOSIS:

Hyperparathyroidism

DISCUSSION:

The "rugger-jersey" spine is characterized by sclerosis subjacent to the vertebral endplates with associated subperiosteal resorption. The central vertebral bodies may be normal or lucent, with poorly defined borders. This finding is characteristic of hyperparathyroidism (HPTH): overactivity of the parathyroid glands that may be primary, secondary, or tertiary. Primary HPTH is caused by intrinsic parathyroid abnormalities (adenoma, hyperplasia, carcinoma) and results in elevated blood calcium levels. Secondary HPTH develops in response to low blood calcium levels, as seen in chronic renal failure and vitamin D deficiency. Tertiary HPTH represents autonomous parathyroid activity following longstanding secondary HPTH. In all cases, increased osteoclastic activity within bone leads to diffuse osteomalacia with fibrous replacement of bone (osteitis fibrosa cystica). Diffuse resorption occurs in subperiosteal, intracortical, endosteal, trabecular, subchondral, subligamentous, and subtendinous locations. Brown tumors (osteoclastomas) are expansile collections of fibrous tissue, disorganized woven bone, and hemorrhage. Lesions appear lytic in the initial phase, but may become sclerotic as the process heals. "Rugger jersey" spine should be distinguished from "sandwich" vertebrae, in which dense sclerosis directly involves the vertebral endplates. The central vertebral bodies may be normal or mildly sclerotic, with well-defined contours. "Sandwich" vertebrae are seen in type II osteopetrosis, fluorosis, myelofibrosis, and systemic stress. Another mimic is vertebral demineralization, in which the vertebral body appears hyperlucent, but the endplates are relatively preserved due to cortical buttressing. Over time, the entire vertebra becomes osteopenic. The intervertebral discs herniate into the weakened endplates and produce a "codfish" deformity.

Reference:

Wittenberg A. The rugger jersey spine sign. *Radiology*. 2004;230(2):491-492.

SCOTTIE DOG

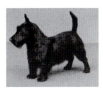

Modality:
XR

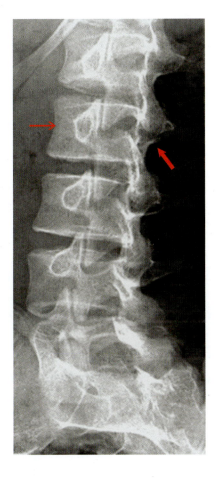

FINDINGS:

Lateral oblique radiograph shows the normal "Scottie dog" appearance at multiple levels, with transverse process (thin arrow) anteriorly and spinous process (thick arrow) posteriorly.

DIAGNOSIS:

Normal spine

DISCUSSION:

On lateral oblique radiography, the normal "Scottie dog" appearance is formed by the transverse process (nose), pedicle (eye), superior articular process (ear), pars interarticularis (neck), ipsilateral inferior articular process (front legs), lamina (body), contralateral inferior articular process (back legs), and spinous process (tail). Isthmic spondylolisthesis, or spondylolysis, affects the pars interarticularis (isthmus) with separation of the vertebral body from the posterior elements. This can be identified radiographically by a lucency or "collar" through the neck of the Scottie dog.

Reference:

Millard L. The Scotty dog and his collar. *J Ark Med Soc.* 1976;72(8):339-340.

SPINOUS PROCESS, STEP(OFF), WIDE CANAL

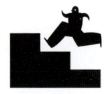

Modalities:
XR, CT, MR

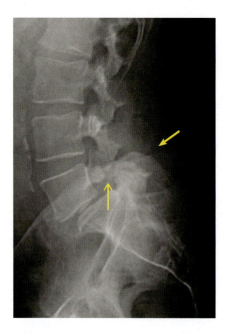 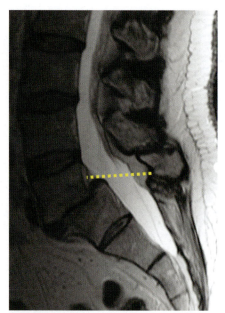

FINDINGS:

- Lateral radiograph shows bilateral L5 pars defects (thin arrow) with stepoff between the L4 and L5 spinous processes (thick arrow).
- Sagittal T2-weighted MR shows grade II anterolisthesis at L5-S1 with widening of the spinal canal (dotted line).

DIAGNOSIS:

Spondylolysis

DISCUSSION:

Spondylolisthesis refers to abnormal displacement of a vertebral body relative to the vertebra below it. Etiologies are categorized using the Wiltse classification: type I (dysplastic), II (isthmic), III (degenerative), IV (traumatic), V (pathologic), and VI (postoperative). The Meyerding classification of anterolisthesis, or anterior vertebral displacement, includes grade I (<25% displacement), II (25%-50%), III (50%-75%), IV (75%-100%), and V (>100%). Degenerative spondylolisthesis is caused by arthrosis at the facet joints without disruption of the pars interarticularis. There is concomitant anterior migration of the vertebra and posterior elements, resulting in grade I anterolisthesis and narrowing of the spinal canal. On lateral images, the spinous process "stepoff" is at the level of the spondylolisthesis. Isthmic spondylolisthesis, or spondylolysis, affects the pars interarticularis (isthmus) with separation of the vertebral body from the posterior elements. This results in grade II or higher anterolisthesis and widening of the spinal canal. On lateral images, the spinous process "stepoff" is above the level of the spondylolisthesis.

Reference:

Ulmer JL, Mathews VP, Elster AD, et al. Lumbar spondylolysis without spondylolisthesis: recognition of isolated posterior element subluxation on sagittal MR. *AJNR Am J Neuroradiol.* 1995;16(7):1393-1398.

T1 HALO

Modality:
MR

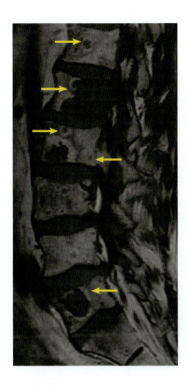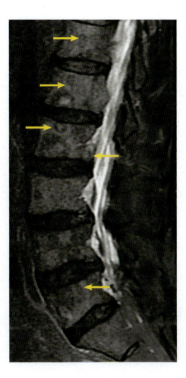

FINDINGS:

- Sagittal T1-weighted MR shows numerous hypointense vertebral lesions, some of which are surrounded by hyperintense fatty marrow (arrows).
- Sagittal T2-weighted MR with fat saturation shows signal drop in the areas of fatty conversion (arrows).

DIAGNOSIS:

Treated inactive metastases

DISCUSSION:

MR is the most sensitive imaging examination for vertebral metastases. Lesions are usually T1-hypointense relative to normal marrow, except for melanotic and hemorrhagic metastases, which can be T1-hyperintense. Active metastases also demonstrate contrast enhancement and/or reduced diffusion. Neoplastic infiltration into the surrounding marrow produces a T2-hyperintense rim of edema ("T2 halo" sign). Other causes of marrow edema, such as infection, inflammation, and trauma, do not typically produce multiple discrete halo signs. Treated inactive lesions can be identified by absence of contrast enhancement, normal or increased diffusion, and low T2 signal reflecting fibrotic/sclerotic changes. Surrounding fatty marrow conversion produces a T1-hyperintense rim ("T1 halo" sign).

References:

Daldrup-Link HE, Henning T, Link TM. MR imaging of therapy-induced changes of bone marrow. *Eur Radiol.* 2007;17(3):743-761.

Shah LM, Hanrahan CJ. MRI of spinal bone marrow: part I, techniques and normal age-related appearances. *AJR Am J Roentgenol.* 2011;197(6):1298-1308.

T2 HALO

Modality:
MR

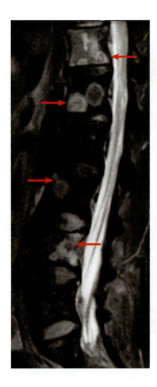 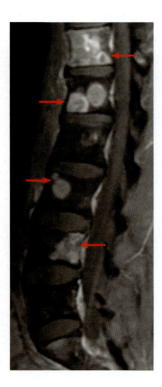

FINDINGS:

- Sagittal T2-weighted MR with fat saturation shows numerous hypointense vertebral lesions with surrounding hyperintense marrow edema (arrows).
- Sagittal contrast-enhanced T1-weighted MR with fat saturation shows avid enhancement of metastases (arrows).

DIAGNOSIS:

Active metastases

DISCUSSION:

MR is the most sensitive imaging examination for vertebral metastases. Lesions are is usually T1-hypointense relative to normal marrow, except for melanotic and hemorrhagic metastases, which can be T1-hyperintense. Active metastases also demonstrate contrast enhancement and/or reduced diffusion. Neoplastic infiltration into the surrounding marrow produces a T2-hyperintense rim of edema ("T2 halo" sign). Other causes of marrow edema, such as infection, inflammation, and trauma, do not typically produce multiple discrete halo signs. Treated inactive lesions can be identified by absence of contrast enhancement, normal or increased diffusion, and low T2 signal reflecting fibrotic/sclerotic changes. Surrounding fatty marrow conversion produces a T1-hyperintense rim ("T1 halo" sign).

References:

Daldrup-Link HE, Henning T, Link TM. MR imaging of therapy-induced changes of bone marrow. *Eur Radiol.* 2007;17(3):743-761.

Shah LM, Hanrahan CJ. MRI of spinal bone marrow: part I, techniques and normal age-related appearances. *AJR Am J Roentgenol.* 2011;197(6):1298-1308.

TOOTHPASTE

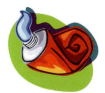

Modality:
MR

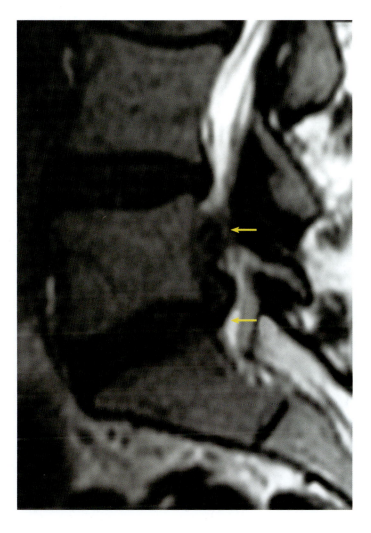

FINDINGS:

Sagittal T2-weighted MR shows an L5-S1 disc extrusion with superior subligamentous migration (arrows).

DIAGNOSIS:

Disc extrusion

DISCUSSION:

Disc extrusion refers to intervertebral disc material that extends beyond the outer ring of the annulus fibrosus, with vertical component exceeding the dimension of the base. Loss of continuity with the parent disc produces a sequestered disc or free fragment. Posteriorly displaced disc material is constrained by the posterior longitudinal ligament, creating a "toothpaste" appearance. Mass effect on the epidural/perineural spaces can impinge on the spinal cord and nerve roots.

References:

Fardon DF, Milette PC; Combined Task Forces of the North American Spine Society, American Society of Spine Radiology, and American Society of Neuroradiology. Nomenclature and classification of lumbar disc pathology. *Spine (Phila Pa 1976)*. 2001;26(5):E93-E113.

van Goethem JW, van den Hauwe L, Parizel PM. *Spinal Imaging: Diagnostic Imaging of the Spine and Spinal Cord*. Berlin: Springer; 2007.

WIDENING OF INTERPEDICULAR DISTANCE

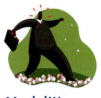

Modalities:
XR, CT, MR

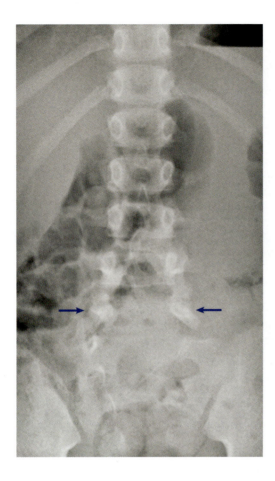

FINDINGS:

AP radiograph shows excessively widened interpedicular distance in the lower lumbar spine (arrows).

DIFFERENTIAL DIAGNOSIS:

- Spinal lesion
- Dural ectasia
- Spinal dysraphism
- Trauma

DISCUSSION:

On frontal radiography, the distance between pedicles gradually increases from the midthoracic to lumbar spine. Excessive widening of interpedicular distance can be seen in the setting of intraspinal tumors, syringohydromyelia, dural ectasia, spinal dysraphism, cord duplication, and trauma with involvement of the posterior elements. Clinical history, physical examination, and cross-sectional imaging (CT and MR) aid in diagnosis.

References:

Eisenberg RL. Clinical Imaging: *An Atlas of Differential Diagnosis*. Lippincott Williams & Wilkins; 2009.

Hinck VC, Clark WM, Hopkins CE. Normal interpediculate distances (minimum and maximum) in children and adults. *Am J Roentgenol Radium Ther Nucl Med*. 1966;97(1):141-153.

WRAPAROUND

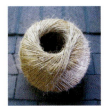

Modalities:
CT, MR

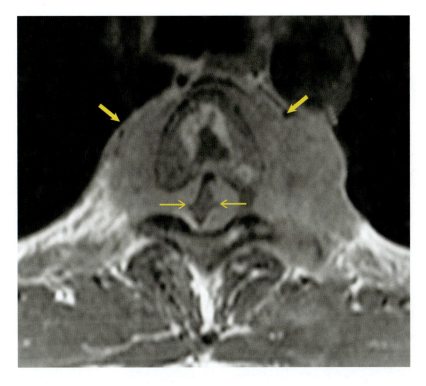

FINDINGS:

Axial contrast-enhanced T1-weighted MR shows enhancing soft tissue in the paravertebral (thick arrows) and epidural spaces (thin arrows) with severe cord compression.

DIAGNOSIS:

Lymphoma

DISCUSSION:

Osseous involvement of disseminated lymphoma is common, while primary bone lymphoma is rare. Lymphoma and other small round blue cell tumors spread in a permeative fashion, infiltrating between bony trabeculae and extending through small penetrating channels into soft tissue. At imaging, homogeneously enhancing tissue can involve the bone marrow, paravertebral, and epidural spaces. Extravertebral disease surrounds the vertebral body without cortical disruption ("wraparound" sign). In contrast, osteomyelitis, multiple myeloma, and metastases contiguously replace bone marrow and invade through the cortex to involve the soft tissues.

References:

Hicks DG, Gokan T, O'Keefe RJ, et al. Primary lymphoma of bone. Correlation of magnetic resonance imaging features with cytokine production by tumor cells. *Cancer.* 1995;75(4):973-980.

Moulopoulos LA, Dimopoulos MA, Vourtsi A, et al. Bone lesions with soft-tissue mass: magnetic resonance imaging diagnosis of lymphomatous involvement of the bone marrow versus multiple myeloma and bone metastases. *Leuk Lymphoma.* 1999;34(1-2):179-184.

WRAPPED DISC

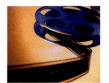

Modalities:
CT, MR

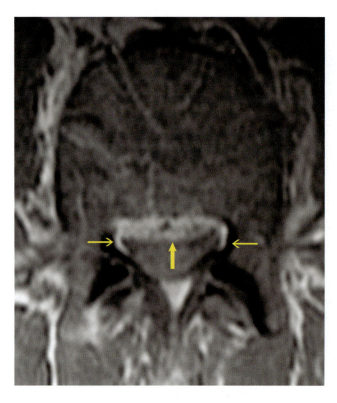

FINDINGS:

Axial contrast-enhanced T1-weighted MR shows a broad-based posterior disc bulge (thick arrow) with enhancement extending into the lateral recesses (thin arrows).

DIFFERENTIAL DIAGNOSIS:

- Disc herniation
- Epidural fibrosis
- Epidural abscess
- Epidural metastasis

DISCUSSION:

Failed back surgery syndrome (FBSS) is defined as persistent pain following back surgery. Major causes include residual or recurrent disc herniation, epidural fibrosis, lateral or central stenosis, arachnoiditis, and altered biomechanics. Surgical removal of herniated disc is a straightforward process, while reoperating on scar tissue exacerbates fibrosis. At imaging, herniated disc is smooth, nonenhancing, contiguous with the annulus fibrosus, and displaces surrounding structures. Scar tissue has a more irregular morphology with infiltration and retraction of the epidural/perineural fat, and is more pronounced above and below the disc space. Appearance ranges from edematous and T2-hyperintense in the early stages, to fibrotic and diffusely low signal in the late stages. The degree of contrast enhancement reflects scar vascularization. In some patients, recurrent disc herniation stimulates a fibroblastic response resulting in ingrowth and encasement by scar tissue, with a "wrapped disc" appearance. Differential considerations include epidural abscess and metastasis. Epidural abscess appears as a discrete rim-enhancing fluid collection, and can be associated with discitis/osteomyelitis causing aggressive bone destruction. Epidural metastasis typically appears as a smoothly elongated, enhancing mass that can span multiple vertebral levels and extend into perineural and paravertebral soft tissues.

References:

Bundschuh CV, Modic MT, Ross JS, et al. Epidural fibrosis and recurrent disc herniation in the lumbar spine: MR imaging assessment. *AJR Am J Roentgenol.* 1988;150(4):923-932.

Hwang GJ, Suh JS, Na JB, et al. Contrast enhancement pattern and frequency of previously unoperated lumbar discs on MRI. *J Magn Reson Imaging.* 1997;7(3):575-578.

ANCHOR

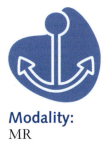

Modality:
MR

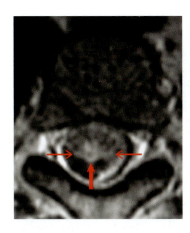 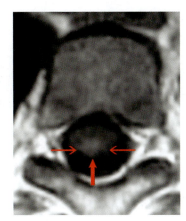

FINDINGS:

Axial T2-weighted and contrast-enhanced T1-weighted MR show hyperintense signal and enhancement in the dorsal (thick arrows) and lateral columns (thin arrows).

DIFFERENTIAL DIAGNOSIS:

- Subacute combined degeneration (late)
- Infectious myelitis
- Demyelinating disease
- Spinocerebellar ataxia

DISCUSSION:

Subacute combined degeneration (SCD), also known as Lichtheim disease, is a vitamin B_{12} (cobalamin) deficiency–related myelopathy. Causes include inadequate B_{12} intake, malabsorption, and other conditions (nitrous oxide intoxication, copper deficiency). Selective demyelination initially involves the dorsal white matter columns, followed by the lateral corticospinal and sometimes lateral spinothalamic tracts of the cervical and thoracic cord. On MR, the "rabbit ears" and "anchor" signs are produced by symmetric edema, reduced diffusion, and/or enhancement in these regions. The differential includes infectious myelitis (HIV-associated vacuolar myelopathy, varicella zoster virus, herpesvirus, Lyme disease, neurosyphilis or tabes dorsalis); multiple sclerosis; and hereditary spinocerebellar ataxias (Friedreich ataxia). However, these entities rarely demonstrate the symmetric and long-segment appearance of SCD.

Reference:

Paliwal VK, Malhotra HS, Chaurasia RN, et al. "Anchor"-shaped bright posterior column in a patient with vitamin B_{12} deficiency myelopathy. *Postgrad Med J*. 2009;85(1002):186.

BAG OF WORMS, HONEYCOMB, ROPE

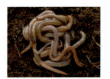

Modalities:
US, CT, MR

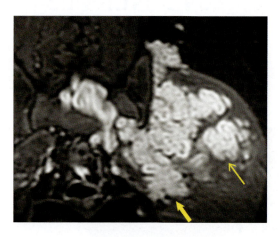

FINDINGS:

Coronal T2-weighted MR shows hyperintense serpiginous masses with infiltration of the left sciatic nerve (thick arrow) and gluteus muscles (thin arrow).

DIFFERENTIAL DIAGNOSIS:

- Plexiform neurofibroma
- Plexiform schwannoma
- Vascular malformation

DISCUSSION:

Peripheral nerve sheath tumors (PNSTs) are proliferations of peripheral nerve sheath cells that can be benign (schwannoma, neurofibroma) or malignant (malignant PNST). Schwannomas, also known as neurilemmomas, are encapsulated lesions composed of myelinating Schwann cells. These are eccentric to, and typically separable from, the underlying nerve. Neurofibromas are unencapsulated lesions involving nonmyelinating Schwann cells, perineural cells, and fibroblasts. These concentrically surround and are intimately associated with the parent nerve. At imaging, PNSTs appear hypoechoic on US, hypodense on CT, iso- to hypointense on T1-weighted MR, hyperintense on T2-weighted MR, and avidly enhancing. Plexiform and diffuse neurofibromas involve several nerve fascicles, producing a "bag of worms" or "honeycomb" appearance when branching, and a "rope" appearance when nonbranching. Rare mimickers include plexiform schwannomas and vascular malformations. Plexiform schwannomas are multinodular masses with a predilection for the head and neck region and subcutaneous tissues. There is an association with neurofibromatosis type II and schwannomatosis. Vascular malformations (VMs) are congenital lesions that can be high-flow (arterial), low-flow (capillary, venous, lymphatic), or mixed. Disorganized clusters of vessels can create the "bag of worms" appearance. Arteriovenous fistulas and malformations demonstrate rapid arterial enhancement and early venous drainage, without an intervening capillary bed. Arteriovenous shunting may occur through a direct communication (AVF) or nidus of vessels (AVM). Venous malformations demonstrate delayed enhancement and are associated with phleboliths. Lymphatic malformations are minimally enhancing masses that can be macrocystic, with multiple septations and fluid-blood levels; or microcystic, with a solid appearance at imaging.

Reference:

Lin J, Martel W. Cross-sectional imaging of peripheral nerve sheath tumors: characteristic signs on CT, MR imaging, and sonography. *AJR Am J Roentgenol.* 2001;176(1):75-82.

BEADED, SACCULATED, SAUSAGE, SERRATED, STACKED COIN

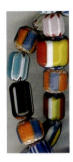

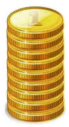

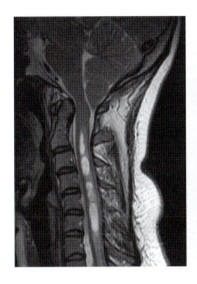

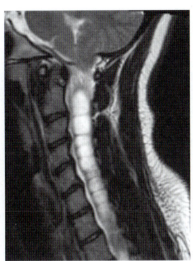

Modalities:
US, CT, MR

FINDINGS:

Sagittal T2-weighted MR in two different patients demonstrates cerebellar tonsillar descent with craniocervical junction stenosis and multilocular cervical cord syrinx.

DIFFERENTIAL DIAGNOSIS:

- Syringohydromyelia
- Cystic cord tumor
- Myelomalacia

DISCUSSION:

Syringohydromyelia refers to a fluid collection within the spinal cord, and may represent dilation of the central canal (hydromyelia) or a cystic collection separate from the central canal (syringomyelia, syrinx). This can be idiopathic or due to obstruction of CSF flow associated with hydrocephalus, Chiari malformation, tethered cord, tumor, trauma, surgery, hemorrhage, infarction, infection, inflammation, and extrinsic compression. At imaging, an intramedullary fluid collection focally expands the cord and follows CSF signal on all sequences. Small lesions have a tubular appearance, while larger lesions are more complex with loculations/septations ("sausage" or "stacked coin" appearance) and cord parenchymal abnormalities. Contrast should be administered to assess for focal enhancement, which raises concern for a cystic cord tumor. Myelomalacia refers to cord atrophy following various insults, with volume loss and T2-hyperintense signal. In advanced stages, cystic degeneration may occur with conversion into syringohydromyelia.

References:

Bou-Haidar P, Peduto AJ, Karunaratne N. Differential diagnosis of T2 hyperintense spinal cord lesions: part B. *J Med Imaging Radiat Oncol.* 2009;53(2):152-159.

Koeller KK, Rosenblum RS, Morrison AL. Neoplasms of the spinal cord and filum terminale: radiologic-pathologic correlation. *Radiographics.* 2000;20(6):1721-1749.

BOWSTRING

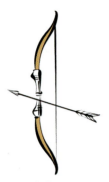

Modalities:
US, MR

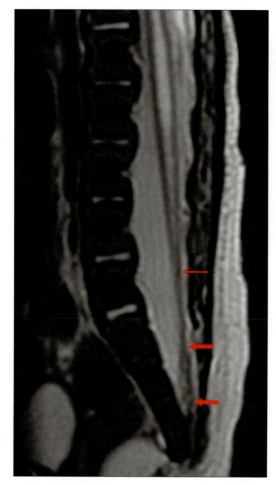

FINDINGS:

Sagittal T2-weighted MR shows syringomyelia and low-lying conus medullaris at the L5 level (thin arrow). The filum terminale (thick arrows) is short, taut, and thickened.

DIAGNOSIS:

Tight filum terminale

DISCUSSION:

The spinal cord forms in utero by primary neurulation (involving neural tube closure and disjunction), and secondary neurulation of the caudal cell mass (involving canalization and retrogressive differentiation). During development, disproportionate growth of the vertebral column and dura relative to the spinal cord causes relative "ascent" of the conus medullaris. Normally, the conus is located at L2-L3 at birth, and reaches the normal adult level (L1-L2) at approximately 2 months of age. The filum terminale and cauda equina nerve roots elongate to accommodate the spinal cord. However, tethering of the cord to surrounding tissues may be caused by congenital, inflammatory, neoplastic, traumatic, and iatrogenic etiologies. This results in a low-lying conus with limitation of nerve root motion. The tight filum terminale syndrome refers to cord tethering associated with a short, thickened filum terminale. The abnormal filum terminale measures over 2 mm at the L5-S1 level and appears taut relative to the curvature of the spine, creating a "bowstring" appearance. There is an association with spinal lipomatous malformations and syringohydromyelia.

Reference:

Raghavan N, Barkovich AJ, Edwards M, et al. MR imaging in the tethered spinal cord syndrome. *AJR Am J Roentgenol.* 1989;152(4):843-852.

BULLSEYE, CENTRAL DOT, FASCICULAR, HALO, TARGET

Modalities:
US, CT, MR

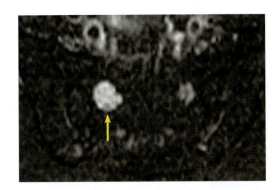

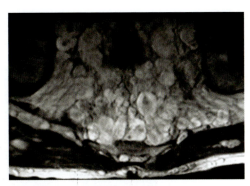

FINDINGS:

- Axial T2-weighted MR with fat saturation shows a hyperintense mass enlarging the right S1 foramen (arrow), with hypointense traversing nerve fascicles.
- Axial T2-weighted MR in a different patient shows innumerable hyperintense masses with central hypointensities throughout the spinal canal, lumbosacral plexi, and pelvis.

DIAGNOSIS:

Peripheral nerve sheath tumors

DISCUSSION:

Peripheral nerve sheath tumors (PNSTs) are proliferations of peripheral nerve sheath cells that can be benign (schwannoma, neurofibroma) or malignant (malignant PNST). Schwannomas, also known as neurilemmomas, are encapsulated lesions composed of myelinating Schwann cells. These are eccentric to and typically separable from the underlying nerve. Neurofibromas are unencapsulated lesions involving nonmyelinating Schwann cells, perineural cells, and fibroblasts. These concentrically surround and are intimately associated with the parent nerve. At imaging, PNSTs appear hypoechoic on US, hypodense on CT, iso- to hypointense on T1-weighted MR, hyperintense on T2-weighted MR, and avidly enhancing. Characteristic imaging features include a fusiform tapered mass with normal entering and exiting fibers, creating a "string" or "tail" appearance in long axis. Smooth outward bulging of perineural fat creates the "split fat" appearance. In cross section, traversing nerve fibers may be identified in a "fascicular" pattern. The "bullseye" or "target" sign corresponds pathologically to central fibrosis and peripheral myxoid tissue. These imaging features suggest benign rather than malignant PNST, which is usually larger, more heterogeneous, and infiltrative. Syndromic PNSTs (multiple neurofibromas in NF1, multiple schwannomas in NF2 and schwannomatosis) have a higher incidence of malignant transformation and may be followed with serial MR and/or PET to evaluate for rapid increases in size, marginal irregularity, internal heterogeneity, and high metabolic activity.

Reference:

Lin J, Martel W. Cross-sectional imaging of peripheral nerve sheath tumors: characteristic signs on CT, MR imaging, and sonography. *AJR Am J Roentgenol*. 2001;176(1):75-82.

BUNDLE, HORSE TAIL

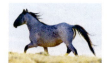

Modalities:
US, MR

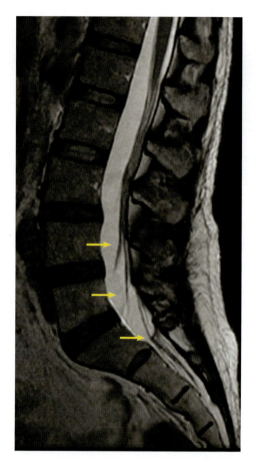

FINDINGS:

Sagittal T2-weighted MR shows a normal conus medullaris terminating at L1-L2, vertical filum terminale, and cauda equina nerve roots fanning out toward the neural foramina (arrows).

DIAGNOSIS:

Normal cauda equina

DISCUSSION:

The distal spinal cord is formed by secondary neurulation of the caudal cell mass and gives rise to the conus medullaris, cauda equina, and filum terminale. The filum terminale (Latin for "terminal thread") is a fibrous structure that extends vertically down from the apex of the conus medullaris, contiguous with the pia mater, and blends inferiorly with the dura mater. The cauda equina (Latin for "horse's tail") is a collection of nerves that originate from the conus and travel inferiorly to innervate the pelvic organs and lower extremities. During development, disproportionate growth of the vertebral column and dura relative to the spinal cord causes relative "ascent" of the conus medullaris. Normally, the conus is located at L2-L3 at birth, and reaches the normal adult level (L1-L2) at approximately 2 months of age. The filum terminale and cauda equina elongate to accommodate the spinal cord. This results in a "bundled" appearance of nerve fibers, which sequentially exit the spinal cord at the neural foramina. At imaging, the cauda equina normally appears smooth and linear. Abnormal nerve root signal, morphology, and/or enhancement should raise concern for pathology. Smooth linear enhancement is seen in bacterial or viral meningitis, inflammatory/autoimmune conditions, and demyelinating disease. Nodular irregular enhancement is seen in leptomeningeal carcinomatosis, fungal or tuberculous meningitis, and granulomatous disease. Postinflammatory arachnoiditis can also produce scarring with nerve root clumping and adhesions. Hereditary hypertrophic neuropathies (Charcot-Marie-Tooth, Dejerine-Sottas) demonstrate fusiform enlargement and abnormal signal in multiple nerve roots. Compression or other injury to the cauda equina can produce saddle anesthesia, bowel/bladder dysfunction, and lower extremity paralysis. This is known as cauda equina syndrome, and requires emergent surgical evaluation.

Reference:

Monajati A, Wayne WS, Rauschning W, et al. MR of the cauda equina. *AJNR Am J Neuroradiol.* 1987;8(5):893-900.

BUTTERFLY, DOUBLE DOT, H, PENCIL, OWL/SNAKE EYES, RING

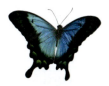

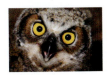

Modality:
MR

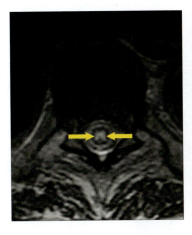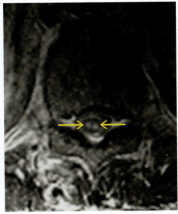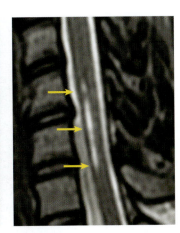

FINDINGS:

- Axial T2-weighted MR shows abnormal hyperintensity throughout the central gray matter (thick arrows).
- Axial T2-weighted MR in a different patient shows punctate hyperintensities in the anterior horns of the gray matter (thin arrows).
- Sagittal T2-weighted MR shows linear hyperintensity within the ventral cord (arrows).

DIAGNOSIS:

Spinal cord infarct

DISCUSSION:

The blood supply to the spinal cord consists of the anterior spinal artery, paired posterior spinal arteries, and radiculomedullary arteries. The anterior spinal artery (ASA) arises from the vertebral arteries and is reinforced by multiple medullary arteries. It courses in the anterior median fissure to supply the anterior two-thirds of the cord, including the anterior horns, spinothalamic tracts, and corticospinal tracts. Vascular disease and mechanical stresses predispose to ASA occlusion with ventral cord infarction, creating a vertical "pencil"-like signal abnormality. In addition, the central penetrating arteries have few collaterals, while the peripheral arteries form an extensive vascular network. Therefore, lacunar infarcts commonly affect the anterior horns of the gray matter with an "owl eyes" appearance on MR. Global hypoperfusion can affect the entire gray matter because of its central watershed location and high metabolic activity. This forms a central "H" pattern with reduced diffusion, T2-hyperintense edema, and/or enhancement. A surrounding T2-hypointense "ring" of preserved white matter is present.

Reference:

Kumral E, Polat F, Güllüoglu H, et al. Spinal ischaemic stroke: clinical and radiological findings and short-term outcome. *Eur J Neurol.* 2011;18(2):232-239.

BUTTERFLY, H

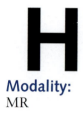

Modality:
MR

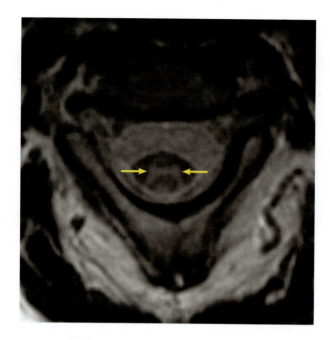

FINDINGS:

Axial T2*-weighted MR shows normal central gray matter (arrows) in the cervical cord.

DIAGNOSIS:

Normal gray matter

DISCUSSION:

The spinal cord is a cylindrical structure that carries descending motor and ascending sensory signals between the brain and peripheral nervous system, as well as coordinating various reflex arcs. It is comprised of peripheral white matter and central gray matter. The white matter consists of myelinated sheets of motor and sensory axons, which are divided into ventral (anterior), lateral, and dorsal (posterior) columns or funiculi. The gray matter consists of neuronal cell bodies, unmyelinated axons, and glial cells. Normal gray matter is mildly hyperintense relative to white matter on T2-weighted MR. Internal architecture is best appreciated on T2*-weighted gradient echo (GRE) or high-field imaging sequences. The normal "H" morphology represents ventral (anterior) and dorsal (posterior) horns that are connected across midline by the gray commissure surrounding the central canal. The ventral horns contain motor neurons and interneurons, while the dorsal horns contain sensory neurons. Wedge-shaped lateral horns are also present at the thoracic and upper lumbar levels, and contain preganglionic sympathetic neurons. Outside the cord, the ventral horns communicate with ventral (pure motor) roots. The dorsal horns communicate with dorsal (pure sensory) roots and dorsal root ganglia, formed by cell bodies of somatic afferent neurons. Spinal nerves are formed by the coalescence of ventral and dorsal roots. After exiting the neural foramina, spinal nerves divide into ventral and dorsal rami, which represent mixed motor and sensory nerves.

References:

Czervionke LF, Daniels DL, Ho PS, et al. The MR appearance of gray and white matter in the cervical spinal cord. *AJNR Am J Neuroradiol.* 1988;9(3):557-562.

Goshgarian HG. Neuroanatomic organization of the spinal gray and white matter. In: Lin VW, Cardenas DD, Cutter NC, eds. *Spinal Cord Medicine: Principles and Practice.* New York: Demos Medical Publishing; 2003.

Jindal G, Pukenas B. Normal spinal anatomy on magnetic resonance imaging. *Magn Reson Imaging Clin N Am.* 2011;19(3):475-488.

C1-C2, COLLAPSE, FESTOON, DRAPED CURTAIN, FLOATING SAC, HEXAGON, LIGHTBULB

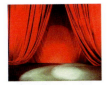

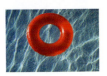

Modality:
MR

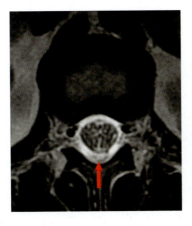 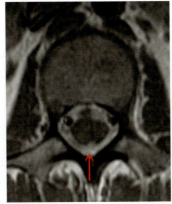 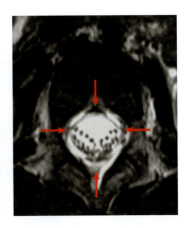

FINDINGS:

- Axial T2-weighted and contrast-enhanced T1-weighted MR show fluid (thick arrow) and engorged epidural veins (thin arrow) surrounding the dural sac.
- Axial T2-weighted MR in a different patient shows partial dural collapse with tethering by meningovertebral ligaments (arrows).

DIAGNOSIS:

CSF hypovolemia

DISCUSSION:

Cerebrospinal fluid hypovolemia is caused by dural tears in the brain or spine with continuous loss of fluid. This can be seen with idiopathic, degenerative, traumatic, or iatrogenic causes. Within the spine, CSF hypotension produces epidural/subdural fluid collections (spinal hygromas) and dural venous engorgement. The "floating dural sac" sign refers to the appearance of dura mater completely surrounded by epidural fluid. More often, dural collapse is limited by tethering from meningovertebral (Hoffmann) ligaments, producing a "festooned" or "draped curtain" appearance. Because false localizing signs can be produced by epidural transudation or migration in areas of loose dural attachment (particularly the C1-C2 region), a careful search should be undertaken for more specific signs such as dural irregularity, contrast extravasation, and extraspinal CSF collections (pseudomeningoceles, perineural cysts). Imaging studies that can identify the site of leakage include radionuclide cisternography and conventional, CT, or MR myelography. Once identified, the leak can be repaired by epidural blood patch, percutaneous fibrin glue injection, or surgery.

References:

Hosoya T, Hatazawa J, Sato S, et al. Floating dural sac sign is a sensitive magnetic resonance imaging finding of spinal cerebrospinal fluid leakage. *Neurol Med Chir (Tokyo)*. 2013;53(4):207-212.

Watanabe A, Horikoshi T, Uchida M, et al. Diagnostic value of spinal MR imaging in spontaneous intracranial hypotension syndrome. *AJNR Am J Neuroradiol*. 2009;30(1):147-151.

CAKE ICING, CHRISTMAS BALLS, FROSTING, GROUND GLASS, SMUDGED, SHEET, SUGARCOATING, ZUCKERGUSS

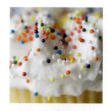

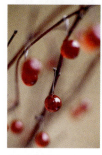

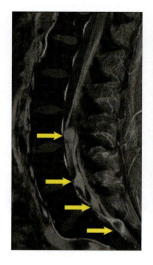

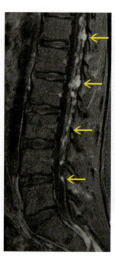

Modality:
MR

FINDINGS:

- Sagittal contrast-enhanced T1-weighted MR with fat saturation in a patient with lymphoma shows thickening and fusiform masses along the cauda equina nerve roots (thick arrows).
- Sagittal contrast-enhanced T1-weighted MR with fat saturation in a patient with neurofibromatosis shows multiple nodules studding the cauda equina (thin arrows).

DIFFERENTIAL DIAGNOSIS:

- Leptomeningeal carcinomatosis
- Multiple primary intradural tumors
- Infectious/inflammatory meningitis
- Neurosarcoidosis

DISCUSSION:

Diffuse nodular leptomeningeal enhancement involving the brain and/or spinal cord is known as Zuckerguss (German for "sugar icing"), and results from CSF dissemination of abnormal cells throughout the neuraxis. This finding may be seen in leptomeningeal carcinomatosis, multiple primary intradural tumors, infectious meningitis (fungal and TB), and inflammatory/granulomatous disease (neurosarcoidosis). Leptomeningeal carcinomatosis may be the result of widespread hematogenous metastases or direct seeding ("drop" metastases) from primary CNS neoplasms. Fungal, tuberculous, and granulomatous meningitis can also demonstrate diffuse nodular thickening of the leptomeninges and cauda equina nerve roots. On MR, CSF may demonstrate a "ground-glass" or "hazy" signal. Irregular thickening of nerve roots produces a "smudged" appearance, and pedunculated masses demonstrate a "Christmas balls" morphology. Rarely, multiple primary tumors (nerve sheath tumors, hemangioblastoma, meningioma, astrocytoma, myxopapillary ependymoma, paraganglioma) can also involve the conus and cauda equina.

Reference:

Krol G, Sze G, Malkin M, et al. MR of cranial and spinal meningeal carcinomatosis: comparison with CT and myelography. *AJR Am J Roentgenol.* 1988;151(3):583-588.

CANDLE DRIPPING/GUTTERING

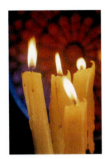

Modalities:
XR, CT, MR

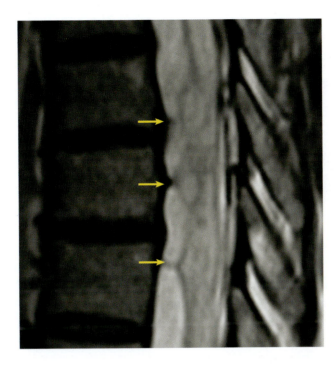

FINDINGS:

Sagittal T2-weighted MR shows abnormal cord signal and contour with multiple ventral adhesions (arrows).

DIAGNOSIS:

Arachnoiditis, type III (adhesive)

DISCUSSION:

Arachnoiditis is a chronic inflammatory condition of the leptomeninges and subarachnoid space. Causes include infection, trauma, chronic compression, and spine surgery or injections. The Delamarter classification consists of three stages: Type I (central, radicular) arachnoiditis affects individual nerves with a thick and blunted "sleeveless" morphology. Clustering of the cauda equina produces a "short caudal sac" with "clumped" nerve roots. In Type II (peripheral) arachnoiditis, meningeal adhesions cause peripheral migration of nerve roots with an "empty sac" appearance. Type III (adhesive, obstructive, obliterative) arachnoiditis involves fibrous scarring, with soft tissue obliteration of the subarachnoid space producing a "candle dripping" contour. Associated CSF obstruction and syringohydromyelia are common. Chronic arachnoiditis is occasionally associated with intrathecal ossification, termed arachnoiditis ossificans. Distinction from other pathologic entities such as leptomeningeal carcinomatosis, intradural neoplasms, infectious meningitis, and granulomatous disease can be difficult. However, these conditions tend to be associated with greater contrast enhancement and intrathecal mass effect.

References:

Delamarter RB, Ross JS, Masaryk TJ, et al. Diagnosis of lumbar arachnoiditis by magnetic resonance imaging. *Spine (Phila Pa 1976).* 1990;15(4):304-310.

Ross JS, Masaryk TJ, Modic MT, et al. MR imaging of lumbar arachnoiditis. *AJR Am J Roentgenol.* 1987;149(5):1025-1032.

CAP

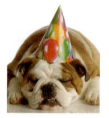

Modality:
MR

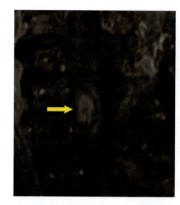
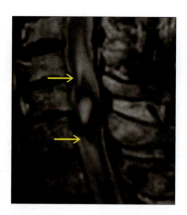

FINDINGS:

- Sagittal contrast-enhanced T1-weighted MR with fat saturation shows an enhancing intramedullary mass (thick arrow) with smooth cord expansion.
- Sagittal T2-weighted MR shows surrounding cord edema and hemorrhage, with susceptibility artifact along the superior and inferior poles (thin arrows).

DIFFERENTIAL DIAGNOSIS:

- Ependymoma
- Hemangioblastoma
- Paraganglioma
- Metastasis

DISCUSSION:

Ependymoma is the most common intramedullary neoplasm in adults, and the second most common in children. There is an association with neurofibromatosis type II (NF2). Tumors originate from ependymal cells lining the central canal and are divided into six subtypes: cellular, papillary, clear cell, tanycytic, myxopapillary, and melanotic. Lesions tend to be centrally located, well-circumscribed, and avidly enhancing. Hemorrhage, cysts, and syringohydromyelia may be seen at the tumor poles. On T2-weighted images, the "cap" sign refers to a hypointense rim of hemosiderin, classically seen in ependymoma or other hypervascular tumors (hemangioblastoma, paraganglioma, metastasis). In contrast, astrocytoma is the second most common intramedullary neoplasm in adults, and the most common in children. There is an association with neurofibromatosis type I (NF1). Tumors tend to arise eccentrically from the cord parenchyma, with an infiltrative and heterogeneous appearance. Hemorrhage and syringohydromyelia are uncommon.

References:

Kim DH, Kim JH, Choi SH, et al. Differentiation between intramedullary spinal ependymoma and astrocytoma: comparative MRI analysis. *Clin Radiol.* 2013.

Smith AB, Soderlund KA, Rushing EJ, et al. Radiologic-pathologic correlation of pediatric and adolescent spinal neoplasms: Part 1, Intramedullary spinal neoplasms. *AJR Am J Roentgenol.* 2012;198(1):34-43.

CAP, CIRCLE, OVAL, MENISCUS

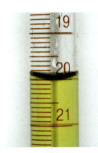

Modalities:
XR, CT, MR

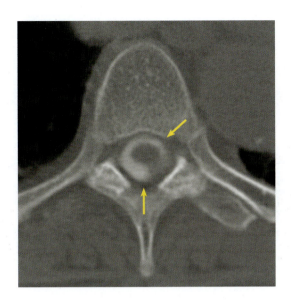

FINDINGS:

Axial CT myelogram shows a filling defect in the left posterolateral spinal canal (arrows). This forms acute angles with the spinal cord and dura, and is sharply outlined by intrathecal contrast.

DIAGNOSIS:

Intradural extramedullary lesion

DISCUSSION:

Myelography involves direct intrathecal injection of contrast with subsequent imaging using fluoroscopy, CT, and/or MR. This helps to evaluate CSF dynamics (leak, obstruction) in the setting of trauma, spinal stenosis, or tumor. The morphology of the contrast column should be evaluated with attention to the dura, spinal cord, and nerve roots. Intramedullary lesions create focal expansion of the cord outline, often with normal CSF dynamics. Intradural extramedullary lesions appear as ovoid filling defects that focally expand the ipsilateral CSF space. Margins form acute angles with the dura, and are outlined by a "meniscus" of contrast. Large masses can displace and compress the cord and nerve roots. The differential includes nerve sheath tumors, meningiomas, arachnoid or epidermoid cysts, and metastases. Arachnoiditis is a chronic inflammatory condition of the leptomeninges and subarachnoid space, and a great mimicker on myelography. Scarring and adhesions produce a wide variety of filling defects. However, there is absence of true mass effect and, in some cases, tenting of the cord and contrast column toward the defect. Finally, extradural lesions form obtuse angles with the dura and can interrupt CSF flow. The differential includes epidural masses, epidural fluid collections, and spinal degenerative disease.

References:

Greenberg MS. *Handbook of Neurosurgery*. 7th ed. New York: Thieme; 2010.

Teng P, Papatheodorou C. Myelographic findings in adhesive spinal arachnoiditis (with a brief surgical note). *Br J Radiol*. 1967;40(471):201-208.

CENTRAL DOT

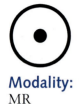

Modality:
MR

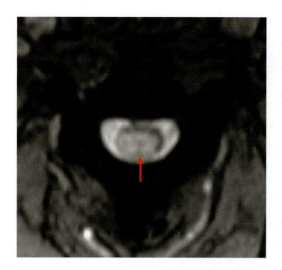

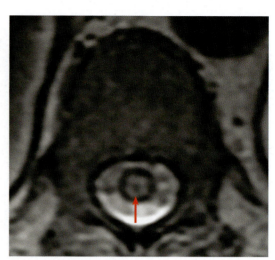

FINDINGS:

Axial T2*-weighted and T2-weighted MR in two different patients show diffuse cord edema with compressed central gray matter (arrows).

DIAGNOSIS:

Transverse myelitis

DISCUSSION:

Transverse myelitis (TM), also known as transverse myelopathy, is a monophasic inflammatory disorder that involves both halves of the spinal cord. The majority of cases are idiopathic but can be associated with vaccination, infectious, toxic/metabolic, neoplastic, autoimmune, demyelinating, vascular, and traumatic etiologies. At imaging, there is transverse cord edema (more than 2/3 of cross section), which can be longitudinally extensive (2-4 vertebral levels). On T2-weighted images, the "central dot" sign refers to central gray matter compressed by uniform cord edema. Mild eccentric or peripheral enhancement may be present. In contrast, multiple sclerosis involves the white matter in a focal and asymmetric fashion (less than 1/2 of cross section, usually 1-2 vertebral levels), with central or leading-edge enhancement in the active phase. Tumors disrupt the normal cord architecture with distortion of the gray matter. Typically, there is solid heterogeneous enhancement with cord expansion and significant surrounding edema (entire cross section, often greater than 3-4 vertebral levels).

References:

Choi KH, Lee KS, Chung SO, et al. Idiopathic transverse myelitis: MR characteristics. *AJNR Am J Neuroradiol.* 1996;17(6):1151-1160.

West TW, Hess C, Cree BA. Acute transverse myelitis: demyelinating, inflammatory, and infectious myelopathies. *Semin Neurol.* 2012;32(2):97-113.

CHRISTMAS TREE, RAILROAD, SERRATE

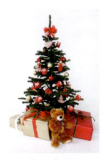

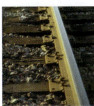

Modality:
NM

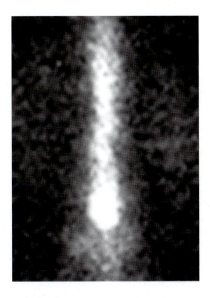

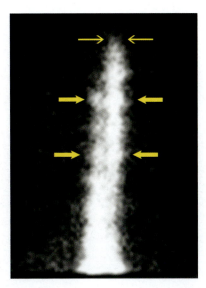

FINDINGS:

^{111}In-DTPA cisternogram, posterior planar images, show intrathecal tracer ascent from the lumbar spine with abrupt cutoff in the thoracic spine (thin arrows) and delayed epidural/perineural opacification (thick arrows).

DIFFERENTIAL DIAGNOSIS:

- Cerebrospinal fluid leak
- Epidural tracer injection

DISCUSSION:

Cerebrospinal fluid hypovolemia is caused by dural tears in the brain or spine with continuous loss of fluid. This can be seen with idiopathic, degenerative, traumatic, and iatrogenic causes. Patients may present with orthostatic headaches, cranial neuropathies, nausea/vomiting, and fatigue. In radionuclide cisternography, intrathecal injection of a radiolabeled pharmaceutical (usually indium-111 diethylene triamine pentaacetic acid) is followed by sequential imaging to evaluate CSF flow. In a normal patient, tracer ascends up the spinal column to the level of the basal cisterns by 1 hour, the frontal poles and sylvian fissures by 2-6 hours, the cerebral convexities by 12 hours, and the arachnoid villi in the sagittal sinus by 24 hours. In the presence of a dural tear, the tracer column is interrupted and fails to ascend beyond the level of the leak. Delayed imaging reveals tracer accumulation in the epidural and perineural spaces, with a "Christmas tree" or "serrated" appearance. The imaging differential includes epidural tracer injection. This should be evident on initial imaging, with absence of intrathecal tracer.

References:

Cheng MF, Pa MH, Wu YW, et al. Radionuclide cisternography in diagnosing spontaneous intracranial hypotension. *Ann Nucl Med Sci.* 2004;17:167-172.

Horikoshi T, Asari Y, Watanabe A, et al. Unsuccessful tracer injection in radionuclide cisternography revisited. *Ann Nucl Med.* 2006;20(4):333-336.

CIGAR, CLUB, GHOST/WEDGE CONUS

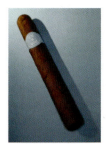

Modalities:
US, MR

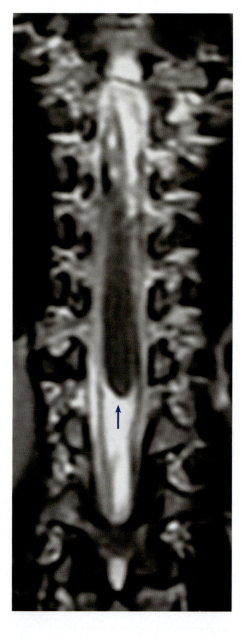

FINDINGS:

Coronal T2-weighted MR shows a foreshortened distal cord terminating at the thoracolumbar junction (arrow), with absent conus and widely separated cauda equina nerve roots.

DIAGNOSIS:

Caudal regression, type 1

DISCUSSION:

Caudal regression, also known as sacral dysgenesis/agenesis, results from embryologic disturbances in primary neurulation or canalization and retrogressive differentiation of the caudal cell mass. Most cases are sporadic or associated with maternal diabetes. Type 1 caudal regression demonstrates a high cord termination and severe sacral anomalies. There is a blunted ("cigar") appearance of the distal spinal cord with absent ("ghost") conus medullaris. The ventral and dorsal cauda equina nerve roots are widely separated with a "double bundle" appearance. Severe associated anomalies can include syringohydromyelia, split cord malformations, open spinal dysraphisms, and visceral malformations. Type 2 caudal regression demonstrates a low-lying conus with cord tethering. Associated anomalies are less severe than in type 1 and include tight filum terminale, lipomatous malformations, and closed spinal dysraphisms. Caudal regression may be part of the VACTERL association (vertebral defects, anal atresia, cardiac defects, tracheo-esophageal fistula, renal anomalies, and limb abnormalities); OEIS complex (omphalocele, exstrophy of the cloaca, imperforate anus, and spinal defects); and Currarino syndrome (sacral hypoplasia, presacral mass, and anorectal malformations).

References:

Barkovich AJ, Raghavan N, Chuang S, et al. The wedge-shaped cord terminus: a radiographic sign of caudal regression. *AJNR Am J Neuroradiol.* 1989;10(6):1223-1231.

Nievelstein RA, Valk J, Smit LM, et al. MR of the caudal regression syndrome: embryologic implications. *AJNR Am J Neuroradiol.* 1994;15(6):1021-1029.

CIRCLE, CROSS, GEOMETRIC, INVERTED TRIANGLE, LINEAR, OVAL, PALM LEAF, POLYGONAL, SPICULATED, SQUARE, STELLATE, TREFOIL, TRIFID, Y

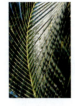

Modalities:
CT, MR

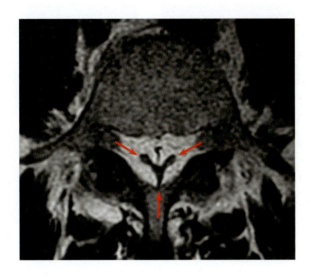

FINDINGS:

Axial T1-weighted MR shows epidural lipomatosis with compression of the thecal sac and anchoring by meningovertebral ligaments (arrows).

DIAGNOSIS:

Epidural lipomatosis

DISCUSSION:

Epidural lipomatosis refers to excessive accumulation of unencapsulated fat in the epidural space, measuring over 7 mm in thickness. This condition can be idiopathic or secondary to steroid use, various endocrinopathies (Cushing disease, hyperprolactinemia, hypothyroidism), HIV-associated lipodystrophy, and morbid obesity. Fat deposition is typically seen in the dorsal thoracic spine, and circumferentially within the lumbar spine. On MR, epidural lipomatosis follows fat signal on all sequences, with signal drop on STIR and fat-suppressed sequences. In advanced cases, there is compression of the thecal sac with tethering by the meningovertebral (Hoffmann) ligaments, which connect the dura mater to the osteofibrous walls of the spinal canal. This forms a variety of geometric configurations, particularly the "polygonal" appearance in the upper lumbar spine and "Y" appearance in the lower lumbar spine. Most cases are asymptomatic, but severe spinal cord and nerve compression can produce neurologic deficits. Treatment options include correction of the underlying cause (steroid taper, hormonal therapy, cessation of HAART medications, weight loss) or surgical decompression.

References:

Borré DG, Borré GE, Aude F, et al. Lumbosacral epidural lipomatosis: MRI grading. *Eur Radiol.* 2003;13(7):1709-1721.

Geers C, Lecouvet FE, Behets C, et al. Polygonal deformation of the dural sac in lumbar epidural lipomatosis: anatomic explanation by the presence of meningovertebral ligaments. *AJNR Am J Neuroradiol.* 2003;24(7):1276-1282.

CLEFT/DOUBLE/SPLIT CORD

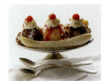

Modalities:
US, CT, MR

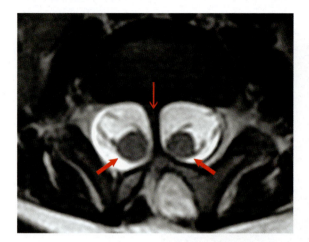

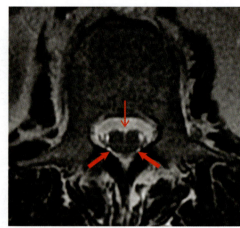

FINDINGS:

- Axial T2-weighted MR shows an osseous septum (thin arrow) separating two dural tubes and hemicords (thick arrows) with unpaired nerve roots.
- Axial T2-weighted MR in a different patient shows a median fibrous septum (thin arrow) with single dural tube and two hemicords (thick arrows).

DIFFERENTIAL DIAGNOSIS:

- Diastematomyelia
- Diplomyelia

DISCUSSION:

Split cord malformations (SCM) are a spectrum of embryologic disorders thought to be caused by abnormal ectodermal-endodermal adhesions with formation of accessory neurenteric tracts. The Pang classification consists of two types. In type I, previously known as diastematomyelia, there is hypertrophy of the neural arch with osteocartilaginous septum creating two separate dural tubes. In type II, previously known as diplomyelia, there is a median fibrous septum with common dural tube. In the majority of cases, two hemicords are present with separate central canals, single ventral/dorsal horns, and unpaired nerve roots. Cord tethering is generally present, due to restriction of motion by the midline septum.

References:

Pang D, Dias MS, Ahab-Barmada M. Split cord malformation: Part I: a unified theory of embryogenesis for double spinal cord malformations. *Neurosurgery*. 1992;31(3):451-480.

Rufener S, Ibrahim M, Parmar HA. Imaging of congenital spine and spinal cord malformations. *Neuroimaging Clin N Am*. 2011;21(3):659-676, viii.

CLUMPED, SHORT CAUDAL SAC, SLEEVELESS

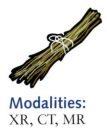

Modalities:
XR, CT, MR

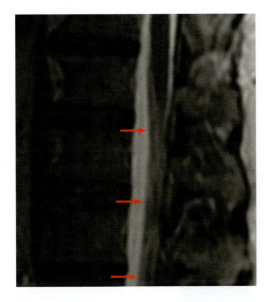
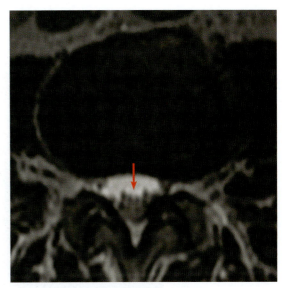

FINDINGS:

Sagittal and axial T2-weighted MR show mild thickening and clustering of cauda equina nerve roots (arrows) within the dorsal spinal canal.

DIAGNOSIS:

Arachnoiditis, type I (radicular)

DISCUSSION:

Arachnoiditis is a chronic inflammatory condition of the leptomeninges and subarachnoid space. Causes include infection, trauma, chronic compression, and spine surgery or injections. The Delamarter classification consists of three stages: Type I (central, radicular) arachnoiditis affects individual nerves with a thick and blunted "sleeveless" morphology. Clustering of the cauda equina produces a "short caudal sac" with "clumped" nerve roots. In Type II (peripheral) arachnoiditis, meningeal adhesions cause peripheral migration of nerve roots with an "empty sac" appearance. Type III (adhesive, obstructive, obliterative) arachnoiditis involves fibrous scarring, with soft tissue obliteration of the subarachnoid space producing a "candle dripping" contour. Associated CSF obstruction and syringohydromyelia are common. Chronic arachnoiditis is occasionally associated with intrathecal ossification, termed arachnoiditis ossificans. Distinction from other pathologic entities such as leptomeningeal carcinomatosis, intradural neoplasms, infectious meningitis, and granulomatous disease can be difficult. However, these conditions tend to be associated with greater contrast enhancement and intrathecal mass effect.

Reference:

Delamarter RB, Ross JS, Masaryk TJ, et al. Diagnosis of lumbar arachnoiditis by magnetic resonance imaging. *Spine (Phila Pa 1976)*. 1990;15(4):304-310.

COIL, KNOT, LOOP, REDUNDANT, SERPENTINE, TANGLED, TORTUOUS

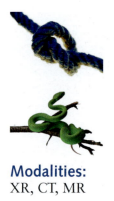

Modalities:
XR, CT, MR

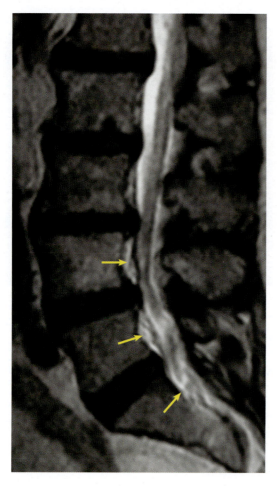

FINDINGS:

Sagittal T2-weighted MR shows lumbar disc bulges with spinal stenosis. The cauda equina nerve roots appear thickened and redundant (arrows).

DIAGNOSIS:

Chronic spinal stenosis

DISCUSSION:

Redundant nerve root syndrome is associated with severe lumbar spinal stenosis. It is thought that mechanical trapping and chronic compression of the cauda equina nerve roots results in a frictional neuritis. On myelography and MR, the nerve roots appear thickened, elongated, and tortuous. This imaging finding has been correlated with more severe neurologic symptoms and poorer response to surgery.

References:

Ehni G, Moiel RH, Bragg TG. The "redundant" or "knotted" nerve root: a clue to spondylotic cauda equina radiculopathy. Case report. *J Neurosurg.* 1970;32(2):252-254.

Ono A, Suetsuna F, Irie T, et al. Clinical significance of the redundant nerve roots of the cauda equina documented on magnetic resonance imaging. *J Neurosurg Spine.* 2007;7(1):27-32.

CORD, FUSIFORM, SPLIT FAT, STRING, TAIL

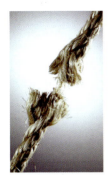

Modalities:
US, CT, MR

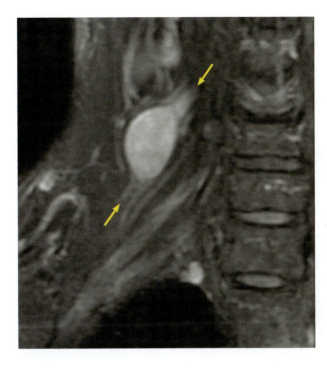

FINDINGS:

Coronal T2-weighted MR MIP shows a fusiform mass arising from the right C5 nerve root with normal entering and exiting fibers (arrows). Inferior to this, the C6-C8 nerve roots course normally toward the interscalene space.

DIAGNOSIS:

Peripheral nerve sheath tumor

DISCUSSION:

Peripheral nerve sheath tumors (PNSTs) are proliferations of peripheral nerve sheath cells that can be benign (schwannoma, neurofibroma) or malignant (malignant PNST). Schwannomas, also known as neurilemmomas, are encapsulated lesions composed of myelinating Schwann cells. These are eccentric to and typically separable from the underlying nerve. Neurofibromas are unencapsulated lesions involving nonmyelinating Schwann cells, perineural cells, and fibroblasts. These concentrically surround and are intimately associated with the parent nerve. At imaging, PNSTs appear hypoechoic on US, hypodense on CT, iso- to hypointense on T1-weighted MR, hyperintense on T2-weighted MR, and avidly enhancing. Characteristic imaging features include a fusiform tapered mass with normal entering and exiting fibers, creating a "string" or "tail" appearance in long axis. Smooth outward bulging of perineural fat creates the "split fat" appearance. In cross section, traversing nerve fibers may be identified in a "fascicular" pattern. The "bullseye" or "target" sign corresponds pathologically to central fibrosis and peripheral myxoid tissue. These imaging features suggest benign rather than malignant PNST, which is usually larger, more heterogeneous, and infiltrative. Syndromic PNSTs (multiple neurofibromas in NF1, multiple schwannomas in NF2 and schwannomatosis) have a higher incidence of malignant transformation, and may be followed with serial MR and/or PET to evaluate for rapid increases in size, marginal irregularity, internal heterogeneity, and high metabolic activity.

References:

Lin J, Martel W. Cross-sectional imaging of peripheral nerve sheath tumors: characteristic signs on CT, MR imaging, and sonography. *AJR Am J Roentgenol.* 2001;176(1):75-82.

Murphey MD, Smith WS, Smith SE, et al. From the archives of the AFIP. Imaging of musculoskeletal neurogenic tumors: radiologic-pathologic correlation. *Radiographics.* 1999;19(5):1253-1280.

DISTORTED H

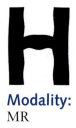

Modality:
MR

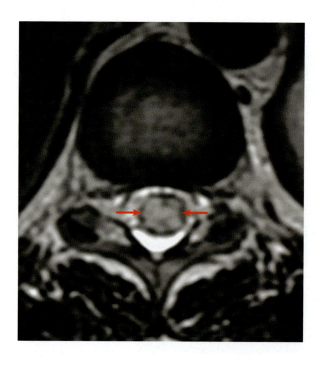

FINDINGS:

Axial T2-weighted MR shows irregular cord expansion with distorted central gray matter (arrows).

DIFFERENTIAL DIAGNOSIS:

- Cord tumor
- Infectious/inflammatory myelitis
- Traumatic myelopathy
- Cord infarct

DISCUSSION:

The spinal cord is a cylindrical structure that carries descending motor and ascending sensory signals between the brain and peripheral nervous system, as well as coordinating various reflex arcs. It is comprised of peripheral white matter and central gray matter. The white matter consists of myelinated sheets of motor and sensory axons, which are divided into ventral (anterior), lateral, and dorsal (posterior) columns or funiculi. The gray matter consists of neuronal cell bodies, unmyelinated axons, and glial cells. Normal gray matter is mildly hyperintense relative to white matter on T2-weighted MR. The "H" morphology represents ventral (anterior) and dorsal (posterior) horns that are connected across midline by the gray commissure surrounding the central canal. The ventral horns contain motor neurons and interneurons, while the dorsal horns contain sensory neurons. Wedge-shaped lateral horns are also present at the thoracic and upper lumbar levels, and contain preganglionic sympathetic neurons. Distortion of the normal "H" pattern can be seen with various cord pathologies (neoplasm, infection/inflammation, trauma, infarction) producing mass effect, edema, and/or hemorrhage in the gray matter. The "distorted H" sign is more apparent for larger cord lesions and with higher field strengths (because of greater spatial and contrast resolution).

References:

Ahmad I, Rosenbaum AE, Yu FS, et al. Intrinsic cervical spinal cord deformation on MRI: "the distorted 'H' sign." *J Spinal Disord*. 1996;9(6):494-499.

Goshgarian HG. Neuroanatomic organization of the spinal gray and white matter. In: Lin VW, Cardenas DD, Cutter NC, eds. *Spinal Cord Medicine: Principles and Practice*. New York: Demos Medical Publishing; 2003.

Held P, Dorenbeck U, Seitz J, et al. MRI of the abnormal cervical spinal cord using 2D spoiled gradient echo multiecho sequence (MEDIC) with magnetization transfer saturation pulse. A T2* weighted feasibility study. *J Neuroradiol*. 2003;30(2):83-90.

DOUBLE BUNDLE

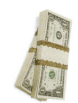

Modalities:
US, MR

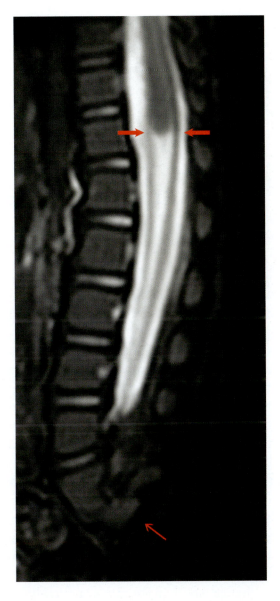

FINDINGS:

Sagittal T2-weighted MR shows sacral dysgenesis (thin arrow) and a high termination of the spinal cord with absent conus. The ventral and dorsal cauda equina nerve roots (thick arrows) are widely separated.

DIAGNOSIS:

Caudal regression, type 1

DISCUSSION:

Caudal regression, also known as sacral dysgenesis/agenesis, results from embryologic disturbances in primary neurulation or canalization and retrogressive differentiation of the caudal cell mass. Most cases are sporadic or associated with maternal diabetes. Type 1 caudal regression demonstrates a high cord termination and severe sacral anomalies. There is a blunted ("cigar") appearance of the distal spinal cord, with absent ("ghost") conus medullaris. The ventral and dorsal cauda equina nerve roots are widely separated with a "double bundle" appearance. Severe associated anomalies can include syringohydromyelia, split cord malformations, open spinal dysraphisms, and visceral malformations. Type 2 caudal regression demonstrates a low-lying conus with cord tethering. Associated anomalies are less severe than in type 1 and include tight filum terminale, lipomatous malformations, and closed spinal dysraphisms. Caudal regression may be part of the VACTERL association (vertebral defects, anal atresia, cardiac defects, tracheo-esophageal fistula, renal anomalies, and limb abnormalities); OEIS complex (omphalocele, exstrophy of the cloaca, imperforate anus, and spinal defects); and Currarino syndrome (sacral hypoplasia, presacral mass, and anorectal malformations).

References:

Barkovich AJ, Raghavan N, Chuang S, et al. The wedge-shaped cord terminus: a radiographic sign of caudal regression. *AJNR Am J Neuroradiol.* 1989;10(6):1223-1231.

Nievelstein RA, Valk J, Smit LM, et al. MR of the caudal regression syndrome: embryologic implications. *AJNR Am J Neuroradiol.* 1994;15(6):1021-1029.

DUMBBELL, HOURGLASS, MUSHROOM

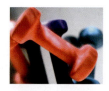

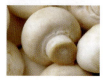

Modalities:
CT, MR

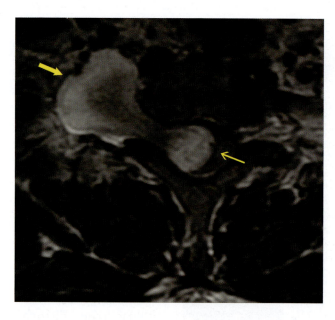

FINDINGS:

Axial T2-weighted MR shows a bilobed mass with intradural (thin arrow) and extradural (thick arrow) components, extending through and widening the right neural foramen.

DIFFERENTIAL DIAGNOSIS:

- Nerve sheath or spinal tumor
- CSF collection
- Bone lesion
- Extraspinal malignancy
- Infection

DISCUSSION:

"Dumbbell" lesions of the spine consist of intradural and extradural components with extension through the neural foramen. The majority are peripheral nerve sheath tumors, which can be benign (neurofibroma, schwannoma) or malignant (malignant PNST). These are T2-hyperintense, enhancing masses with smooth foraminal expansion and pedicle erosion. Other spinal tumors (neuroblastic tumors, ependymoma, hemangioblastoma, meningioma, hemangioma) can infrequently extend through the foramina. Nonenhancing CSF collections include meningeal (arachnoid) cyst, perineural cyst, lateral meningocele, and pseudomeningocele. Bone tumors (plasmacytoma, chordoma, aneurysmal bone cyst) and other skeletal lesions (synovial cyst, ganglion cyst, lateral disc herniation, neurenteric cyst) can also extend eccentrically into the foramen. Infections (particularly tuberculosis) can cause vertebral destruction and paraspinal abscesses. Finally, extraspinal malignancies (regionally invasive tumor, metastasis, lymphoma) can involve the foramina and paraspinal soft tissues.

Reference:

Kivrak AS, Koc O, Emlik D, et al. Differential diagnosis of dumbbell lesions associated with spinal neural foraminal widening: imaging features. *Eur J Radiol.* 2009;71(1):29-41.

EMPTY/FEATURELESS SAC

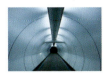

Modalities:
XR, CT, MR

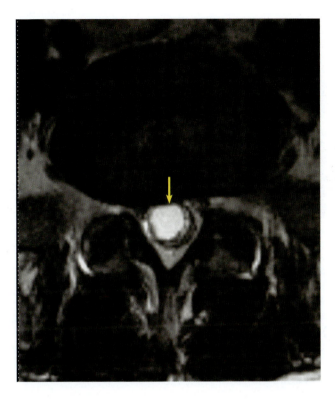

FINDINGS:

Axial T2-weighted MR shows peripheral migration of the cauda equina nerve roots toward the margins of the thecal sac (arrow).

DIAGNOSIS:

Arachnoiditis, type II (peripheral)

DISCUSSION:

Arachnoiditis is a chronic inflammatory condition of the leptomeninges and subarachnoid space. Causes include infection, trauma, chronic compression, and spine surgery or injections. The Delamarter classification consists of three stages: Type I (central, radicular) arachnoiditis affects individual nerves with a thick and blunted "sleeveless" morphology. Clustering of the cauda equina produces a "short caudal sac" with "clumped" nerve roots. In Type II (peripheral) arachnoiditis, meningeal adhesions cause peripheral migration of nerve roots with an "empty sac" appearance. Type III (adhesive, obstructive, obliterative) arachnoiditis involves fibrous scarring, with soft tissue obliteration of the subarachnoid space producing a "candle dripping" contour. Associated CSF obstruction and syringohydromyelia are common. Chronic arachnoiditis is occasionally associated with intrathecal ossification, termed arachnoiditis ossificans. Distinction from other pathologic entities such as leptomeningeal carcinomatosis, intradural neoplasms, infectious meningitis, and granulomatous disease can be difficult. However, these conditions tend to be associated with greater contrast enhancement and intrathecal mass effect.

References:

Delamarter RB, Ross JS, Masaryk TJ, et al. Diagnosis of lumbar arachnoiditis by magnetic resonance imaging. *Spine (Phila Pa 1976).* 1990;15(4):304-310.

Ross JS, Masaryk TJ, Modic MT, et al. MR imaging of lumbar arachnoiditis. *AJR Am J Roentgenol.* 1987;149(5):1025-1032.

FIFTH/TERMINAL VENTRICLE

Modalities:
US, MR

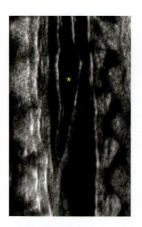
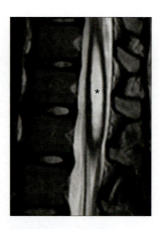

FINDINGS:

Sagittal US and T2-weighted MR show a central cystic structure within the conus medullaris (asterisks).

DIFFERENTIAL DIAGNOSIS:

- Ventriculus terminalis
- Transient central canal dilation
- Syringohydromyelia
- Cystic neoplasm
- Myelomalacia

DISCUSSION:

The ventriculus terminalis (VT), or "fifth ventricle," is an ependyma-lined residual lumen within the conus medullaris that forms during canalization and retrogressive differentiation of the caudal cell mass. This represents a normal variant in infants and children, and usually regresses by 5 years of age. At imaging, VT appears as a well-circumscribed, ovoid cavity with signal characteristics identical to CSF. The differential diagnosis includes transient dilation of the central canal, which occurs in healthy newborns and disappears in the first weeks of postnatal life. The absence of nodularity, septation, and enhancement distinguishes VT from cystic cord tumors. Syringohydromyelia typically extends proximally and is associated with CSF flow obstruction. Myelomalacia refers to cord atrophy following various insults, which may undergo cystic degeneration. VT is usually asymptomatic, but can occasionally undergo benign cystic expansion and require drainage. In adults, atypical imaging features including septations, perilesional edema, and associated vascular malformations can confound the diagnosis. If there are progressive neurologic symptoms, surgery may be required.

References:

Coleman LT, Zimmerman RA, Rorke LB. Ventriculus terminalis of the conus medullaris: MR findings in children. *AJNR Am J Neuroradiol*. 1995;16(7):1421-1426.

Suh SH, Chung TS, Lee SK, et al. Ventriculus terminalis in adults: unusual magnetic resonance imaging features and review of the literature. *Korean J Radiol*. 2012;13(5):557-563.

FLAME, RIM

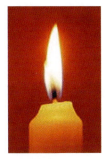

Modality:
MR

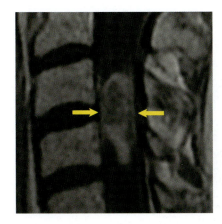
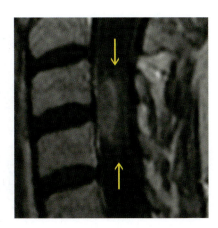

FINDINGS:

Sagittal contrast-enhanced T1-weighted MR shows an enhancing intramedullary mass, with increased enhancement at the periphery (thick arrows) and patchy enhancement along the superior and inferior poles (thin arrows).

DIAGNOSIS:

Intramedullary metastasis

DISCUSSION:

Enhancing intramedullary masses may represent primary cord tumors or metastases from CNS and non-CNS primaries. Primary cord tumors include ependymoma, astrocytoma/glioma, and hemangioblastoma. Non-CNS primaries include lung, breast, melanoma, genitourinary, gastrointestinal, head and neck carcinoma, and lymphoma. Distinction between these entities is difficult on imaging, yet crucial for effective treatment. Recently, two signs have been described as highly specific for non-CNS metastases. The "rim" sign refers to increased enhancement at the periphery of an enhancing mass. The "flame" sign represents ill-defined patchy enhancement along the superior and/or inferior poles of an otherwise well-defined lesion. Multiplicity of lesions and involvement of other compartments (intracranial, leptomeningeal, epidural, vertebral, extraspinal) further support the diagnosis of metastasis. Less typical features such as low-level enhancement, cystic/necrotic changes, and intratumoral hemorrhage should bring primary cord neoplasms higher in the differential. Both primary and metastatic tumors tend to be eccentrically located, with cord expansion and architectural distortion ("distorted H" sign). There is diffuse and long-segment surrounding edema (entire cross section, often greater than 3-4 vertebral levels).

References:

Rykken JB, Diehn FE, Hunt CH, et al. Intramedullary spinal cord metastases: MRI and relevant clinical features from a 13-year institutional case series. *AJNR Am J Neuroradiol.* 2013;34(10):2043-2049.

Rykken JB, Diehn FE, Hunt CH, et al. Rim and flame signs: postgadolinium MRI findings specific for non-CNS intramedullary spinal cord metastases. *AJNR Am J Neuroradiol.* 2013;34(4):908-915.

FLAME, WEDGE

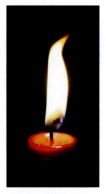

Modality:
MR

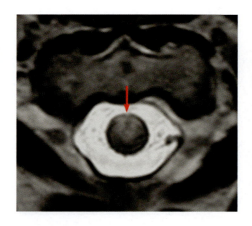

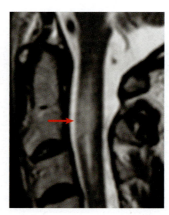

FINDINGS:

Axial and sagittal T2-weighted MR show patchy hyperintensity in the ventral cervical cord (arrows).

DIFFERENTIAL DIAGNOSIS:

- Demyelinating disease
- Infectious/inflammatory myelitis
- Vascular disease
- Cord tumor
- Traumatic myelopathy

DISCUSSION:

Cord edema is seen in a wide variety of pathologies including demyelination, infection/inflammation, vascular, neoplastic, and traumatic. Multiple sclerosis tends to involve the white matter in a focal and asymmetric fashion (less than 1/2 of cross section, usually 1-2 vertebral levels). Plaques characteristically have a "flame" or "wedge" shape, with central or leading-edge enhancement in the active phase. Transverse myelitis demonstrates uniform cord edema (more than 2/3 of cross section), which can be longitudinally extensive (2-4 vertebral levels). Mild eccentric or peripheral enhancement may be present. Infectious myelitis demonstrates rapidly progressive edema and enhancement, which can be complicated by abscess formation. Granulomatous disease demonstrates a more gradual time course, with patchy or nodular enhancement. High-flow vascular malformations are associated with venous hypertension and ischemia (Foix-Alajouanine syndrome), producing long-segment "flame"-like central cord edema, peripheral T2 hypointensity, and pial venous engorgement. Cord tumors usually show solid heterogeneous enhancement, parenchymal expansion/distortion, and significant edema (entire cross section, often greater than 3-4 vertebral levels). Traumatic cord contusions may be accompanied by hemorrhage, fractures, and soft tissue injury.

Reference:

DeSanto J, Ross JS. Spine infection/inflammation. *Radiol Clin North Am.* 2011;49(1):105-127.

FLOWER PETAL, PAINTBRUSH, SCALLOPED, STALAGMITE

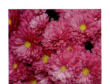

Modalities:
XR, CT, MR

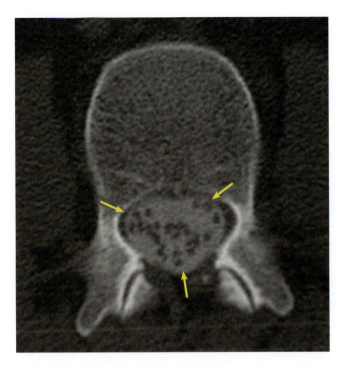

FINDINGS:

Axial CT myelogram shows multiple clusters of cauda equina nerve roots (arrows) within the spinal canal.

DIAGNOSIS:

Arachnoiditis

DISCUSSION:

Arachnoiditis is a chronic inflammatory condition of the leptomeninges and sub-arachnoid space. Causes include infection, trauma, chronic compression, and spine surgery or injections. On myelography, arachnoiditis is a great mimicker with widely variable imaging appearances. Early in the disease process, scattered streaks and droplets of contrast collect between clusters of nerve roots. Later on, fibrous adhesions obliterate the subarachnoid space with "flower petal," "candle guttering," "oval," "paintbrush," "scalloped," or "stalagmite"-shaped filling defects. The spinal cord and contrast column retain their normal orientation or are tented toward the defects, rather than being displaced away as would be expected with a true mass. The Wilkinson classification consists of four groups that are correlated with the physiologic severity of obstruction: I (unilateral focal defect along nerve root), II (annular defect with minimal contrast passage), III (complete transverse obstruction), IV (funnel-shaped cutoff incorporating nerve roots).

References:

Delamarter RB, Ross JS, Masaryk TJ, et al. Diagnosis of lumbar arachnoiditis by magnetic resonance imaging. *Spine (Phila Pa 1976)*. 1990;15(4):304-310.

Teng P, Papatheodorou C. Myelographic findings in adhesive spinal arachnoiditis (with a brief surgical note). *Br J Radiol*. 1967;40(471):201-208.

Wright MH, Denney LC. A comprehensive review of spinal arachnoiditis. *Orthop Nurs*. 2003;22(3):215-219.

HOURGLASS, PAINTBRUSH

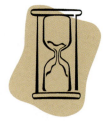

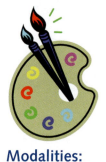

Modalities:
XR, CT, MR

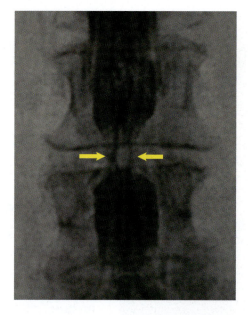

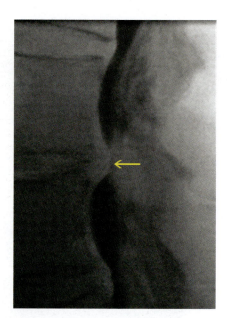

FINDINGS:

AP and lateral myelography show multilevel facet arthrosis and disc bulges, producing lateral (thick arrows) and anterior (thin arrow) impressions on the contrast column.

DIFFERENTIAL DIAGNOSIS:

- Spinal disease
- Epidural lesion
- Arachnoiditis

DISCUSSION:

Myelography involves direct intrathecal injection of contrast with subsequent imaging using fluoroscopy, CT, and/or MR. This helps to evaluate CSF dynamics (leak, obstruction) in the setting of trauma, spinal stenosis, or tumor. The morphology of the contrast column should be evaluated with attention to the dura, spinal cord, and nerve roots. Extrinsic compression of the dura can partially or completely interrupt CSF flow. The differential diagnosis includes epidural masses, epidural fluid collections, and spinal degenerative disease. Spinal stenosis with facet arthrosis and disc bulges produces lateral and anterior impressions on the contrast column, known as the "hourglass" and "paintbrush" appearances. Arachnoiditis is a chronic inflammatory condition of the leptomeninges and subarachnoid space, and a great mimicker on myelography. Scarring and adhesions produce a wide variety of filling defects. However, there is absence of true mass effect and, in some cases, tenting of the cord and contrast column toward the defect.

Reference:

Greenberg MS. *Handbook of Neurosurgery*. 7th ed. New York: Thieme; 2010.

INVERTED PEAR, KEYHOLE, OVAL

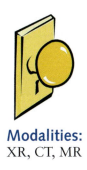

Modalities:
XR, CT, MR

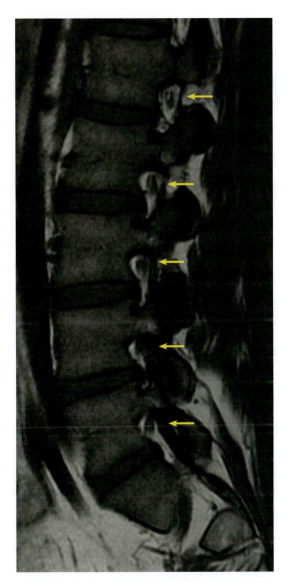

FINDINGS:

Sagittal T1-weighted MR shows normal lumbar foramina with nerve roots (arrows) exiting superiorly and surrounded by fat.

DIAGNOSIS:

Normal neural foramina

DISCUSSION:

The neural foramina normally demonstrate a "keyhole" morphology with superior and inferior margins formed by the pedicles above and below; anterior margin formed by the posterior vertebral cortices and intervertebral disc; and posterior margin formed by the facet joint. This anatomy is best appreciated on sagittal oblique images in the cervical spine, and sagittal images in the thoracic and lumbar spine. Cervical nerves exit in the lower portions of the foramina, at or slightly below the level of the disc. Thoracic and lumbar nerves exit in the upper portions of the foramina, just below the superior pedicle. Foraminal stenosis can be caused by degenerative, traumatic, neoplastic, infectious, and congenital etiologies. Degenerative spine disease is the most common and includes disc pathology, spondylolisthesis, facet arthropathy, and ligamentum flavum redundancy. MR is the examination of choice to evaluate spinal canal and foraminal stenosis, and assess for cord/nerve root compression. T1-weighted images are helpful in assessing the vertebral marrow and epidural/perineural fat, while T2-weighted sequences are used to evaluate the spinal canal, cord, and nerve roots.

References:

Lee S, Lee JW, Yeom JS, et al. A practical MRI grading system for lumbar foraminal stenosis. *AJR Am J Roentgenol.* 2010;194(4):1095-1098.

Park HJ, Kim SS, Lee SY, et al. A practical MRI grading system for cervical foraminal stenosis based on oblique sagittal images. *Br J Radiol.* 2013;86(1025):20120515.

INVERTED V, RABBIT EARS

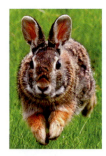

Modality:
MR

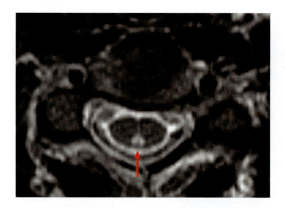

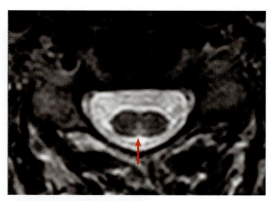

FINDINGS:

Axial T2-weighted MR in two different patients shows symmetric hyperintense signal in the dorsal columns (arrows).

DIFFERENTIAL DIAGNOSIS:

- Subacute combined degeneration (early)
- Infectious myelitis
- Demyelinating disease
- Spinocerebellar ataxia

DISCUSSION:

Subacute combined degeneration (SCD), also known as Lichtheim disease, is a vitamin B_{12} (cobalamin) deficiency-related myelopathy. Patients present with progressive lower-extremity weakness, paresthesias, and gait disturbances. Causes include inadequate B_{12} intake (strict vegetarians); malabsorption (pernicious anemia, gastrointestinal infection/inflammation, surgery); and other conditions (nitrous oxide intoxication, copper deficiency). Selective demyelination initially involves the dorsal white matter columns, followed by the lateral corticospinal and sometimes lateral spinothalamic tracts of the cervical and thoracic cord. On MR, the "rabbit ears" and "anchor" signs are produced by symmetric edema, reduced diffusion, and/or enhancement in these regions. The differential includes infectious myelitis (HIV-associated vacuolar myelopathy, varicella zoster virus, herpesvirus, Lyme disease, neurosyphilis or tabes dorsalis); multiple sclerosis; and hereditary spinocerebellar ataxias. However, these entities rarely demonstrate the symmetric and long-segment appearance of SCD.

References:

Kumar A, Singh AK. Teaching NeuroImage: inverted V sign in subacute combined degeneration of spinal cord. *Neurology.* 2009;72(1):e4.

Naidich MJ, Ho SU. Case 87: Subacute combined degeneration. *Radiology.* 2005;237(1):101-105.

LOBULAR, OVOID, SAUSAGE

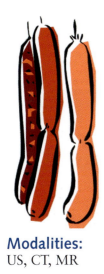

Modalities:
US, CT, MR

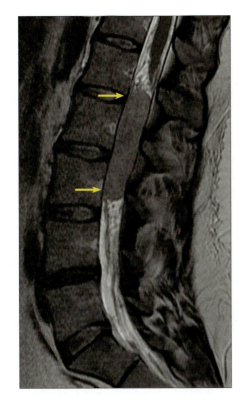 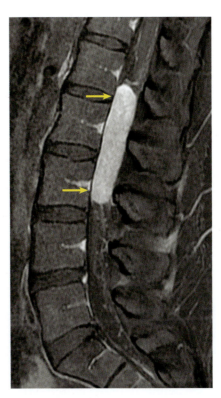

FINDINGS:

Sagittal T2-weighted and contrast-enhanced T1-weighted MR with fat saturation show a homogeneously enhancing filar mass (arrows) that splays the cauda equina nerve roots.

DIAGNOSIS:

Myxopapillary ependymoma

DISCUSSION:

Myxopapillary ependymoma, which comprises 13% of all spinal ependymomas, arises from ependymal glia of the distal neural tube. The classic appearance is a well-circumscribed ovoid "sausage"-shaped mass involving the filum terminale and/or conus medullaris. Due to the high mucin content, signal is T1 iso- to hyperintense and T2-hyperintense. Lesion hypervascularity results in avid enhancement, flow voids, and tumoral hemorrhage. Large tumors can splay the cauda equina nerve roots and remodel surrounding bone.

References:

Koeller KK, Rosenblum RS, Morrison AL. Neoplasms of the spinal cord and filum terminale: radiologic-pathologic correlation. *Radiographics*. 2000;20(6):1721-1749.

Soderlund KA, Smith AB, Rushing EJ, et al. Radiologic-pathologic correlation of pediatric and adolescent spinal neoplasms, part 2: intradural extramedullary spinal neoplasms. *AJR Am J Roentgenol*. 2012;198(1):44-51.

TETHERED CORD

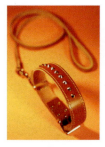

Modalities:
US, MR

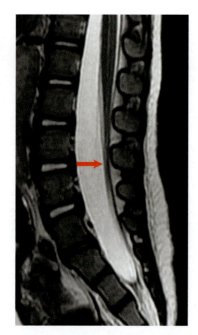
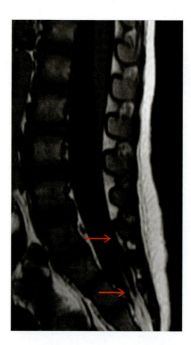

FINDINGS:

- Sagittal T2-weighted MR shows a low-lying conus at L3-L4 (thick arrow).
- Sagittal T1-weighted MR shows a fatty filum terminale (thin arrows).

DIAGNOSIS:

Tethered cord

DISCUSSION:

The spinal cord forms in utero by primary neurulation (involving neural tube closure and disjunction), and secondary neurulation of the caudal cell mass (involving canalization and retrogressive differentiation). During development, disproportionate growth of the vertebral column and dura relative to the spinal cord causes relative "ascent" of the conus medullaris. Normally, the conus is located at L2-L3 at birth, and reaches the normal adult level (L1-L2) at approximately 2 months of age. The filum terminale and cauda equina nerve roots elongate to accommodate the spinal cord. However, tethering of the cord to surrounding tissues may be caused by congenital, inflammatory, neoplastic, traumatic, and iatrogenic etiologies. This results in a low-lying conus with limitation of nerve root motion. Associated malformations include tight filum terminale, dorsal enteric remnants, lipomatous malformations, sacral neoplasms, split cord malformations, and other spinal dysraphisms.

References:

Agarwalla PK, Dunn IF, Scott RM, et al. Tethered cord syndrome. *Neurosurg Clin N Am.* 2007;18(3):531-547.

Raghavan N, Barkovich AJ, Edwards M, et al. MR imaging in the tethered spinal cord syndrome. *AJR Am J Roentgenol.* 1989;152(4):843-852.

TRUMPET

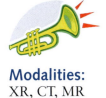

Modalities:
XR, CT, MR

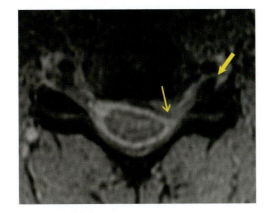
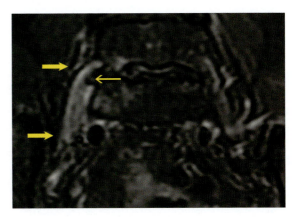

FINDINGS:

- Axial T2*-weighted MR shows a left lateral disc herniation (thin arrow) with compression of the exiting cervical nerve. The extraforaminal nerve is focally enlarged (thick arrow).
- Coronal STIR MR in a different patient shows L4-L5 right lateral osteophyte (thin arrow) compressing the L4 nerve root, with long-segment extraforaminal edema (thick arrows).

DIAGNOSIS:

Nerve root compression

DISCUSSION:

Spinal nerve compression has various causes including degenerative, traumatic, neoplastic, infectious, and congenital etiologies. Degenerative spine disease is the most common, with typical sites of impingement including traversing nerve roots in the lateral recesses; exiting nerve roots within the neural foramina; and extraforaminal nerve roots beyond the foramina. On MR, compressed nerves may demonstrate contour deviation, focal enlargement ("trumpet" sign), edema, and enhancement. This appearance is thought to reflect a combination of mechanical deformation, chemical irritation, and direct compression. Morphologic alterations can also be appreciated on conventional or CT myelography. Treatment options include conservative management with analgesics, selective nerve root block, or surgery.

Reference:

Postacchini F. *Lumbar Disc Herniation*. Berlin: Springer; 1999.

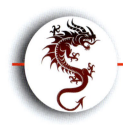

Index

Sign Name

Diagnosis

Modality

CT (computed tomography)

MR (magnetic resonance)

NM (nuclear medicine)

US (ultrasonography)